Psychological Interventions from Six Continents

This book presents psychological assessment and intervention in a cultural and relational context. A diverse range of contributors representing six continents and eleven countries write about their therapeutic interventions, all of which break the traditional assessor-as-expert-oriented framework and offer a creative adaptation in service delivery. A Collaborative/Therapeutic Assessment model, including work with immigrant communities, and Indigenous modalities underscore individual and collective case illustrations highlighting equality in the roles of the provider and the receiver of services. The universality and uniqueness of culture are explored as a construct and through case material. Some chapters describe a partnership with a Eurocentric scientific model, while others adopt a purely community method, preserved with Indigenous language and subjective methodology. This volume brings together diverse therapeutic collaborative ideas, and recognizes relational, community, and cultural psychologies as integral to mainstream assessment and intervention literature. This book is essential for psychologists and clinicians internationally and graduate students.

Barbara L. Mercer, PhD, is the former Assessment Program Director and clinical supervisor at WestCoast Children's Clinic, a community psychology clinic in Oakland, California. She has worked in community mental health throughout her career. She has presented and written about foster care, culture, trauma, and collaborative assessment.

Heather Macdonald, PsyD, has been a licensed clinical psychologist since 2010 and has focused her practice on psychological assessment. She has produced numerous scholarly publications on the interface between culture, social justice, relational ethics, clinical practice, post-colonial thought, and psycho-political theory.

Caroline Purves, PhD, has administered psychological assessments for over 30 years, working with clients of all ages and a variety of ethnicities and backgrounds in the US, Canada, and England.

Psychological Interventions from Six Continents

Culture, Collaboration, and Community

Edited by Barbara L. Mercer, Heather Macdonald, and Caroline Purves

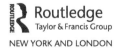
Routledge
Taylor & Francis Group

NEW YORK AND LONDON

Cover image: Original Painting by Helen Milroy

First published 2023
by Routledge
605 Third Avenue, New York, NY 10158

and by Routledge
4 Park Square, Milton Park, Abingdon, Oxon, OX14 4RN

Routledge is an imprint of the Taylor & Francis Group, an informa business

British Library Cataloguing-in-Publication Data
A catalogue record for this book is available from the British Library

Library of Congress Cataloguing-in-Publication Data
A catalog record has been requested for this book

ISBN: 978-0-367-64348-5 (hbk)
ISBN: 978-0-367-64347-8 (pbk)
ISBN: 978-1-003-12406-1 (ebk)

DOI: 10.4324/9781003124061

Typeset in Times New Roman
by MPS Limited, Dehradun

Search for what is good and strong and beautiful in your society and elaborate from there.

—Michel Foucault (Raskin, 1984)

Contents

Figures

Acknowledgments

We are grateful to our authors, first of all. Some are inspired and resourceful clinicians we worked alongside long ago, some we shared conferences with, others were referred by colleagues, and some we had read or searched for and were impressed by their work in far-off locales. These authors are not solely academics; they have busy clinical lives full of commitments, so they completed their chapters amidst many other obligations.

We were raised, schooled by, and created programs with the clinic, where we all worked for many years, WestCoast Children's Clinic now in Oakland, California. This clinic began as a small nonprofit training and child guidance clinic and has become a thriving community clinic with community programs and a local and national advocacy voice for youth. This clinic reflects the impact that is possible through gradual steps and a commitment to a shared community vision.

We are indebted to our mentors, Dr. Stephen Finn, Dr. Deborah Tharinger, Dr. Constance Fischer, and to Dr. Philip Erdberg, our Rorschach bodhisattva, for believing in and nurturing our growth and our mission and for waiting compassionately until we understood. The psychologists who generously referred clinicians to us for this volume, Dr. Filippo Aschieri, Dr. Patrizia Bevilacqua, and Dr. Joseph Gone, greatly enriched our work. Many thanks to Dr. James Allen, whose work in combining Indigenous intervention with Collaborative Assessment was a guiding inspiration to our volume.

We also want to thank Routledge/Taylor & Francis for collaborating with us, especially on the beautiful cover art provided by one of our authors, Dr. Helen Milroy, of Australia. To Edie Wells for creating image and design ideas, and Mark Bailie for his careful reading and thoughtful notes, many thanks.

About the Editors and Contributors

The editors have developed programs, supervised, and worked as clinicians in an assessment, psychotherapy, and training component of a community mental health clinic over the last 30 years. They have presented papers internationally and published articles and books related to psychological and collaborative assessment, community psychology, race, and culture.

Contributors to the book have written, presented, and trained in the field of assessment and intervention; they have authored books and articles, presented at the Society for Personality Assessment, Conference of Neuropsychology, and the Rorschach and the International Rorschach Conference, and led research projects. Each contributor has extensive experience in the field with psychological assessment and community psychology, Therapeutic Assessment, and research. Contributors are from North America (Canada and United States), Latin America (Argentina and Mexico), Europe (the Netherlands and Italy), Asia (India and Japan), Africa (South Sudan and Zimbabwe), and Australasia (Australia). Highlighted themes include interventions related to Indigenous populations, immigrant populations in European countries and the United States, in-depth psychological assessments in Latin America, adolescents diagnosed with *Hikikomori* (shut-ins) in Japan, cultural norms related to mental health in India, and culturally sensitive interventions and transpersonal work in Africa and Australia.

Contributors

James Allen, PhD is a professor at the University of Minnesota Medical School, Duluth Campus in the Department of Family Medicine and Biobehavioral Health. As a partner with the Memory Keepers Medical Discovery Team–American Indian and Rural Health Equity, he collaborates in research describing cultural strategies for health in Indigenous communities. For over 25 years, Dr. Allen has been continuously supported through NIH initiatives to develop community intervention to promote protective factors from suicide and substance misuse among Alaska Native youth, and to describe Indigenous community resilience processes that create protection and facilitate recovery and well-being.

Daniela Escobedo-Belloc, MD is currently working on a PhD focused on borderline personality disorder, attachment theory, and economic games at the Universidad de Nuevo León. She is a licensed psychologist in México, and her clinical work has focused on both psychotherapy and psychological assessments. She is the former president of the Mexican Society of Rorschach and Psychodiagnostic Methods.

Jonathan Brakarsh, PhD, is a child psychologist, director of the Say and Play Therapy Centre in Zimbabwe, founder of the Post-Covid Treatment Network-Africa, and author of books used in 30 countries to help children navigate the challenges in their lives: *The Journey of Life Series*, *Say and Play*, and *Singing to the Lions.*

Marta Breda is a psychologist who works in the fields of childhood and disabilities. She completed a psychology placement at Cooperativa Crinali in Milan, Italy, and contributed to the cooperative's latest book, *Sviluppi della clinica transculturale nelle relazioni di cura* (edited by Maria Luisa Cattaneo and Sabina Dal Verme, 2020).

Jane Chidzungu is a teacher, trainer, public speaker, and experienced mental health and psycho-social professional. She has done work in mentoring and supporting community-based facilitators. She is skilled in collaborative work with key stakeholders, including local political and traditional leaders at the community level. Jane contributed to the article "Community Intervention During Ongoing Political Violence: What Is Possible? What Works?" (*American Journal of Peace Psychology* 2013). She is a senior trainer who contributed to the piloting of Singing to the Lions, a psychosocial support tool that is designed to help children and youth lessen the impact of violence and abuse in their lives.

The Cooperativa Crinali is a social cooperative in Milan, Italy. The Crinali Transcultural Assessment Group is a part of this cooperative, and it is supervised by Dr. Patrizia Bevilacqua (psychologist, psychotherapist, and university lecturer).

Hilde De Saeger, PhD, is a licensed psychologist and psychotherapist in the Netherlands and Belgium. She works at the Viersprong, a specialized clinic for the assessment and treatment of adults and adolescents with severe personality pathology and conduct disorders. Her work mostly consists of assessment and providing trainings and supervision on Therapeutic Assessment, both nationally and internationally. Dr. De Saeger has published several papers on psychological assessment.

Nicole Fratellani is a psychologist who works with children with special educational needs and disabilities in schools in Milan. She previously collaborated with the child neuropsychiatry unit at San Paolo Hospital as well as with San Vittore Prison in Milan, Italy, providing support to foreign inmates. She is a member of the Crinali Transcultural Assessment Group in Milan.

Francesca Grosso is a psychologist who specializes in psychodiagnostics. She collaborates with the Università Cattolica del Sacro Cuore in Milan as a group tutor for the Psychology Degree. She is a member of the Crinali Transcultural Assessment Group in Milan.

Kakli Gupta, PsyD., is a psychotherapist based in Bangalore, India. Dr. Gupta holds a doctorate in clinical psychology from California, USA and a master's degree in psychology from the University of Delhi. She has received training in play therapy and therapeutic assessments. Dr. Gupta has a private practice in which she works with children, adolescents, and adults. She also provides therapy and training as well as supervision to other mental health professionals in India.

Shaun Hains, PhD, is an Indigenous and Native Canadian in the Department of Social Transformation at Saybrook University. She is a member of the Métis Nation of Alberta with Algonquin, Iroquois, Sioux, Dené, and Anishinaabe descent. Growing up in the wilderness of Northern Ontario she began to lead as an academic and a hereditary chief in 2015. Her awards include the following: Emory L. Cowen Dissertation Award from the Society for Community Research and Action, Division 27 of the American Psychology Association, 2002; National Aboriginal Teacher of the Year Award from the Canadian Teachers' Federation in 2013; and Aboriginal Teacher of the Year Award from the Alberta Teachers' Association in 2012. Her definition of Indigenous research was shared and later published by the Social Sciences and Research Council of Canada in their summary paper, *SSHRC's Dialogue on Research and Aboriginal Peoples*. Dr. Hains published works include: *An emerging voice: A study using traditional Aboriginal research methods.* Saybrook University (2001); Defining of a peace process within Indigenous research, Indigenous ethics, and their implications in psychology. *Journal of Indigenous Research*; Indigenous utmost care. *Journal of Indigenous Research, 9*, (2021).

Shraddha Kashyap, PhD was born in Kenya. She has Indian heritage and migrated to Australia in 2002 where she completed her PhD in clinical psychology at the University of Western Australia in 2018 and was awarded a Fulbright Scholarship to conduct research at the Bellevue/New York University Program for Survivors of Torture. Following this, she was a postdoctoral research fellow in the Refugee Trauma and Recovery Program at the University of New South Wales, Sydney, and began working with Helen Milroy as a postdoctoral research associate at the University of Western Australia School of Indigenous Studies in May 2020. As a clinician and researcher, Shraddha understands the importance of community participatory-based research and is passionate about working alongside Aboriginal and Torres Strait Islander peoples to help build an evidence base to promote culturally safe mental health care practices.

John Chuol Kuek, PhD, LMFT, CCTPII, is the director of Integrated Services at La Maestra Community Health Centers in San Diego, California. He is a visiting lecturer and doctoral dissertation member at the University of San Diego. He is the author of two books, *South Sudanese Community Insights: A Cross-Generational Cross-Cultural Rescue Model for Families and Family Counselors* (2012) and *Culture, Trauma and Transpersonal Psychology: A Contemporary Study of South Sudanese* (2015). Dr. Kuek also co-authored one of the first articles on the broken educational system in the Republic of South Sudan: "Hunger for an Education: A Research Essay on the Case of South Sudan and the Voices of Its People" (*FIRE: Forum for International Research in Education*, 2014). Dr. Kuek was born in South Sudan and immigrated to the United States in 1995. In addition to specializing in the assessment and treatment of South Sudanese persons, he is also very active in bringing peace to the Republic of South Sudan. He is the founder of the organization Relief Organization for South Sudan in the United States that is active with the United Nations as well as non-governmental organizations that provide medical and mental health, and educational services to South Sudanese citizens.

Heather Macdonald, PsyD, has been a licensed clinical psychologist since 2010. Her clinical professional background includes working with young children, adolescents, and adults in a variety of settings with a wide range of identified concerns. Prior to working at the Samaritan Center in Seattle, Washington, where she now practices, Dr. Macdonald worked at the Danielsen Institute at Boston University and taught psychology at Lesley University in Cambridge, Massachusetts. She completed her master's degree in psychology at Seattle University and her doctorate at Pacific University in Forest Grove, Oregon. She has published numerous articles, one monograph, and two edited volumes. Her most recent edited book, published in 2019, is *Race, Rage, and Resistance: Philosophy, Psychology, and the Perils of Individualism* (edited with David Goodman and Eric Severson; published by Routledge's Taylor & Francis Group).

Barbara L. Mercer, PhD, developed and was the director of the Assessment Program and a clinical supervisor at WestCoast Children's Clinic, a community child psychology clinic in Oakland, California, from 1986–to 2018. She has worked in community mental health throughout her career. She has presented at international conferences on child research, child treatment, and assessment topics related to cross-cultural assessment, foster care, trauma, community psychology, and training and supervision. She has published in journals and is an editor of and a contributing author to *Assessment of Children in the Urban Community* (edited with Tricia Fong and Erin Rosenblatt, 2016; published by Routledge). She is currently a psychologist in Seattle, Washington.

Helen Milroy is a psychiatrist and professor in Western Australia. She is a descendant of the Palyku people of the Pilbara region of Western Australia (WA) but was born and educated in Perth. Helen has made a personal and professional commitment to improving the lives of Aboriginal and Torres Strait Islander children and families. She is currently Professor and the Stan Perron Chair of Child and Adolescent Psychiatry at the Perth Children's Hospital and the University of Western Australia and holds several leadership positions. These include being a Commissioner for the Australian Football League, a former commissioner with the National Mental Health Commission (2017–2021), and from 2013 to 2017 Helen was a commissioner for the

Royal Commission into Institutional Responses to Child Sexual Abuse. Helen was awarded the Australian Mental Health Prize in 2020 and was named WA Australian of the Year 2021.

Eugenia Mpande is a mental health and psychosocial professional, counselor, and mental health activist in Zimbabwe. She has devoted much of her 20 years in the profession to extensive work with individuals (adults and children), families, community groups, and members of civil society organizations who have lived through both traumatic and traumagenic experiences. Over the years, she has developed trauma-informed care programs and materials for communities, volunteer facilitators, and frontline workers. She has specialist skills in collective trauma healing and transcultural mental health. Eugenia has contributed to several publications, including the paper *Trauma and Mental Health in Zimbabwe* for a 2011 American Friends Service Committee workshop on healing, a 2013 article in the *American Journal of Peace Psychology* titled "Community Intervention During Ongoing Political Violence: What Is Possible? What Works?" 2020. *Special Bulletin on Reparation for Victims of Torture in Africa* published by the Centre for the Study of Violence and Reconciliation, and a community-led prevention and response measure related to organized violence and human rights abuses during the COVID-10 lockdown in *Zimbabwe Pan-African Reparation Perspective, Special Bulletin on Reparation for Victims of Torture in Africa Published by the Centre for the Study of Violence and Reconciliation (CSVR).*

Lightwell Mpofu is a program development practitioner in Zimbabwe who has a strong interest in psychosocial support, human rights, and peacebuilding. He has been a part of several community publishing initiatives on different generative themes both in Zimbabwe and abroad. He has also written a poetry anthology, *Faces to Hearts* (2018).

Noriko Nakamura, PhD, is a licensed clinical psychologist and Therapeutic Assessment practitioner. She is co-director of the Nakamura Psychotherapy Institute in Tokyo (since 1989) and is the founder of Exner Japan Associates, which teaches and conducts research on the Rorschach Comprehensive System. Dr. Nakamura is also a founding member of the Japan Rorschach Society for the Comprehensive System and was its president for 12 years. She has served as vice president and president of the International Rorschach Society and is a co-founder/ director of the Asian-Pacific Centre for Therapeutic Assessment.

Ilaria Oltolini is a trainee clinical psychologist at the Università Cattolica del Sacro Cuore in Brescia, Italy, is tutor coordinator at the university's Milanese campus and teaches in a local prison. Since completing her master's degree, she has specialized in psychodiagnostics and clinical neuroscience. She is a member of the Crinali Transcultural Assessment Group in Milan.

Lic. Ernesto Pais is a licensed psychologist in Buenos Aires, Argentina. His clinical work is focused on psychotherapy and psychological assessments. He is an associate professor of clinical practice and integrative psychological assessment at the Universidad Abierta Interamericana, where he runs the University Center for Collaborative and Therapeutic Assessment. Dr. Pais is the co-author of papers and congress presentations on psychological assessment. He is fully certified in Therapeutic Assessment with adults.

Monique Platell, PhD, was born and raised in Perth, Western Australia. Monique is a research fellow in the School of Population and Global Health at the University of Western Australia. Completing her PhD in 2020, her thesis explored factors influencing adolescents' mental health service access in Perth, Western Australia. Leading this research, she developed her passion for mental health advocacy, ensuring that all in the community have equitable access to mental health services to promote happy and healthy lives. Dr. Platell's current research position is under the Thoughtful Schools Program, which looks to educate Western Australian schools in becoming adversity and trauma-informed to support their students.

Caroline Purves, PhD, began her studies at the University of British Columbia, completed her master's degree at San Francisco State College, and earned her doctorate at the California School of Professional Psychology. She did further training at the Tavistock Clinic in London. Prior to her return to California, she practiced in London and British Columbia. Before her retirement, she was a supervisor and group leader at the WestCoast Children's Clinic in Oakland, California, and had an ongoing private practice in the Bay Area. Dr. Purves has been particularly interested in using the collaborative model with involuntary clients such as incarcerated youth and parents seeking reunification with their children and has written and presented internationally on these topics. Exploring how to develop accessible feedback to children and adults has been of continuing interest to her, both in her work and in her teaching and supervising.

Benedetta Rubino is a psychologist specializing in psychodiagnostics. She is involved in projects related to the mental health of refugees and asylum seekers and is a member of the Crinali Transcultural Assessment Group in Milan.

Stefania Sharley, psychologist and trainee psychotherapist, works with children with special educational needs and disabilities. She completed a psychology placement with Cooperativa Crinali and contributed to their latest book, *Sviluppi della clinica transculturale nelle relazioni di cura* (Cattaneo & Dal Verme, 2020). In 2020, as a participant in Italy's Civilian Service program, she was involved in projects aimed at promoting child protection in Cambodia.

Lucy Y. Steinitz, PhD, worked for 25 years in US social services until she and her husband had a midlife crisis that they solved by moving their family to Africa, where they lived for 17 years. Most of her work was focused on families affected by HIV and AIDS, especially orphans. In 2014, Dr. Steinitz and her husband moved back to the United States, where she now works on peace, justice, and protection issues with Catholic Relief Services.

Inge Van Laer is a licensed psychologist in the Netherlands and Belgium. She works at the Viersprong, a specialized clinic for the assessment and treatment of adults and adolescents with severe personality pathology and conduct disorders. Her expertise lies in working with adolescents and their families. Dr. Van Laer trains and supervises other psychologists on Therapeutic Assessment with adolescents and their families.

Foreword

This is a book about culture. More definitively, it is an account of the many ways the work of community psychology unceasingly resides within a contextual landscape. Context is the vital crossroads by which the psychological well-being of an individual intersects and is nourished by strengths within the social-ecological surround of setting. These strengths include the familial, collective, and historical narratives composing a setting's cultural bedrock. *Psychological Interventions from Six Continents: Culture, Collaboration, and Community* illuminates this truth. The book provides a deep description of work in the cultural context. Of equal importance, it centers *collaboration* as foundational to this work. These pages provide a rich portrait of the global reach of relational methodologies applied to research, and to implementing interventions guided by this research.

Central to the work described within this volume are horizontal relationships based in the commitment to equality. Its narrative describes the work of psychologists who understand their own usefulness comes out of relating to the other as equal. This profound acceptance of otherness necessarily incorporates an accompanying deep respect for different ways of knowing, and through this, appreciation of different structures of understanding and meaning. Respect is conveyed through the dialogue of equality. In each of the stories to follow, the relational methods compel formulation and implementation of intervention in culturally congruent ways.

Accordingly, the book opens with a meditation on the relationship of the provider of psychological services to those they hope to serve. The chapter that follows elevates an understanding of the importance of cultural uniqueness in the multiplicity of cultural systems and philosophies that create the diversity of global paradigms for psychological well-being. Each ensuing case study then portrays a way to intervene to promote well-being that arises from premises valuing uniqueness expressed in underrepresented ethnocultural viewpoints on their own merits. These case studies include a thoughtful cultural adaptation of existing interventions along with autochthonous approaches, or interventions borne only of that place. Notably, psychological assessment is presented through a similar lens. The case studies emphasize local, culture-based collaborative assessment models foundationally situated in the commitment to equality. This commitment drives purposeful attentiveness to each nuance of cultural context, bringing its knowledge systems and meaning structures into the assessment process.

The efforts described in these pages are each guided by diverse implementations of a community-based participatory research perspective. As a perspective, and not a method, each of the participatory approaches described is adaptive as it seeks to better match practices of its setting. The perspective joined with collaboration privileges indigenous theory describing the knowledge, practices, and meaning systems local to setting.

Core to all the accounts is a parallel story where a commitment to equality also necessitates an abiding concern for social justice. Within this concern, culture operates as a fundamental set of defining characteristics both in psychological understanding and meaningful social action. A woven thread emerges out of this volume of diverse communities each claiming ownership of their own knowledge and meaning making. Their collective voices provide an invitation to a psychology that is conscious of its own current ethnocentrism, and to psychological practice that incorporates true collaboration.

James Allen
University of Minnesota Medical School, Duluth Campus

Introduction: Culture, Collaboration, and Community

Barbara L. Mercer, Heather Macdonald, and Caroline Purves

Collaborative/Therapeutic Assessment in the United States

Our book is about how culture gives context to collaborative psychological assessment and psychological intervention practices around the world. To address this challenging topic, we present ten chapters from authors across the globe who speak about work in their communities and their cultural influences. Our intent is to open up similarities that bind us, at the same time to describe the world's unique cultural contexts, and in so doing push the boundaries of psychological assessment and intervention, to expand our ideas and our capacity for listening and learning. We reflect our core philosophy of valuing the applied, lived experience of psychological work and healing applied to each locale's culture and community.

Trained first as psychotherapists and later practiced in traditional Western psycho-diagnostic assessment, we gravitated toward nontraditional psychological assessment modalities that would incorporate a more person-centered relational approach, as we sought alternatives for accomplishing more fully collaborative therapeutic interventions through a personality assessment. Over the last several decades we have worked in city or nonprofit community clinics and social service environments, and from that perspective have embraced the rich diversity of our own locale. This both ignited and continues to fuel our desire to learn more about the cultures within our and other countries and their unique approaches to mental health. We are three women. We are of Canadian, Russian Jewish, and Scottish origins. We are all White. We have all spent not insignificant portions of our lives and careers traveling, working, and living in different countries and continents. We have absorbed and come to value many aspects of other cultures' ways of being.

The origin and inspiration for this book came from our work in a community child psychology clinic in Oakland, California, whose clients pay for mental health assistance with public funding insurance called Medi-cal.

DOI: 10.4324/9781003124061-1

Most have fewer financial resources than families who can afford private practice rates. Our clients arrived from multiple social systems with most referrals for psychological assessment and therapy coming from social workers who were the official public guardians of children and youth in foster care, from teachers who were concerned about their students, and from parents who qualified for low-cost mental health services. Whether or not their systems were familiar to our therapists/providers, it was incumbent upon us to understand youth as connected to the people and groups in their lives. Community psychology must reside within the contextual landscape from which those seeking assistance must not be separated nor made invisible to their individual, familial, or collective historical narratives.

As we evolved a systemic approach with our families, we began to recognize the unique adaptability of the collaborative model for our work in the community. The idea for this book grew from our work training increasing numbers of students from other cultures, and a commensurate desire to expand our understanding of mental health and psychology in other countries.

In conducting psychological assessments with children, we early on began to implement the innovative model of Collaborative/Therapeutic Assessment that departed from the expert-driven, "top-down" modalities. We trained and worked with Dr. Stephen Finn (2007, 2008; Finn & Tonsager, 1997, 2002), founder of the Therapeutic Assessment Institute, who served as a consultant in live sessions to inform our work with our youth and families. He showed us how traditional testing and psychological assessment could become inherently *therapeutic* and an *intervention*. Our work with foster children, with transcultural clientele, and with immigrants from Latin America and other countries, more and more came to reflect networks and increasingly complex systems, for example, grounded in public funding, multi-tiered social service, legal, and family systems.

Over half (55%) of the children seen in the clinic are in foster care and as such been separated from their biological parents. Forty-four percent of the families are African American, 33% of the clients are White, 12% are of Hispanic origin, 0.9% are Native American/Alaska Native, and 5% are Asian Pacific Islander (with 5% identifying as biracial or not reporting). (Kelley Gin, Personal Communication, August 2021). Many of the children have experienced abuse, neglect, socioeconomic and racial discrimination, immigration fears and trauma, and community violence, as well as abandonment by or loss of their biological parents and have been placed in the foster care system. Therapists and assessors often go to meet and assess children in their homes and in their neighborhoods.

If we looked solely at the "reason for referral" and "behavior," we missed vital aspects of our clients' experience. If we assessed them through the lens of purely standardized results, rigid administration, diagnosis, and a formal expert stance, we missed the person, their daily lives' struggles, their strengths and potentials, and the essential relational impact of the assessment. Issues of family, racial identity, ethnic and cultural values and practices, intergenerational and personal histories, and traumas, seeking refuge from wars, migration, economics, and their collective support networks or lack thereof, all demanded that we pay attention.

In our treatment and narratives, we sought a language that illuminated the uniqueness of our communities. In our psychological assessments, we challenged our trainees to divest themselves of the academic language they learned in graduate training (we asked "Where is the person in your report?"). The Collaborative/Therapeutic Assessment model, which emphasizes knowledge, understanding, and transparency during the process, by placing the "symptom" in a biographical, historical, and cultural narrative, provided for us an appropriate methodology. The clinic's clients are African-American or biracial, White, Latinx, Asian American, Native American, or families immigrating (documented and undocumented) from other countries—Latin American, African, Asian Pacific, South Asian, and Middle Eastern locales. Our assessments included relational aspects of identity and of hierarchy. ("How do our clients perceive us? as well as "How do we view them?").

At the end of an assessment, we gave feedback about it to the child/ youth that took the form of a story we wrote based on their struggles and their strengths. These "tales" or fables often provided a better, more clear understanding for both the parent and the child, even more so than the formal report. For a child who lost her mother and was being raised by her grandmother, we had stories like "The Rainforest Vet" (in which the assessor is the *veterinarian*) who gives Fearless the Tiger and Grandma Tiger a recipe for Feelings Soup, a soup they could cook together that's made from their important memories and feelings. "You can put all those feelings that are jumbled up inside of you into that soup," the assessor wrote. Also, there was "The Story of Marcus Who Never Cried," no matter how sad he felt or what he had been through. Or, "The Diary of a Grumpy Kid" whose brother did "scary" things and whose parents fought and got divorced.

As more doctoral students from other countries and more ethnically and racially diverse students came to graduate school, to internship, and to doctoral programs and wrote dissertations, they raised questions about assessment, cultural context and cultural equivalence, and the inclusion of cultural and Indigenous psychology that could not be ignored.

At international personality assessment conferences—where Western psychological principals predominated—we noted a growing interest in intersectionality when connecting with clinicians from other countries, even though Indigenous psychology or culturally adapted assessment measures were rarely mentioned.

After leaving Oakland, many of our students and staff returned to their own countries or moved to other countries (e.g., India or Zimbabwe) and opened a psychological practice or worked in rural areas or Indigenous reservations using alternative interventions. The Therapeutic Assessment model, as well as relationally focused projective measures (Crisi, 1998, 2018, George et al., 1999), have now spread throughout the world. These new models are both richly qualitative and supported by research in development and outcome. Clinicians are employing it with adults, children, and families across the planet.

Live trainings occur yearly in Japan and Italy under the supervision of Therapeutic Assessment's developer, Stephen Finn, where therapists come from all over the world to participate. And even the ongoing Coronavirus pandemic has seen these trainings continue through the wonder of the Internet.

Finn's (2007) proposal that we be "in our client's shoes" is our starting point. This collaborative approach in psychological assessment has been our portal to broader, more inclusive thinking about psychological interventions as a cooperative, transparent relationship between those delivering and those receiving service. This meant that the tenets of collaborative and therapeutic assessment could be expanded to *interventions* with *assessment* as a component. Therefore, we seek to learn more about how other cultures work to realize their aspirations for mental health and well-being. The chapters in this book are only a brief sampling of such practices. By reading books and articles, and reaching out to professionals around the world, we have encountered myriad innovative projects steeped in collaboration, in a sharing of cultural voices and values. We hope these pages will expand your notions of assessment and therapeutic interventions, help to pique your interest in these voices and values, and in so doing contribute to their visibility and viability for the mental health and psychology mainstream.

Culture in Mind: Thoughts About Culture and Mental Health Services

Frantz Fanon, the French West Indian psychiatrist and philosopher who worked with Algerian and French soldiers in Algeria in the 1950s, observed the posttraumatic effects of colonial violence on the human psyche. He formulated a model for community psychology and systems of mental health, believing that people suffering from mental health disorders would fare better if they were integrated into their family and community instead of being assigned to a rigid category, isolated, or institutionalized. He also understood that community-based psychology was a model that could address the vital intersection of people's psychological health with their social and economic situations. Community and social work models in the mental health field along with increasing collaborative psychological assessment seek a widening paradigm where knowledge and meaning are shared and "co-created."

At this sociocultural moment in the United States, we are facing alarming polarizations about race and economic inequities that demand urgent discussion. How we, as clinicians and writers in the United States, conceptualize "culture" may differ from those in another country or continent. And while our cultural concerns in the United States about social and racial challenges, mental health, and psychological intervention may well align with practitioners and writers from other countries, the processes by which they are addressed cannot.

Psychologies in India likely differ from psychologies created for Indigenous people in Canada or Australia. Historical impact, such as that of "abusive and coercive residential schooling in Canada" (Teo & Wendt, 2020, p. 373), may bear similarities with the forced permanent separation of children and families in Australia; but the impact on mental health and well-being may differ radically depending on locale. James Allen (2002), in his work with Inuit Alaska Natives, noted the rich variation of Indigenous people in North America with their "vast differences in customs, religion and social organization" (p. 216). He cites from a 1991 Bureau of Indian Affairs publication the statistic that there are over 500 federally recognized tribal entities with over 200 spoken languages. In India in South Asia, there are currently 28 different states and 8 unions with nearly as many languages and cultural beliefs.

Therefore, it is important for treatment, research, and training in each locale to hold their own knowledge and perspective. In reaching out to psychologists across the globe and learning about psychological assessment and intervention from other perspectives, we realized that with some clinicians, their culture is the climate or fabric that gives background texture to their collaborative work with clients. With other clinicians, we learned that psychological services needed adaptation taking holistic cultural practices and world views in mind in order to give relevant treatment. Finally, we understood that Western and Eastern locales contain a hybrid of ideas and intervention strategies, but may purposefully seek ways to create and implement their own cultural treatments. At this time, the crises of a pandemic as well as of migration have connected us across the globe in ways we could not have imagined. Yet in this time of loss, we have been able to connect over the Internet to talk with and learn about each other. Physical and emotional well-being have never been more manifestly bound together, connected to all of us in some, often meaningful way.

The countries and cultures of our planet have become increasingly linked, leading to a desire and necessity for a more spacious awareness and dialogue. Through voluntary and forced migrations adding to already existing cultural groups within countries, this traditional model is no longer sufficient to help psychologists understand their clients. In this context, the idea of the learned psychologist using much-studied "tests" to "solve" or determine the "inner workings" of the client is not enough to both help the client and to generate helpful feedback to others involved. Literature on mainstream Western psychology and community and cultural psychology are rarely integrated so readers and practitioners must be cognizant enough to search both fields of study for information on therapeutic philosophy, treatment, and research.

One of our authors wondered that working with colleagues around the globe during this time must be a hard thing to do. He likened it to a "Quijotada" ("against all odds"), to Cervantes Don Quijote de la Mancha (Ernesto Pais, personal communication, 18 August 2021). That is to say, at moments our venture has seemed like that of the infamous knight errant, romantic, and impractical. Over 20 years ago, Hermans and Kempen (1998) called our accelerated process of globalization and interconnectedness a challenge to contemporary psychology. They proposed an approach for thinking about culture that is neither homogeneous, dichotomous, nor geographically located. Their hope, perhaps idealized and radical in these times, is to regard our communities as interculturally connected. Global connection and the diaspora have enriched our lives, yet made the task of belonging challenging or arduous. When we began to visualize this volume, full of energy as we researched and gathered the writings of committed clinicians around the world, we gained more knowledge, a greater awareness of blind spots, and an acknowledgment of the complexities inherent in how we identify and define culture.

Historical Origins

In the United States, psychological assessment (in mainstream practice) has been informed to a significant degree by behavioral and evidence-based modalities originating from European culture, from German academic research laboratories; whereas Latin American psychology, primarily psychoanalytic, has its underpinnings in European philosophical traditions. Indigenous psychologies may comprise a mingling of a particular Indigenous culture and Western methods or, in contrast, advocate a discreet or untainted treatment preserving the Indigenous language, definitions, and applications. Thomas Teo (2013) states the evident premise that psychological theories by definition reflect the culture from which they emerge. Therefore, Indigenous, cultural, or critical psychologies are essential as concepts, and practices of mental health can be vastly different from Western practices (Teo & Wendt, 2020).

By the same premise, Western or Eurocentric psychologies should be assessed for their values and their ability to reach the people they serve.

Traditional empirical research with standardized norms and statistical outcomes can be effective and progressive if its approach is not objectifying or applied interpretively for power over others. However, as practitioners we need to continue to be aware of biases that may be built into the structure of statistical analyses that derive standardized scores or even the ways we interpret our assessments or design our interventions. Several of the studies we explored, including some in this book, initiated Indigenous programs partnered with supplementary research design from traditional Western clinicians and specialists.

Integrative or Sovereign

We have seen a phenomenological approach in Native American treatment approaches in the United States and Canada in which terminology is subjective and idiographic, not nomothetic—that is, not comparable to standardized norms or universal scientific principles of human nature. Subjectivity need not preclude objectivity and can bring a needed holistic meaning into service delivery. Harvard's Joseph P. Gone (2019) states, "Our culture is our treatment" (p. 174). Eduardo Duran, working with Native clients in Montana, avows that "we must go beyond this paradigm and find different ways of measuring human potential as well as to treat and diagnose maladies afflicting the soul" (Eduardo Duran, personal communication, June, 2020). While he notes that Native cultures have included non-Native treatments, or offered only non-Native mental health providers, he wonders whether non-Native clinicians are able to shed enough skepticism or find sufficient openness to integrate Native healing methods in providing service (Duran & Duran, 1995). He states, "We cannot decolonize as long as we continue to measure ourselves by standards based on racism ... which have their genesis in correlational stats" (Eduardo Duran, personal communication 2020). Supportive of this injunction, we hold two viewpoints of cultural thought in mind. As one of our authors states: "Our community does it differently" (Lucy Steinitz, personal communication, 2020). From another perspective, we see ways we are interdependent, how we import and incorporate each other's ideas and practices into our own.

Throughout this book, these thoughtful authors illuminate uniqueness. Each country or therapeutic process presents differences in style and in the location of services, whether private practice or public setting. Approaches reflect choices of scientific or phenomenological qualitative approaches. The authors utilize some form of psychological assessment whether using traditional tests and treatments in a collaborative manner, innovative measures, or a mixture of both. They write of historical and sociopolitical contexts or concentrate on their own culturally rich interventions. We see a focus on individual treatment or a solely collective intervention. Despite differences, common themes involve collaborative work between provider and receiver of service, co-creation of service between clinicians and their community, transparency of treatment in the offering of a design for emotional health and well-being, participation throughout the process, and, finally, the owning and dissemination of the resulting knowledge. The basic tenets of these complementary models encourage exchange of information, allowing the client to fully participate in the process. All of these psychological interventions "break the traditional frame" and offer some disruption or creative adaptation in psychological assessment, service delivery, and ideas about relationships and psychology in the context of culture and community. Our intention is not to define culture but to open and widen our perspective.

In section I, Chapter 1, titled "Beginnings: Psychological Service Delivery" (by Barbara L. Mercer) investigates the meaning of mental health service delivery and gives an overview of cultural psychology, asserting that although culture is implicit in every locale, "culture" stipulates that one delivery style does not necessarily apply to all. Chapter 2, "Paradigms for Well-Being: Ways of Knowing and Psychological Services" (also by Barbara L. Mercer) highlights several unique cultural systems and philosophies that illustrate the variations and potentialities of psychological assessment and treatment.

Psychological Interventions from Six Continents

Two methodological threads are the textural substructures of this volume. The first is derived from the Therapeutic Assessment model created and developed by Constance Fischer (1970, 1985) and Stephen Finn. The method presented here by six of our authors is called Therapeutic Assessment (TA; relying on a specific certification and an empirically based set of steps) as well as what is termed the Collaborative/Therapeutic Assessment (C/TA), which preserves the core ideas and collaborative techniques of TA. Both TA and C/TA encourage practitioners to adapt their assessments to particular settings, for example, with foster families, in a community or school setting, immigration, an Indigenous research project, or assessment practices in a particular country.

Readers will see this collaborative approach in section II, which contains descriptions of various Collaborative/Therapeutic Assessment models. Chapter 3, "Assessment, Training, and Social Justice, in Community Psychology" (by the editors of this volume) looks at doctoral assessment training in Oakland, California, the delivery of services during a time of racial injustice and national turmoil, and an assessment feedback using culturally based images and language. Chapter 4, "Assessment of Japanese Children: *Hikikomori* "(by Noriko Nakamura), reviews the author's therapeutic assessment approach with a particular youth, delving into the culturally embedded problem of "shut-ins." Chapter 5, "Growing Empathy With Complex Clients in Developing Countries: Collaborative/ Therapeutic Assessment in Latinoamérica" (by Ernesto Pais and Daniela Escobedo-Belloc), takes us through two depth-oriented cases, each with a complex presenting problem and astute interventions. Chapter 6, "Culture and Psychological Assessment in India" (by Kakli Gupta) writes of the author's personal journey as a young Western-trained Indian psychologist and her creative use of therapy-oriented assessments. These authors all write of cases where a relational assessment process led to therapeutic understanding and change.

In Section III, titled "Collaborations and Immigration," the clinicians use the Collaborative/Therapeutic assessment approach as well as a holistic, transpersonal, and culturally attuned method. (See John Chuol Kuek in Chapter 9). In Chapter 7, "Collaborative Assessment from a Transcultural Perspective: Cooperative Crinali's Experience in Milan, Italy" (by members of the Cooperativa Crinali) the authors show a sensitive use of immigrant native language speakers as mediators on an assessment team. Chapter 8, "Different Cultures Wear Different Shoes!" Therapeutic Assessment with a 17-Year-Old Moroccan Immigrant Boy" in the Netherlands (by Hilde De Saeger and Inge Van Laer) provides reflections on Therapeutic Collaborative interventions and gives an empathic view into the life of a Moroccan youth and his mother. The last contribution in this section, Chapter 9, "Psychological Assessment of South Sudanese Persons in Mental Health Treatment in the United States" (by John Chuol Kuek), highlights a culturally attuned and trauma-informed perspective on immigration and a transpersonal approach to trauma recovery—both in the United States and in South Sudan—with a guide for mental health practitioners from a culturally based understanding of symptoms.

Section IV, titled "New Measures, Alternative Interventions, and Indigenous Inclusion," introduces the second thread of our volume and a paradigm and developing direction for psychological intervention. These chapters combine and integrate new assessment measures adapted for Indigenous clientele and combine outcome measures with workshops based in cultural values and developed for work with trauma. They propose an Indigenous paradigm, one that Kim and Berry (1993) describe as "the scientific study of human behavior or mind that is native, that is not transported from other regions, and that is designed for its people" (p. 2). According to these authors, this process emphasizes contextual understanding rooted in a particular setting. The historical, political, and cultural context of each region becomes this embedded context. It is also important to note that some Indigenous approaches do not incorporate *scientific* studies *per se* but adopt other paths toward healing and well-being. Thomas Teo (Teo & Wendt, 2020) notes that even

Indigenous as a concept or terminology is debated and varies in definition. He states that Indigenous psychologies may show "differing forms of life" and also "highlight the power and violence that stems from societal privileges" (p. 373). Indigenous psychologies are essential to the field of psychology because their core conceptualizations and practices offer depth and alternatives in their differences from Western approaches.

Some of the intervention models in this section are *autochthonous*—born in their own locale, independent of imported origins—with a focus on reclaiming ownership of knowledge and meaning making and on creating research and treatment related to local culture, behaviors, and training of providers (Georgas & Mylonas, 2006). However, the intervention models described here incorporate some interface with assessment measures, theories, or practices working in tandem with community consultants, guides, and providers.

Chapter 10, "Singing to the Lions: Culturally Relevant Intervention in Zimbabwe and Beyond" (by Jonathan Brakarsh, Lucy Steinitz, Jane Chidzungu, Eugenia Mpande, and Lightwell Mpofu), introduces a creative workshop model for working with children dealing with trauma. Their model has been used in other countries in Africa, Asia, and the Middle East. Chapter 11, "Indigenous Inclusion and Intervention: The Flight of Eagles" (by Shaun Hains), describes North American Indigenous practices in working with Native and non-Native children and youth within a public-school system and introduces Indigenous ethics and intervention as a valid research and practice model. Chapter 12, "Indigenous Psychology in Australia: Aboriginal Mental Health" (by Helen Milroy, Monique Platell, and Shraddha Kashyap), promotes the reclamation of Aboriginal knowledge, practices, and cultural survival in the context of the colonization of and discrimination against Aboriginal people. The authors explore the interface of Western mental health and Aboriginal cultural ideas and providers, offering some new validated measures and tools for well-being embedded in Aboriginal culture and values.

Some Final/Finer Notes

Case Material and Relevant Contexts

We wanted our volume to focus on hands-on interventions, as well as theoretical, historical contexts, and therapeutic assessment and intervention models. Each chapter contributes hypothetical case material or personal accounts with permission from the clients. We wanted to provide the experience of the client and provider in a cultural context. Many of our chapters and authors address work with children and families, but adults are also included in some case material. All authors highlight a collaborative process as an essential therapeutic intervention.

Grammar and Spelling

Part of cultural variation is the English language itself. In the spirit of cultural variance, we want to preserve both the US and UK systems, based on the author's preferred usage. English is not the first language of some of our authors. Some chapters may have been written in a first language and translated into English. In some cases, we kept some stylistic expressions or ways of speaking that may differ from standard English. We have tried to use terms for communities that have emerged from the communities, and authors themselves. This can vary with, for example, Native American, American Indian, Indigenous, Aboriginal, Latinx, Latinoamérica, Hispanic, and White (the "W" capitalized in APA format). *Elder* is capitalized in Indigenous cultures.

References

Allen, J. (2002). Assessment training for practice in American Indian and Alaskan Native settings. *Journal of Personality Assessment, 79*(2), 216–225.

Crisi, A. (1998). *Manuale del test di Wartegg: Norme per la raccolta, la siglatura e l'interpretazione* [Wartegg test manual: Rules for collection, scoring and interpretation]. Magi Edizioni.

Crisi, A. (1998). *The Crisi Wartegg System (CWS): Manual for administration, scoring, and interpretation.* English Adaptation and Additional Content by Jacob A. Palm. (2018), Routledge.

Duran, B., & Duran, E. (1995). *Native American postcolonial psychology.* State University of New York Press.

Finn, S. E. (2007). *In our client's shoes: Theory and techniques of therapeutic assessment.* Erlbaum.

Finn, S. E. (2008). The many faces of empathy in experiential, person-centered, collaborative assessment. *Journal of Personality Assessment, 91*, 20–23.

Finn, S. E., & Tonsager, M. E. (1997). Information-gathering and therapeutic models of assessment: Complementary paradigms. *Psychological Assessment, 9*, 374–385.

Finn, S. E., & Tonsager, M. E. (2002). How therapeutic assessment became humanistic. *The Humanistic Psychologist, 30*, 10–22.

Fischer, C. T. (1970). The testee as co-evaluator. *Journal of Counseling Psychology, 17*, 70–76.

Fischer, C. T. (1985). *Individualizing psychological assessment.* Laurence Erlbaum Associates.

Georgas, J., & Mylonas, K. (2006). Cultures are like all other cultures, like some other cultures, like no other culture. In U. Kim, K.-S. Yang, & K.-K. Hwang (Eds.), *Indigenous and cultural psychology: Understanding people in context* (pp. 197–221). Springer Science.

George, C., West, M., & Pettem, O. (1999). The Adult Attachment Projective: Disorganization of adult attachment at the level of representation. In J. Solomon & C. George (Eds.), *Attachment disorganization* (pp. 462–507). Guilford.

Gone, J. P. (2019). "The thing that happened as he wished": Recovering an American Indian cultural psychology. *American Journal of Community Psychology, 64,* 172–184. https://doi.org/10:1002/ajcp.12353

Hermans, H. J. M., & Kempen, H. J. G. (1998). Moving cultures: The perilous problems of cultural dichotomies in a globalizing society. *American Psychologist, 53*(10), 1111–1120.

Kim, U., & Berry, J. W. (1993). *Indigenous psychologies: Experience and research in cultural context.* Sage.

Raskin, J. (1984, July 27). A last interview with French philosopher Michel Foucault. *Washington City Paper.*

Teo, T. (2013). Backlash against American psychology: An indigenous reconstruction of the history of German critical psychology. *History of Psychology, 16*(1), 1–18.American Psychological Association. https://doi.org/10.1037a0020386.

Teo, T., & Wendt, D. C. (2020). Some clarifications on critical and indigenous psychologies. *Theory and Psychology, 30*(3), 371–376.

Section I

Psychological Service Delivery

Chapter 1

Beginnings: Psychological Service Delivery

Barbara L. Mercer

Should Psychology Be Delivered "To" or "With"?

Service delivery is the part of a health system where patients receive the treatment and supplies they are entitled to (Transparency International, 2020).

People have a different experiential, affective sense of self and relationships, as well as vastly different internalized world views that give profoundly different meanings to everyday experiences and relationships (Roland, 1988, p. 4).

> Cultures are like all other cultures, like some other cultures, like no other culture. (Georgas & Mylonas, 2006, p. 201)

The history of psychological assessment highlights an ongoing and often tense dialogue between empirical, theoretical, and "lived" humanistic understanding, between actuarial/evidence-based and clinical methods (Mercer, 2016). Meehl (Dawes et al., 1989; Meehl, 1954) argued for the superiority of actuarial data and the abandonment of the clinical approach. Even a noted clinical researcher who contributed to the early development of in-depth psychological testing, Klopfer (1954), cautioned that more than superficial feedback could be destructive to the patient. Psychoanalytic assessment (Lerner, 2007) emphasized understanding the experience of the person being assessed, the assessment relationship, and writing in plain and interesting language. Fischer (1985/1994), Finn (2007), Tharinger et al. (2007), and Handler (2006) further developed the therapeutic collaborative assessment process as an integration of statistical rigor within the interpersonal context.

One of the main models of psychological assessment and intervention put forth in this book originated in the Therapeutic/Collaborative Assessment process that contrasts its service delivery style with *traditional assessment*. Stephen Finn (2007) defines traditional assessment as the model where

DOI: 10.4324/9781003124061-3

psychological tests are administered to clients primarily for the purposes of diagnosis, treatment planning, treatment evaluation and/or increased understanding. The main emphasis in traditional assessment is typically on the standardized data that is carefully collected by the "expert" assessor who then compares test scores to nomothetic norms in order to derive conclusions that will be useful in understanding, communicating about, and treating a certain 'patient' or in monitoring the progress of treatment. (pp. 3–4)

Scholars as early as the 1970s (Brown, 1972; Fischer, 1970) criticized this approach as a dismissal of clients' resources and dignity and one that focused only on their psychopathology. The pioneering work of Constance Fischer (1970) demonstrated that humanistic and inter-subjective values and practices could be incorporated into psychological assessment. Fischer laid out the basic principles of what would later come to be referred to as a "new paradigm of psychological assessment" (p. 4). She viewed the assessment session as an interpersonal situation that is reflective of a person's characteristic and relational approach (Aschieri et al., 2016). She was not trained this way, however.

Fischer (Finn et al., 2012) described being admonished by her su-pervisors during one of her assessment trainings after her 19-year-old psychotic testee said she was "frightened by the giggling and talking that she heard coming from the one-way mirror." [Fischer explained to the testee that] "my teachers were watching me to see if I was doing the test correctly. I had been told not to talk with the patient, just to test" (p. x), not to be interactive, and above all not to make the process transparent.

The growing focus of conferences, books, and articles that combine statistics with case studies (Viglione, 2003), neuropsychology with collaboration (Engleman, 2007; Smith, 2007), and analytic with struc-tural data (Lerner, 2007) indicate that collaborative ideas and cultural contexts are yielding a new era of assessment in the United States and Europe. However, in a search for references to *community psychology* in the *Journal of Personality Assessment*, not a single article emerges. Dana (1996)) and Allen (Allen & Dana, 2004) have challenged our status quo assumptions with articles on the cross-cultural use of the Rorschach and the Minnesota Multiphasic Personality Inventory (Butcher & Hass, 2009) and have argued for the development of an empirical basis for multicultural assessment. The publication of inter-national norms for the Exner Comprehensive System (Meyer et al., 2011) has further awakened our understanding of a cross-cultural interpretive framework and the consideration of social context as es-sential to test validation.

Collaborative-style psychological assessment often incorporates traditional and scientific methods purposed for diagnosis and treatment planning, but more importantly, it is *contextualized* and is inherently a *therapeutic intervention.* In reviewing these complex ideas, we intend to show the intersection of our own familiar context with those of other cultural psychologies.

Cultural Psychologies: Review of Concepts and Definitions

Cross-Cultural Psychology, Cultural Psychology, and Indigenous Psychology

Collaborative Assessment deviates from the traditional model by following a more transparent and relational process, but *cultural psychology* inhabits an even more discrete field in psychological literature. There is yet further distinction in the cultural psychology field between *"cross-cultural" comparative* psychology and cultural and Indigenous psychologies. Eurocentric psychological studies tend to research comparisons among cultures; the results often find variability at a statistically insignificant level, with a predilection for commonality, and subsequently, advocate for a standardized or uniform service delivery. The literature centers around whether approaches to psychological traits and values are *etic* (an outsider evaluation of cultural comparisons) vs. *emic* (an insider perspective and culture specific).

Cross-cultural psychology augments this process of cross-cultural research comparisons by arriving at or comparing generalized trait characteristics for different countries or ethnic groups. Examples of questions asked from this perspective are: Do Greeks support religiosity and family values in a similar way to Russians or Danes? (Georgas & Mylonas, 2006); Is the Japanese concept of *amae* particular to the Japanese? (Yamaguchi & Ariizumi, 2006); Do Koreans and Americans perceive behaviors in similar ways? (Wang et al., 2020); and, Are there country or cultural differences in attributional processes? (Zajenkwska et al., 2020).

Cultural psychology, by further contrast, begins with a notion proposed by James Allen (1998) that "the convention of cross-cultural uniformity as null hypothesis needs re-examination" and "can bring implicit value judgment and disservice to ethnic minority clients" (p 19). Cultural variance, Allen posits, should be adopted as the null hypothesis. As mental health professionals, when we meet with clients we take a history, viewing the individual's historical context as relevant to current symptoms or problems. Yet reports or interventions are then often decontextualized. In psychological writing and practice, we rarely expand to the broader, historical perspective. Therefore, he asserts, "An important starting point for multicultural assessment practice is culturally appropriate delivery of assessment service" (Allen, 2002, p. 220).

Indigenous psychology delves more deeply into contextual elements and expands our psychological paradigms. Many authors, scholars, and researchers have noted how local, Indigenous, and Eurocentric ideas have been successfully combined for assessment and intervention service delivery. Allen (1998) notes as an example the reclaiming of local knowledge through Elders and community while bringing in traditional scientific outcome measures, then returning to community dissemination of knowledge and results.

Eduardo Duran (2019) writes eloquently and forcefully of healing soul wounds in Native communities resulting from trauma and dislocation. Duran wonders whether Western psychologists, with their skepticism of native healing practices, can trust enough to effectively utilize nontraditional interventions and approaches. In *Native American Postcolonial Psychology* Duran and Duran (1995) write: "The study of cross-cultural knowledge is a difficult endeavor at best. A post-colonial paradigm would accept knowledge from differing cosmologies as valid in their own right, without having to yield to a separate cultural body for legitimacy" (pp. 5–6). At the same time, in Eduardo Duran's depth-oriented therapy for healing with clients, he is able to incorporate Jungian-oriented dream work and sand tray therapy with children in uncovering and healing trauma.

Joseph Gone's (2007, 2019) description of work derived from his own people, the Gros Ventre, at the Fort Belknap Reservation such as Indian shamanic healing and storytelling, retains Native languages and practices without mention of Western influence or linguistic reinterpretations. As the Plains Indian shaman Traveling Thunder relayed to Gone in a riveting interview: "We never was happy, you know, living as a Whiteman" (2007, p. 294). In other studies, Gone (Gone et al., 2019) employs scientific research tools to investigate the link between Indigenous historical trauma and negative health outcomes. This research link between historical trauma and current symptoms of suffering often utilizes scientific measures combined with local interventions in culturally sensitive ways. In addition, the symbols woven through Gone's review of Gros Ventre healing modalities suggest that these approaches can be administered with awareness by non-Native providers or even in non-Native settings with some clients.

In James Allen's examination of service delivery construct and measurement equivalence in Alaska Native and Alaskan Indian communities (1998), he references the Fischer/Finn model of collaborative assessment as a useful template. This approach to assessment can be used whether the assessor is a Native or non-Native psychologist.

The *Therapeutic Assessment* process involves a collaborative formulation of questions that a person would like answered about themselves and concludes with feedback that invites the person to give or correct their own impressions about the results. This model has been expanded in Alaska to a community-based participatory research approach (CBPR) that includes community members (e.g., Elders and youth) to create their own research questions at the outset, devise the strategy for investigation, and direct the dissemination of findings (Rasmus et al., 2019).

The Indigenous model put forth by Kim, Berry, and colleagues, in their comprehensive *Indigenous Psychologies: Understanding People in Context* (Kim et al., 2006), describes *Indigenous psychology* as "the scientific study of human behavior or mind that is native, that is not transported from other regions, and that is designed for its people" (Kim & Berry, 1993, p. 5). These authors go on to say that "Although both indigenous and general psychology seek to discover universal facts, principles, and laws of human behavior, the starting point of research is different. General psychology ... assumes that current psychological theories are universal" (Koch & Leary, 1985 as cited in Kim et al., 2006). "Indigenous psychology, however, questions the universality of existing psychological theories and attempts to discover psychological universals in social, cultural, and ecological context (Kim & Berry, 1993). "Indigenous psychology represents an approach in which the content (i.e., meaning, values, and beliefs) context (i.e., family, social, cultural, and ecological) are explicitly incorporated into research design" (Kim et al., 2006, p. 3).

Kim's model identifies the importance of psychological phenomena in context and the use of the first-person subjective voice as an essential part of understanding human functioning. Therefore, indigenous studies must not be merely "ethnic or anthropological studies". This model neither includes nor precludes a particular method, thus allowing, but not suggesting, an integration of more Western "traditional" measures or methods into local practices.

The term *Indigenous psychology* reveals further complexities in any global consideration of psychological assessment and intervention. A number of authors (Berry, 2000; Diaz-Loving, 1999; Poortinga, 1999) discuss parallel and integrative methods of investigating psychology in different cultures, advocating for cultural interpretations as primary but leading to potentially universal constructs. The two Greek psychologists cited above (Georgas & Mylonas, 2006) encourage a partnership between comparative cross-cultural psychology and cultural/Indigenous psychology. Kim (Kim & Berry, 1993; Kim et al., 1999) emphasizes the need for psychologists from non-Western countries to be creative in thinking and developing psychological concepts and methods based on their own culture with the option of integrating Western scientific methods. One of the goals for Indigenous psychologies is that universal facts become discoverable through understanding a culture rather than being assumed or imposed *a priori.*

A cultural framework of Indigeneity almost always involves a historical narrative—such as colonization, civil war, oppression and suppression of culture, language, and human rights—and an emic framework (based on the internal elements of the culture or language) for the reclamation of cultural knowledge, values, and practices. A core belief in most Indigenous psychologies involves the claiming of one's own historical and cultural system of knowledge, thus imparting power and identity. Some Indigenous psychologists work collaboratively with Western-trained therapists, whereas others seek psychological assistance only from tribal or spiritual leaders. Many Indigenous psychologies integrate Eurocentric techniques (e.g., Jungian or play therapy) or research methods (e.g., outcome measures or culturally adapted assessment materials) into their own cultural language and framework.

Implicit Contexts and Meanings

Western traditional psychological theories—as well as *whiteness*—are central to an ideology that is intrinsic throughout psychological discourse rather than explicitly named in research and practice. The United States contains myriad cultures and ethnic communities that bear no equivalence to a prevailing cultural norm. European cultures also have their own historical and multicultural contexts. Teo (2013) discusses the development of *critical psychology* in Germany, Latin America, and South Africa as a *liberation psychology* and an important contrast to more "traditional" approaches. Cultural mores and differences may appear subtle (e.g., greeting style, eye contact, pace of conversation, openness to conversation about particular topics) or more pronounced (e.g., ideas about time, an individualistic vs. a collective or holistic, cultural and familial way of being, behavioral focus vs. clinical understanding). I believe that highlighting cultural and historical contexts, so often neglected, or hard to talk about, should be the starting point for a multicultural perspective in psychological assessment and intervention. Even so, as clinicians, we must remind ourselves to keep separate, or to bracket, our own milieux within which our own biases all too comfortably reside.

Georgas and Mylonas (2006), highlight the etymology of the terms *autochthonous* and *indigenous*. Autochthonous is defined as "a resident from the onset in the land of one's family." (They define "auto" in Greek as meaning "he, she, it, they or those"; chthonos meaning land). Indigenous is defined as "one who has been born in a specific place, who belongs there as a native inhabitant, who resides in one's place of birth and descent." (p. 197). Discussion of Indigenous communities is most often employed when these communities are, by contrast to other nations, forced to become settlers in their own land or having their country colonized. The goal of Indigenous psychology is to reclaim ownership of knowledge and meaning making, "to make psychological research more culturally sensitive, more autochthonous—that is, more independent of its imported origins and more focused on addressing local issues, customs, behaviors, and local training" (Adair, 1999; Georgas & Mylonas, 2006, p. 199).

Historical Roots

The literature of Indigenous psychology most often derives from the context of colonization. The definition of *colonialism* in the context of Native communities in the United States and Canada and the settling of lands, languages, and culture in Australia and Aotearoa/New Zealand, refers predominantly to Western European countries' colonization of lands in the Americas, Africa, Asia, and Oceania; the main European countries responsible for this form of colonization included Spain, Portugal, France, the Kingdom of England (later Great Britain), the Netherlands, Belgium, and the Kingdom of Prussia (now Germany) (Wikipedia, 2021). When one country colonizes another, it usually exploits the land, resources, and its populace for economic gain. The completion of the act of colonization is achieved when the occupying country creates its own government to which the occupied populace must be subservient.

Historically, exceedingly few countries have been neither a colonizing power nor colonized, and many of those were forced to fight back against colonization or invasion (e.g., Ethiopia). Thailand developed close personal and diplomatic ties with Britain; and many powers have tried and failed to colonize Afghanistan, due to various combinations of its rugged terrain, tribal culture, and shifting political and religious alliances. (World Population Review, 2021).

Other countries have experienced a *de facto* colonization by which their lands and people were exploited for economic gain but the occupying power did not establish its own government. For example, the British government did not officially rule Iran, but for much of the 20th century, it held sway over its government's policies by virtue of securing the right to develop its most valuable resource—petroleum (World Population Review).

Migrations to the Americas, Europe, and Asia, either forced or by preference, have introduced hundreds of cultural groups and practices such that few if any can claim a monocultural identity. But, this does not mean that we must develop a unique psychology for every cultural group. Our global history and interconnection invite us to seek a cultural psychology that asks us to be conscious of our own histories, ethnocentrism, and to incorporate a collaborative and culturally sensitive service delivery.

Evolving Paradigms

Indigenous psychologies as a service/delivery *philosophy* need not be limited to Native peoples but is an essential *attitude* for all cultural, Native, and ethnic groups within the larger or governing culture's context, and its ideas can be considered as a *paradigm* for a larger context. Teo (2013), in advocating for this type of approach, asserts that "all psychologies have culture-centric dimensions" (p. 10). Teo prefers to define *Indigenization* as the process through which a local culture develops its own form of psychology from within that culture *or* imports aspects of psychologies developed elsewhere and combines them with local concepts (Teo, 2013; see also Pickren & Rutherford, 2010). For the purposes of this book, however, I and my co-editors do not define the importing of traditional, Western ideas as indigenization. However, Teo's premise that no culture is a pure rendering but imports and mingles with other racial, cultural, and philosophical elements, is a crucial one. The *ideas* of Indigenous psychology offer a valuable contribution to the field of cultural psychology.

Authors who explore colonization and post-colonization expand these ideas, questioning the notion of a purely geographical national culture and seeing that many nations subject to colonization and subsequent diaspora generate in their citizens a different understanding of acculturation, not necessarily a sub summation, but rather an amalgam of values, meanings, and identities.

Indigenous psychologies have much to inform a Western tradition. Bhatia, the Indian psychologist states that "a truly meaningful collaboration between Western and Third World psychologists will, [however] need to begin with the acknowledgment of their shared history within the context of Orientalism in colonial times and cultural imperialism in the postcolonial era" (Bhatia, 2002, p. 395).

In Australia, Aboriginal authors, like those in our book, contend that culturally validated assessment tools combined with cultural responsiveness are essential. They echo the importance of giving clients within a mainstream delivery service access to incorporating Indigenous mental health providers and their ideas for symptom assessment and treatment.

Joseph Gone, offering the American-Indian perspective from the other side of the world asserts, "A decolonization approach ... will collaborate with community experts and leaders toward local innovations in counseling and therapeutic services based on tailored responses to community needs" (Gone, 2021, p. 267). He references, for example, a Blackfeet Indian culture camp bringing Indigenous therapeutic traditions to treat addiction in the Blackfeet Nation. Suggesting an approach that honors Eduardo Duran's work with Indigenous communities (2019), Gone alludes to the importance of coordination with spiritual leaders or openness to including prayer in therapy sessions. He notes that because knowledge is the focus of professional inquiry and expertise, a decolonization approach as a generic framework, rather than a method, *per se*, legitimizes local knowledge and recovers communal meaning. He discusses the emergence of Indigenous Research Methodologies (IRM) as a critical source that aims to "respect, value, engage and serve Indigenous people" (p. 52). At the same time, he advocates for the blending of academic and Indigenous community knowledge systems as a vital participatory research strategy. (Gone, 2019). This research methodology is presented in Sean Hains's chapter on the introduction of Indigenous practices into the public school system in Alberta. Duran reinforces both treatment and research for Native approaches which includes an "alchemical" mixture of psychotherapeutic and Native practice. He embraces faith in feeling, subjectivity, and spirituality in treatment, and in assigning to the community any participatory research, engagement, and control, preferring to call it *liberation research* (2019, p. 152).

The Collaborative/Therapeutic approach highlighted by many of our clinicians has been a foundation in our own work and expanded our perspective to be open to how other community practices might inform and enrich our own service delivery. The sensitive Collaborative/ Therapeutic Assessment approaches in this volume show how a relational model can be individualized to a country in South America or Europe or Asia. Psychological interventions can be rigorous while taking in a person's historical truth and social context. In many of our chapters, clinicians share like-minded psychological ideas within their own particular country or cultural milieux. Authors from countries and psychologies from around the world, while culturally distant from one other, assert that if our disparate traditions are to find any collaborative purpose, we must incorporate into our service delivery what the field of phenomenology has to offer: How it can help us learn from the experience of others as it helps to focus on a person's *lived* experience in the world (Neubauer et al., 2019). Douglas Adams, author of *Hitch-Hikers Guide to the Galaxy*, took a journey around the world with Zoologist Mark Carwardine to search for the world's rare animals. He opined: "Human beings, who are almost unique in having the ability to learn from the experience of others, are also remarkable for their apparent disinclination to do so." (Adams & Carwardine, 1990, p. 116). As scientists, researchers, and providers, let us continue to listen and respond to the experience of our communities.

Culture, Collaboration, and Community

The editors of this volume have connected with practitioners from six continents to bring to light assessments and interventions from current practices around the globe. Each author offers an amalgam of traditional academics rooted in their own cultural context. To say that there are more diverse communities and peoples than we can ever hope to cover is an understatement. Supported by these theoretical underpinnings, we hope to give the reader an experience of service delivery from ten diverse global and cultural locales.

The next chapter highlights cultural constructs and practices from a sampling of these global communities. The underlying principle of this volume and its contributors promotes collaborative models and techniques that embody what was described early on by Fischer (1970) as the "testee" or person seeking service, whether it be an assessment or a needed intervention, as a "co-evaluator." The Māori assessor participates in this therapeutic relationship calling it a *sharing in* inviting in, and *walking "alongside of"* (Waitoki, 2016, p. 183), and the testee is not a passive recipient of an impersonal process. Waitoki (2012) described the relationship between provider and receiver of therapeutic work as "sharing-power" (p. 150). A common thread and question in our chapters is: Who owns and disseminates the knowledge? This relational and client-centered approach, developed by Finn, has been transported to Latin America, Europe, and Asia, and the Therapeutic Collaborative model is integrated with each country's cultural values.

References

Adair, J. G. (1999). Indigenization of psychology: The concept and its practical implementation. *Applied Psychology*, *48*, 403–418.

Adams, D., & Carwardine, M. (1990). *Last chance to see*. Ballantine Books.

Allen, J. (1998). Personality assessment with American Indians and Alaska Natives: Instrument considerations and service delivery style. *Journal of Personality Assessment*, *70*(1), 17–42.

Allen, J. (2002). Assessment training for practice in American Indian and Alaska Native settings. *Journal of Personality Assessment*, *79*(2), 216–225. https://doi.org/10.1207/S15327752JPA7902_05

Allen, J., & Dana, R. H. (2004). Methodological issues in cross-cultural and multicultural Rorschach research. *Journal of Personality Assessment*, *82*(2), 189–206.

Aschieri, F., Fantini, F., & Smith, J. D. (2016). Collaborative, therapeutic assessment: Procedures to enhance outcome. In S. Malzman (Ed.), *The Oxford handbook of treatment processes and outcomes in psychology*. Oxford University Press. (pp. 1–32). https://doi.org/10.1093/oxfordhb/978019973 9134.013.23

Berry, J. W. (2000). Cross-cultural psychology: A symbiosis of cultural and comparative approaches. *Asian Journal of Social Psychology*, *3*, 197–205.

Bhatia, S. (2002). Orientalism in Euro-American and Indian Psychology: Historical representations of "Natives" in colonial and postcolonial contexts.

History of Psychology, 5(4), 376–398. Educational Publishing Foundation. https://doi.org/10:1037/1093-4510.5.4.376

Brown, E. C. (1972). Assessment from a humanistic perspective. *Psychotherapy: Theory, Research, and Practice*, 9, 103–106.

Butcher, J. N., & Hass, G. (2009, March). *Considering culture, race & ethnicity in personality assessment* [Paper presentation]. Society for Personality Assessment Annual Convention, Chicago, IL, United States.

Colonialism (2021). *Wikipedia*. https://en.wikipedia.org/wiki/Colonialism.

Dana, R. H. (1996). Culturally competent assessment practice in the United States. *Journal of Personality Assessment*, 66(3) 472–487.

Dawes, R. M., Faust, D., & Meehl, P. E. (1989). Clinical versus actuarial judgment. *Science*, 243, 1668–1674.

Diaz-Loving, R. (1999). The indigenization of psychology: Birth of a new science or rekindling of an old one? *Applied Psychology*, 48, 433–449.

Duran, B., & Duran, E. (1995). *Native American postcolonial psychology*. State University of New York Press.

Duran, E. (2019). *Healing the soul wound: Trauma-informed counseling for Indigenous communities* (2nd ed.). Teachers College Press.

Engleman, D. H. (2007, March). *Advantages of collaboration in a complicated adolescent neuropsychological assessment* [Paper presentation]. Society for Personality Assessment Annual Convention, Washington, DC, United States.

Finn, S. E. (2007). *In our clients' shoes: Theory and techniques of therapeutic assessment*. Taylor & Francis Group.

Finn, S. E., Fischer, C. T. & Handler, L. (2012). *Collaborative therapeutic assessment: A casebook and guide*. John Wiley & Sons.

Fischer, C. T. (1970). The testee as co-evaluator. *Journal of Counseling Psychology*, 17, 70–77.

Fischer, C. T. (1994). *Individualizing psychological assessment*. Lawrence Erlbaum Associates. (Original work published 1985).

Georgas, J., & Mylonas, K. (2006). Cultures are like all other cultures, like some the cultures, like no other culture. In U. Kim, K.-S. Yang, & K.-K. Hwang (Eds.), *Indigenous and cultural psychology: Understanding people in context* (pp. 197–221). Springer Science+Business Media. https://doi.org/10.1007/0-387-28662-4_9

Gone, J. P. (2007). "We never was happy living like a Whiteman": Mental health disparities and the postcolonial predicament in American Indian communities. *American Journal of Community Psychology*, 40, 290–300. https://doi.org/10.1007/s10464-007-9136-x

Gone, J. P. (2019). Considering indigenous research methodologies: Critical reflections by an Indigenous knower. *Qualitative Inquiry*, 24(1), 45–56. Sage publications. https://doi.org/10.1177/1077800418o787545

Gone, J. P. (2021). Decolonization as methodological innovation in counseling psychology: Method, power, and process in reclaiming American Indian therapeutic traditions. *Journal of Counseling Psychology, American Psychological Association*, 68(3), 259–270. https://doi.org/10.1037cou0000500

Gone, J. P., Hartman, W. E., Pomerville, A., Wendt, D. C., Klem, S., & Burrage, R. L. (2019). The impact of historical trauma on health outcomes for indigenous populations in the USA and Canada: A systematic review.

American Psychological Association, 74(1), 20–35. https://doi.org/10.1037/amp0000338

Handler, L. (2006). Therapeutic assessment with children and adolescent. In S. Smith & L. Handler (Eds.), *Clinical assessment of children and adolescents: A practitioner's guide* (pp. 53–72). Lawrence Erlbaum Associates.

Kim, U., & Berry, J. W. (1993) Contributions to indigenous and cultural psychology. In U. Kim, K.-S. Yang, & K.-K. Hwang (Eds.), *Indigenous and cultural psychology: Understanding people in context* (pp. 3–25). Springer Science +Business Media.

Kim, U., Park, Y. S., & Park, D. H. (1999). The challenge of cross-cultural psychology: The role of indigenous psychologies. *Journal of Cross-cultural Psychology, 31*(1), 63–75.

Kim, U., Yang, K.-S., & Hwang, K.-K. (2006). *Indigenous and cultural psychology: Understanding people in context*. Springer Science-Business Media.

Klopfer, W. G. (1954). Principles of report writing. In M. D. Ainsworth, W. G. Klopfer, & R. R. Holt (Eds.), *Developments in the Rorschach technique: Vol. 1, Technique and theory* (pp. 601–610). Harcourt, Brace & World.

Lerner, P. (2007). When we were comrades together: A note on the language of assessment. *Journal of Personality Assessment, 85*(3), 271–278.

Meehl, P. (1954). *Clinical versus statistical prediction: A theoretical analysis and review of the evidence*. University of Minnesota Press.

Mercer, B. L. (2016. Assessment of children in a community mental health clinic. In B. Mercer, T. Fong, & E. Rosenblatt (Eds.), *Assessing children in the urban community* (pp. 19–30). Routledge/Taylor & Francis.

Meyer, G. J., Viglione, D. J., Mihura, J. L., Erard, R. E., & Erdberg, P. (2011). *Rorschach Performance Assessment System: Administration, coding, interpretation, and technical manual*. Rorschach Performance Assessment System.

Neubauer, B. E., Witkop, C. T., & Varpio, L. (2019). How phenomenology can help us learn from the experience of others. *Perspectives on Medical Education, 8*, 90–97. https://doi.org/10.1007/s40037-019-0509-2

Pickren, W. E., & Rutherford, A. (2010). *A history of modern psychology in context*. Wiley.

Poortinga, Y. H. (1999). Do differences in behavior imply a need for different psychologies? *Applied Psychology, 48*, 419–432.

Rasmus, S., Tricket, T., Charles, B., Simeon, J., & Allen, J. (2019). The *qasgiq* model as an Indigenous intervention: Using the cultural logic of contexts to build protective factors for Alaska Native suicide and alcohol misuse prevention. *Cultural Diversity & Ethnic and Minority Psychology, 25*(1) 44–54. 10.1037/cdp0000243

Roland, A. (1988). *In search of self in India and Japan: Toward a cross-cultural psychology*. Princeton University Press.

Smith, S. R. (2007, March). *Collaborative therapeutic neuropsychological assessment: What has been learned one year later?* [Paper presentation]. Society for Personality Assessment Annual Convention, Washington, DC, United States.

Teo, T. (2013). Backlash against American psychology: An indigenous reconstruction of the history of German critical psychology. *History of Psychology, 16*(1), 1–18.

Tharinger, D. J., Finn., S. E., Wilkinson, A. D., & Schaber, P. M. (2007). Therapeutic assessment with a child as a family intervention: Clinical protocol and a research case study. *Psychology in the Schools, 44,* 293–309.

Transparency International. (2020). Delivery of healthcare services. https://ti-health.org/delivery-of-healthcare-services/

Viglione, D. J. (2003). *New ventures in Rorschach interpretation: Systematic methods for case studies* [Paper presentation]. Society for Personality Assessment Annual Convention, San Francisco, CA, United States.

Waitoki, W. (2012). The development and evaluation of a cultural competency training programme for psychologists working with Māori: A training needs analysis (Thesis, Doctor of Philosophy (PhD)). University of Waikato: Hamilton, New Zealand. Retrieved from https://hdl.handle.net/10289/6654

Waitoki, W. (2016). The baskets of knowledge: A curriculum for an indigenous psychology. In W. Waitoki & M. Levy (Eds.), *Te manu kai i te mātauranga: Indigenous psychology in Aotearoa/New Zealand* (pp. 283–299). The New Zealand Psychological Society.

Wang, J., Han, K., Ketterer, H., Weed, N. C., Ben-Porath, Y. S., Kim, J.-H., & Moon, K. (2020). Evaluating the measurement invariance of MMPI-2-RF Restructured Clinical Scale 4 (antisocial behavior) between American and Korean clinical samples: Exploring cultural and translation issues affecting item responding. *Journal of Personality Assessment, 103*(4), 465–475.

World Population Review. (2021). *World Population Review.* https://worldpopulationreview.com/country-rankings/countries-never-colonized

Yamaguchi, S., & Ariizumi, Y. (2006). Close interpersonal relationships among Japanese: *Amae* as distinguished from attachment and dependence. In U. Kim, K.-S. Yang, & K.-K. Hwang (Eds.), *Indigenous and cultural psychology: Understanding people in context* (pp. 163–174). Springer Science+Business Media.

Zajenkowska, A., Russa, M. B., Radoslaw, R., Park, J., Jasielska, D., & Skrzypek, M. (2020). Cultural influences on social information processing: Hostile attributions in the United States, Poland, and Japan. *Journal of Personality Assessment, 103*(4), 489–497.

Chapter 2

Paradigms for Well-Being: Ways of Knowing and Psychological Services

Barbara L. Mercer

This chapter offers a sampling of psychological assessment frameworks and intervention service delivery methods from around the world. Projects highlighted here complement the chapters in this volume and focus on collaborative and nontraditional interventions outside a purely Eurocentric framework, or explorations of cultural identity and topics. In this overview gathered from the literature of descriptions of psychology in North American Native Communities, India, Aotearoa/New Zealand, and Africa, I focus on cultural paradigms that widen and challenge our perspective; this reflects my understanding of assessment and intervention practices presently transforming assessment, intervention, and research across the globe. John Lewis, the United States Civil Rights activist and Congressman frequently declared, "When people tell me nothing has changed, I say come and walk in my shoes and I will show you change." (2015). Communities have much to impart about their ways of being in the world, and change begins with our listening.

Culture and Assessment Service Delivery in North American Native Communities

American Indian and Alaska Native Communities

Personality assessment with American Indians and Alaska natives has identified key issues and problems with the traditional assessment service delivery style—the conceptual and personality construct equivalence and definitions of "cultural identity" (Allen, 1998). Added to these noted limitations are examples of poor interpretive utilization of test findings, linguistic equivalence, and metric equivalence. One such body of research has led to the finding of a culturally distinct explanation for a category of depression resulting in a redesigned American Indian Depression Scale-Hopi Version (Manson et al., 1985). The mind/body split in mainstream practice within the United States does not directly translate in Hopi constructs. The Hopi construct that most closely resembles *mental*

DOI: 10.4324/9781003124061-4

illness—mood swings, hallucination, for example, is *worry sickness. Unhappiness* in Hopi culture is linked to *death in the family and loss of crops. Turning one's face to the wall* includes withdrawal and suicidal ideation (see Allen, 1998). Cultural identity literature examines the definition of self-reported cultural identity vs. how someone might be perceived by service providers, for example, speaking the dominant language. The Northern Plains Bicultural Immersion Scale (NPBI); (Allen & French, 1994) assesses immersion in a tribal identity, which creates a more flexible, interactive approach that makes use of a four-factor scale to measure the level of immersion in Indian and European culture, language, and practices.

A National Institute of Mental Health grant (Rasmus et al., 2019) supported a team of Native and non-Native psychologists to work with Alaska Natives in the Yup'ik community to identify research and intervention needs. The model grew out of an earlier community-based participatory research (CBPR) study in Southwest Alaska, where youth and Elders formed action groups to identify local Arctic peoples' needs and strengths for use in interviewing, implementing, and disseminating findings for the pursuit of a culturally healthy life to contribute to individual well-being. Their results concluded that being "useful by helping others," especially Elders, and "being proud of our village" are key to well-being.

University researchers were brought to a meeting with Yup'ik culture Elders and official tribal and community leadership in the Yukon Kuskokwim Delta. In the model, there were no "chiefs"; everyone brought their own experience and knowledge and role. Depending on the nature of the needs, some knowledge sources found broader applicability. The latest Western science and clinical practices were integrated and remained supportive of the cultural process. The Elders identified the focus population—youth aged 12–18—with a desirable outcome of increased strength and protection, as well as defined reasons for "life and sobriety." Suicide was noted as the leading cause of death for Alaska Native men between the ages of 15 and 25, and alcohol was associated with 60% of those suicides, as well as being responsible for many accidents and deaths. A Yup'ik Elder described the project as follows:

> *Qasgirarmeq* (*qas gee raar neq*) has a meaning to encircle. In coming together around our youth in the ways of our ancestors, we are strengthening our collective spirit in an effort to cast the spirit of suicide and substance abuse out from our communities, forever.
>
> (Rasmus et al., 2019, p. 2)

Integral to Yup'ik culture prior to the advent of missionaries in the second half of the 20th century was the *qasgiq* (phonetic: kuz-gik), a round, semi-subterranean structure used as a primary living space that was also central to community gatherings. This circular housing community was considered improper by European standards so forcibly restructured into single-family homes by the missionaries, giving some health and technological improvements but severely fragmenting the social structure. Today, the qasgiq has been restored and has become not only a "place" but an action, a collective process. Some communities call a qasgiq when a collective issue arrives that needs attention and resolution (Rasmus et al., 2019).

The Yup'ik qasgiq process involved the integration of Native practice with a Western-based conceptual logic model and theory of change resulting in "Tools for Life" (Rasmus et al., 2019, p. 2), or *Qungasvik* (qoo ngaz vik). These tools included resources, strengths, resilience, and knowledge; symbols and strategies marshaled for intervention; bringing together Elders and community members; and interventions—cultural activities related to hunting and fishing, ice safety, and building workgroups with mentors and youth for tool making and food gathering. The outcome of these activities was cycled back to the qasgiq for report and evaluation. Finally, the most relevant outcomes related to life and sobriety protection were selected and made available for health interventions with other Yup'ik communities.

Native Communities in Montana and Wyoming

"Our culture is our treatment." (Gone, 2019a, p. 174).

Joseph P. Gone, Harvard professor (2007, 2019a, 2019b, 2021), has written extensively about North Central Plains American Indians, specifically ethnographic inquiry and interviews with the Aaniih (Gros Ventre) people on his home reservation of Fort Belknap, Montana. He writes of the complex problems American Indian communities face in recovering their own cultural psychology, in contrast to the supremacy of biomedicine and empirical discourse, as well as his hope for the linking of Indigenous and professional understanding.

Gone's contributions reveal an estimable breadth and contrasting approaches to his subject, beginning with a narrative of the 18th-century shaman Bull Lodge, conserved by Gone's great-grandfather. In a wholly Indigenous context, Gone (2021) shares his great-grandfather's journals detailing Bull Lodge's healing career of visions, and sacrifices of his own flesh to extract poisons and sickness from his patients. Gone interviews a modern traditional healer Traveling Thunder (2007, 2019a), who tells him "we never was happy, you know, living like a Whiteman" (2007, p. 294) and prescribes an Indigenous approach to alcohol treatment, depression, and self-determination as a *strong and clean mind* and the power of *thought-wish* (2019a, p. 181) to create reality and sobriety.

Gone's riveting accounts of Bull Lodge and Traveling Thunder contrasts with a later article, (Langa & Gone, 2019), the case of an American Indian woman in relation to her DSM-5 diagnosis (*Diagnostic and Statistical Manual of Mental Disorders,* 5th ed.; American Psychiatric Association, 2013). These authors argue that the latest DSM-5 removal of the *bereavement exclusion* and its evolution of the PTSD diagnosis reduces the definition of a trauma *stressor* to "*threatened death, loss of serious injury or sexual violence*" (p. 216) and "*loss of a loved one if not violent or accidental*" (p. 271) and ignores the relational context of patient's extreme stress and traumatic loss due to family deaths (mother and a brother). The resulting Major Depressive diagnosis likewise ignores her depression related to bereavement as a needed focus for her treatment. Most striking in the authors' account is that several providers prescribed medications that made the patient feel worse and offered psychiatric treatment with negligible interpersonal focus. The client was a self-identified "modern" acculturated Iroquois woman in her late 40s, living in a metropolitan area, not connected with a Native community. However, she was able to divulge early traumatic material only to a Native interviewer. After her assessment, and by participating in a healing lodge, she finally found relief by unburdening herself to a friend, after which she felt "like myself again" (p. 15). Although she had had few contacts with Native American peoples prior to her treatment, she felt a strong shared cultural connection in the healing lodge.

These examples of Indigenous and Western approaches accentuate the gulf as well as a potential link between the two perspectives. The traditional Native starting point is the *unquestioned existence* of historical events that created a loss of culture and its healing practices. Gone proposes in a fascinating discussion *Indigenous Research Methodologies: Critical Reflections by an Indigenous Knower* (2019b), that *Indigenous Research Methods* (IRM) ideally include a mixture of Indigenous and mainstream research. He sees spiritual oral tradition embedded in Indigenous daily life as an essential bridge with academic literacy but accountable to Indigenous knowledge. Gone's goal is to recover an American Indian cultural psychology and provide services that do not "simultaneously and surreptitiously reproduce colonial power relations" (2019b, p. 172) but can make American Indian cultural ideas accessible to modern practitioners and academicians.

In his *Healing the Soul Wound*, Eduardo Duran (2019), traces this wound to the conquest of tribes by colonizers, their removal to reservations, to dishonored treaties, loss of cultural support, and the destruction of Native American families by relocating children to boarding schools, and its resultant loss of culture and language. These events created a loss of identity and spirituality, dissociation and self-hatred, and led to drugs and alcoholism, violent crimes against one another, and suicide. He pointedly speaks of the "drunken Indian" myth that is viewed by society as an *individual* pathology rather than a collective loss of culture and sense of self. He sees treatment as dependent on strengthening culture and connection to tribal leaders to increase autonomy. He guides the reader through his therapy of "soul healing"—a synthesis of ritual, community intervention, dream work, sand tray, and narrative work. His assessment work begins with an acculturation assessment of the way in which the person relates to their tribal or Native life-world.

Duran sees the possibilities of shaman and psychotherapist working together only if the Western therapist can accept Native teachings as part of the work. Related meta principles and community research questions put forth by Wallerstein and Duran (2006) are as follows: Who has control of the goals and knowledge? What is the level of involvement of the research parties and for what reasons? Who consents to the research, and who owns the data in terms of interpretation and dissemination? Rather than a set of research methods, these authors' orientation—community-based partici- patory research—is a dynamic process focused on relationships between academic and community partners incorporating the role of research in social change.

India: Acculturation and Colonial Influence

Service delivery in India, or with Indian individuals living in other countries, requires an imperative to thinking in terms of what Sunil Bhatia calls "the construction of identities through the intermingling, mixing, and moving of cultures" (Bhatia & Ram, 2001, p. 11). Colonization and globalization have led to a hybridization of both cultural values and meaning that may make conflation of nation and culture problematic. Bhatia posits that diasporic communities, such as that of Indians, retain a strong identification with their home country while navigating their new identity. He asserts that the diaspora that requires communities to continually navigate between their homeland and host land cultures—to cope with contrasting constructs can engender inner conflict as well as offer an expanded duality.

The following are compelling quotes from Indian psychoanalyst Sudhir Kakar (1996). He synthesizes elements of Indian identity from his own experience with deep sensitivity.

> My father had always been brilliant in his studies, effortlessly standing first in his class at school and in due course, he received a scholarship to study economics and political science at the college in Lahore ... My father's family did not have enough money to finance years of study in England. The examination of the Indian Civil Service, for which one ideally prepared in England, was beyond my father's cultural capabilities. To enter the service, the young man had

to be at least the second if not the third generation out of the bazaar to possess the natural ease with Western manners and social sang-froid that upper-class English interviewers looked for in Indian recruits who were to be moulded into passible imitations of themselves. (p. xi–xii)

The following two excerpts depict the task of holding Eastern and Western cultures in mind:

When I now look at the yellowing newsprint of [my] … early stories, I am struck by their intensity of longing for the life of provincial Indian towns where I grew up. For though my head was filled with the intellectual excitement of the West, India was still an over-powering emotional presence and these stories, crude in many ways, convey a deep and persistent undercurrent of nostalgia, almost sensual in character, for the sights, smells, tastes and sounds of the country of my childhood (p. xvii).

Like many other young men of my class who had discovered the West in India and who later went abroad to study, I too began to discover India while living in the West, understanding its history, culture and mythology primarily through the eyes of Western scholars. (p. xvii)

The effects of the colonial experience beneath the British Crown following the Indian uprising in 1857, and the ultimate break from British rule through Indian independence in 1947, including the violent Hindu-Muslim partition, have produced complex cultural, philosophical, and religious forces within Indian culture. Although the British described India as its "jewel in the crown," they preferred to project their own image of political, economic, scientific, technological, educational, and legal systems into India. They valued an individual, context-free market economy over contextualization (Roland, 1988). Thus, while the urban elite in India, business and trading classes, and the intelligentsia gained economic and educational advantages, their culture and their access to greater advancement and recognition were often subsumed by British centrality. While Eastern thinkers and philosophers influenced Western ideas for academicians and truth seekers, it was the Indian people who had the task of acculturation in two cultures. In modern society, Western countries actively seek urban Indian citizens for business, technology, and medical expertise. Indians living within their own country or abroad are challenged to navigate and hold both the individualistic and the collectivistic, as well as other cultural values. India is a prime example of how a geographical nation cannot fully capture an individual's complex relationship between their own national and historical culture and their construction of Self (Hermans & Kempen, 1998; Roland, 1988). These are essential but too often invisible threads in thinking about the delivery of psychological services.

Indigenous Psychologies in Aotearoa/New Zealand

The bird that consumes the miro berry owns the forest; the bird that consumes knowledge owns the world.
— Māori proverb (In Waitoki, 2016.)

The Māori way in Aotearoa/New Zealand and the Aboriginal path in Australia are comprised of collective ideals, connections with family, community, and the natural world. The following Māori passage captures the idea of *Kaupapa* Māori (collective vision) and mātauranga (Māori knowledge): "We can improve the way in which humankind exists and lives in the world through new strategies of indigeneity, rekindling kinship between people, and between people and the natural world" (Royal, 2012, p. 37).

In November 2020, a Māori woman, Nanala Mahuta, was elected Aotearoa/New Zealand's minister of foreign affairs. She stated that she hoped for a "reimagining what prosperity looks like" by transferring values from the Indigenous community of *manaakitanga* [Māori for looking after people] and *kaitakitanga* [guardianship of the environment]; (Cave, 2020, p. A7) to the Aotearoa/New Zealand community at large.

Psychological assessment and intervention in Aotearoa and Australia contain these underlying principles. New Zealand psychologist Waikaremoana Waitoki (2016) links these values to her account of a psychological assessment and therapy with Ripeka, a woman who has survived traumatic experiences of abuse and suffers from depression, hearing voices, and a mood disorder. She invites us to understand this woman through the eyes of a Māori psychologist. Waitoki asks:

> what would happen when we understood interconnectedness of whakapapa [genealogy] and tikanga [Māori customs and traditional values] to Ripeka's past, present and future and how they could be used to guide pathways forward? We asked what would happen when we viewed Ripeka and her whānau through a lens of unrelenting hope and unrealized potential, ... what value are we able to add as Māori psychologists to Ripeka's life, and to that of her whānau? (p. 283).

It is through the whānau, Waitoki states it is through the whānau (family wellbeing) that values and traditions from the ancestors are adapted to the modern world to infuse hope and realization of potential.

Here is an example from Ripeka's therapy with Hukarere, in Waitoki's "The Baskets of Knowledge: A Curriculum for Indigenous Psychology":

> Hukarere invited Ripeka to bring something of her grandmother that they could use in therapy. [Ripeka tells Hukarere]: My Nan had a love for the land, and especially the river. She came to me one day and showed me a stone; it was a big piece of stone, from the River ... She told me to hold it; and as I held it, I felt this energy force, the mauri of the stone. She told me a story of the three baskets of knowledge and the two sacred stones.
>
> (Waitoki, 2016, p. 291)

Waitoki calls this *walking alongside* Ripeka. She describes the above process as welcoming of her spirit (*mihi to her wairua*) with love and respect (*aroha*) to acknowledge her trauma and the way in which it has taken her vital energy (*mauri*). Waitoki states:

> I am going to work differently with a client if I have an epistemological world view that understands hearing voices or contact with ancestors as a totally acceptable part of reality, not always positive, sometimes traumatic, but possible. In comparison, if I believed voice hearing was merely a psychological coping strategy for trauma or a by-product of a chemical brain imbalance I am not going to work with the client as effectively and may even alienate them. (2016, p. 289).

The phrase "baskets of knowledge" refers to the core notion of indigenous knowledge that holds the memory and knowledge of ancestors and culture (in a *kete* or basket) and translates it to psychological work.

This approach rooted in ancient Māori tradition is not dissimilar to what therapists in the West have adopted more recently as trauma-informed care. I cite this approach in detail because the Māori language itself is filled with power and energy. It reflects what the 2011 Waitangi Tribunal (a commission charged with reclaiming Māori cultural identity and investigating and making recommendations on Māori claims related to 19th-century British Crown land rights and Māori knowledge breaches) called "the unique Māori way of viewing the relational phenomena of the world, understanding the seen and unseen that exists, has existed, and may yet exist" (Waitoki, 2016, p. 284). As prominent Māori psychiatrist Mason Durie (2012) points to the importance of the Māori life practice: "Simply learning about 'things Māori' is not the same as being guided by an evolving knowledge system called mātauranga Māori" (p. 23).

Africa: Historical and Current Narratives

Among the myriad ethical issues confronting service providers in African countries are multicultural diversity in cultural and religious practices, contextual histories, and of course, language. Indigenous service providers can be trained, and all practitioners should have a multicultural worldview (Foxcraft, 2011). Economic and educational inequality, poverty, natural disaster, famine, and disease play recurring roles against the seemingly unremitting backdrops of severe economic and physical hardship. Africa's cultural trauma is a paramount assault: the history of apartheid, the violence of war or armed conflict, forced migration, child abuse and child trafficking, torture, imprisonment, and murder.

According to data from the Uppsala Conflict Data Program, there were 21 active civil wars on the continent in 2018 (Karssen, 2020). And, while his article in the Africa Portal Roundup Newsletter speaks to the development of objectives toward a "Roadmap of Practical Steps to Silence the Guns," by the African Union Peace and Security Council, Africa's many conflicts continue to "become ever more complex ... drawing in a wide array of local, regional, and international actors," and posing a challenge to the much-needed initiative.

Spirituality, Religion, and Mythology

Africa is the second largest and also the second most populated continent in the world. This vast continent of over 1.3 billion people has 54 sovereign countries with the addition of Somaliland, a self-proclaimed independent territory (World Population Review, 2020), and is widely accepted as the geographic location where our species originated. Africa's history is ancient, rich, and complex. This complexity combines revered cultural strengths and practices with extreme cultural trauma. Nigerian-born Harvard professor Jacob Olupona speaks of the spirituality of Africa as a powerful and indispensable medium for working with emotional and physical ills. In an interview with Anthony Chiorazzi (2015) Olupona is quoted in the *Harvard Gazette*:

> African spirituality is truly holistic. For example, sickness in the indigenous African worldview is not only an imbalance of the body, but also an imbalance in one's social life, which can be linked to a breakdown in one's kinship and family relations or even to one's relationship with one's ancestors.

Theologians and health and mental health providers have documented the origin of Indigenous African religions and native beliefs prior to the

Christian and Islamic colonization of African countries. One's religious traditions were informed by ethnic identity and where one's family came from. Olupona identified 32 different traditions from East, Central, West Africa, and the diaspora. For instance, the Yoruba religion has historically been centered in southwestern Nigeria, the Zulu religion in southern Africa, and the Igbo religion in southeastern Nigeria (Chiorazzi, 2015). Christianity and Islam represent approximately 40% of the African population. Christianity is more dominant in the south, while Islam is more dominant in the north. Indigenous African practices tend to be strongest in the central states of Africa, but some form of their practices and beliefs can be found almost anywhere in Africa.

Nevertheless, since 1900 the number of Christians in Africa has grown from approximately 7 million to over 450 million today. Islam has experienced a similar rapid growth. Olupona (2014) states that both Christianity and Islam have adapted to meet African needs and practices, although Africa still struggles to maintain its Indigenous religious identity against a view of African practice as being more than superstitions and witchcraft. African people who still wholly practice African Indigenous religions represent only a fraction of what it was only a century ago, when Indigenous religions dominated most of the continent. However, there are many self-identified Christians and Muslims who incorporate Indigenous religious rituals and practices. Olupona and other African practitioners speak to the ways that Christianity and Islam are mixed with African religious practices.

While diminishing the prevalence of African Indigenous religions, the growth of Christianity and Islam on the African continent has been extraordinary. And while Indigenous practices tend to be strongest in the central states, some form of their practices and beliefs can be found almost anywhere in Africa. Olupona and other African practitioners speak to the ways that Christianity and Islam are mixed with Indigenous religious practices noting that they are imbued with animism, shamanism, and the spirit world. Olupona (2014) describes the seeking of spiritual help through the direction and relief from healers, medicine men and women, charms (adornments often worn to ensure good luck), amulets (adornments often used to ward off evil), and diviners (spiritual advisers).

Whether living in Africa or as part of the diaspora in the United States, Europe Cuba, Haiti, or Brazil, Africans routinely accommodate other religions with traditional ones. An example of this is the Gullah Geechee communities on the North Carolina/Georgia seaboard. Indeed, the distinctive religious practices of the Gullah/Geechee communities contain influences from several cultures, including Christianity, Islam, and West African traditions. The Gullah *ring shout* (College of Coastal Georgia, 2021) is similar to ecstatic religious rituals still performed in West and Central Africa. Olupona (2014) reckons this spiritual flexibility is due to the oral nature of not fully codified African traditions. (He recounts his own Anglican upbringing by what means he navigates his simultaneous Yoruba and Christian identities.) While standardized interview formats, research methods, and assessment tools are often utilized in some African intervention service deliveries, they are invariably infused with culturally sensitive variations that bring a strong transpersonal and spiritual approach to providing service. Olupona sees African religion as integral to all life in Africa and convincingly argues that the African "spiritual space is no longer bound by the African continent" (p. 120).

A wholly Indigenous healing approach in South Africa described by Thornton (2017) involves the *sangoma* (he roughly translates as "indigenous healer") for the treatment of mental illness and emotional turmoil. The concepts of "exposed being" and "augmented self" describe the collaborative intensity—the mutuality of "sharing the illness and the suffering"—as curative, not dissimilar to the "wounded healer" of Jungian therapy. The process can involve a secret society of healers. music, dance rituals, and/or dreams and trance-like states (as altered consciousness).

The advent of illness deviates from identifying a specific cause as *outside* the sufferer (a Western concept), to focusing instead on the *protection of the personhood* through magic or warding off from further harm (bad luck or disease), as well as *augmentation* or *increasing the energy* of the vulnerable patient's Self. Thornton differentiates this *protective* process from a *therapeutic* one because, unlike traditional therapeutic methods, it does not seek to link symptom to cause nor link diagnosis to cure. The fundamental premise is that a person is open or vulnerable to negative influences, e.g., agents of evil, that luck is random but "lumpy," and often favors the "lucky" (p. 218). Therefore, the patient must be assisted in avoiding bad luck through *infused* strength.

While there is no "cure" *per se*, there is a transition from a state of illness to a state of wellness. It's a *balancing* of parts rather than making someone *whole*. Citizens cannot be stripped of their social being and can be strengthened within a healing relationship. Thornton attributes this philosophy in part as necessary to combat South African apartheid policies in which there is no entitlement to public health.

Community Approach to Healing in the Wake of Political Violence

In Chapter 10 of this volume, Jonathan Brakarsh and coauthors describe a Zimbabwean community-crafted workshop called Singing to the Lions that works with groups of children who have experienced trauma ranging from social and political trauma to bullying to cataclysmic natural disasters. Using metaphors, this innovative program helps children face fears and gain access to their strengths and powers. This program's community trainers—who are part of a nongovernmental organization called Tree of Life—partnered with Western-trained researchers to design, implement, and evaluate a community-based healing model for working with victims of organized violence and torture (Mpande et al., 2013). Their program operated routinely nearing the times of elections when ruling parties suppressed opposition or activism by intimidation and violation of human rights ("Can we discuss past traumas when current safety is not assured?") (Mpande, et al., 2013. p. 197).

Their community meetings employed traditional group meetings with "concepts of story-telling, healing of the spirits, reconnecting with the body, and reestablishing a sense of community and self-esteem" (Reeler et al., 2009, 180). The authors note that this process was developed from traditional circle processes in the Native American community for coping with challenging community issues.

The Tree of Life workshop and research project was adapted for work in rural areas of Zimbabwe with trauma survivors, and it demonstrated that even during periods of continuing conflict in a climate of risk and threat, participants can begin to utilize a collective psychological model for healing and empowerment. The partnering of community members who develop and lead the workshops with academics who assist in designing and evaluating the program is a progressive model for the joining of traditional Western science with traditional healing community practices. When a project is owned and implemented by the community, traditional science can support the research and thus serve the production of community knowledge.

Community-Based Participatory Assessment and Research: Liberia, Haiti, Bosnia, Sri Lanka

Liberia's Civil War (1989–1997), began when the National Patriotic Front of Liberia, led by Charles Taylor, fought to overthrow the government of Samuel Doe (note, a second Civil war spanned from 1999 to 2003). Ethnic tensions fueled the war, with even a West African peacekeeping group coming under attack before the conflict ended in 1997 with the election of Charles Taylor as president. During 1997–1998, Women's Rights International, (a project of the Tides Center), a US-based nongovernmental organization, partnered with the Women's Health and Development Program (at the Mother Patern College of Health Sciences) in Monrovia to examine women's experiences during the war and to consider ways to support Liberian women in dealing with the effects of war trauma. (Swiss et al., 1998; Jennings et al., 2003; Jennings & Swiss, 2000).

The research was designed by Liberian women, who decided which aspects to explore through small group discussions with women in the marketplace, high school girls, and women and girls living in displaced person's camps or urban neighborhoods in Monrovia. The women chose the survey topics, wrote the questions, carried out the interviews, and guided the interpretations of collected data. One context-specific example was that women were taken from their families and forced to cook for a fighter/soldier, subjecting them to involuntary control and at risk for sexual assault. Wording the questions carefully enabled the interviewers to more accurately identify and document the participants' experiences, resulting in more openness.

The challenges of conducting research in the middle of a war necessitated protecting the safety of both the research team and the survey participants. Dangers were mitigated by organizing the survey's primary theme around *women's health* and insisting there be absolutely no questions that might, however inadvertently, betray the identities of participants, or allude to location or even the most benign seeming details of events. They even traveled to rural areas inconspicuously in an old station wagon to avert confiscation of surveys at armed checkpoints.

Women's Rights International continued to work with this group of Liberian nurses and midwives to create a story methodology for communicating the *central tendency position* outcome (central findings) of their research with women in rural villages who could not read or write.

This story addresses trust and shame after being gang raped: *secret keeping:*

> Once there was a girl living with her mother. She grew up into a beautiful girl. The girl and her parents remained in their village until the other village engaged them in a tribal fight. Everybody scattered and the girl found herself in the bush alone. While in the bush she was raped by three of the fighters from the other village. (Women's Rights International, USA, and the Women's Health and Development Program at Mother Patern College of Health Sciences, Liberia 1998, p. 6)

It illustrates how even seeking help can be dangerous:

> When things started to quiet down, the girl went to the oldest Zoe who was her aunt. The aunt made medicine for her and told her she will be okay. Few days later the girl started to hear news of the rape in the town. She became confused as to how it spread. The girl was forced to leave the village because of the shame and disgrace she felt. (Women's Rights International, USA, and the Women's Health and Development Program at Mother Patern College of Health Sciences, Liberia 1998, p. 6)

Through the discussion of several different types of parables, the village women were able to talk about their own often conflicted responses, as well as the responses and feelings of their tribes.

The Liberian team also constructed stories (*The One God Sent to Stop the Boys from Killing Me*) based on compsite statistical characters created from the average characteristics and most frequent experiences reported in the survey (Jennings, P., Swiss, S, & Turay-Kanneh, R., 2003) These stories and statistical vignettes were also used to introduce the survey findings to the Truth and Reconciliation Commission of Liberia in 2008 (under the government and mandate of Ellen Johnson Surleaf.)

A similar participatory model was employed by Women's Rights International in Haiti in partnership with a leadership program of high school girls called Fanm Kouraj (Regan & Jennings, 2005) to focus on the challenges of teen pregnancy, domestic violence, and child abuse and trafficking, through theater pieces along with audience discussions that were also broadcast on community radio stations. Other research documenting war violence was conducted in collaboration with the U.N. Commission on Human Rights in the former Yugoslavia (Swiss & Giller, 1993), and in Sri Lanka with The Asia Foundation and Vehilihini Development Center (Swiss et al., 2019). These projects accentuate ethical considerations in participatory research and provide guidelines on how to conduct nongovernmental organization collaborations (Swiss et al., 2019).

These and other missions in Community Based Participatory Research (CBPR) are a growing and welcome trend in mental health, public health, and human rights research and intervention. They embody the belief and philosophy that dissemination, language, and ownership should originate with the community and its people.

References

Allen, J. (1998). Personality assessment with American Indians and Alaska Natives: Instrument considerations and service delivery style. *Journal of Personality Assessment, 70*(1), 17–42.

Allen, J., & French, C. (1994). *Northern Plains Bicultural Immersion Scale: Preliminary manual and scoring instruction.* University of South Dakota.

American Psychiatric Association. (2013). *Diagnostic and statistical manual of mental disorders* (5th ed.). https://doi.org/10.1176/appi.books.9780890425596

Bhatia, S. & Ram, A. (2001). Rethinking 'acculturation' in relation to diasporic cultures and postcolonial identities. *Human Development, 44*(1), 1–18.

Cave, D. (2020, November 15). With progressive politics on march in New Zealand, Maori minister blazes new trails. *New York Times.* https://www.nytimes.com/2020/11/15/world/asia/new-zealand-progressives-nanaia-mahuta.html

Chiorazzi, A. (2015, October 6). The spirituality of Africa. *Harvard Gazette.* https://news.harvard.edu/gazette/story/2015/10/the-spirituality-of-africa/

College of Coastal Georgia. (2021). Georgia's Gullah-Geechee heritage: Music & language. https://libguides.ccga.edu/gullahgeechee/audio

Duran, E. (2019). *Healing the soul wound: Trauma-informed counseling for indigenous communities* (2nd ed.). Teachers College Press.

Durie, M. (2012). Interview: Kaupapa Māori: Shifting the social. *New Zealand Journal of Educational Studies, 47*(2), 21–29.

Foxcraft, C. D. (2011). Ethical issues related to psychological testing in Africa: What I have learned (So far). *Online Readings in Psychology and Culture, 2*(2). 1–17. https://doi.org/10.9707/2307-0919.1022

Gone, J. P. (2007). "We never was happy living like a Whiteman": Mental health disparities and the postcolonial predicament in American Indian communities. *American Journal of Community Psychology, 40*, 290–300.

Gone, J. P. (2019a). "The thing that happened as he wished": Recovering an American Indian cultural psychology. *American Journal of Community Psychology, 64*, 172–184. https://doi.org/10:1002/ajcp.12353

Gone, J. P. (2019b). Considering Indigenous research methodologies: Critical reflections by an Indigenous knower. *Qualitative Inquiry, 24*(1), 45–56. Sage publications. https://doi.org/10.1177/1077800418o787545

Gone, J. P. (2021). Decolonization as methodological innovation in counseling psychology: Method, power, and process in reclaiming American Indian therapeutic traditions. *Journal of Counseling Psychology, 68*(3), 259–270. https://doi.org/10.1037/cou0000500

Hermans, H. J. M., & Kempen, H. J. G. (1998). Moving cultures: The perilous problems of cultural dichotomies in a globalizing society. *American Psychologist, 53*(10), 1111–1120.

Jennings, P. J., & Swiss, S. (2000). Statistical information on violence against women during the civil war in Liberia. In *Statistics, development and human rights: Proceedings of the International Association of Official Statistics, Session I-PL 5, Montreux, Switzerland.* United Nations Digital Library.

Jennings, P. J., Swiss, S. & Turay-Kennah, R. (2003). "The one god sent to stop the boys from killing me": Using storytelling to communicate survey findings about Liberian women living in displaced-persons camps. *Feminism & Psychology, 13*(3), 295–301.

Kakar, S. (1996). *Indian identity.* New Delhi: Penguin Books.

Karssen J. (2020, February 7). Africa Portal Silencing the guns in Africa: Achievements and stumbling blocks. https://www.africaportal.org/features/silencing-guns-africa-achievements-and-stumbling-blocks/

Langa, M. E., & Gone, J. P. (2019). Cultural context in DSM diagnosis: An American Indian case illustrative of contradictory trends. *Transcultural Psychiatry, 57*(4), 567–580. https://doi.org/10.1177/1363461519832473

Lewis, J. [@repjohnlewis]. (2015, March 7). When people tell me nothing has changed, I say come walk in my shoes and I will show you change. #Selma50 [Tweet] Twitter. https://twitter.com

Manson, S. P., Shore, J. H., & Bloom, J. D. (1985). The depressive experience in American Indian communities. A challenge for psychiatric theory and diagnosis. In A. Kleinman & B. Good (Eds.), *Culture and depression: Studies in the anthropology and cross-cultural psychiatry of affect and disorder* (pp. 331–368). University of California Press.

Mpande, E., Higson-Smith, C., Chimitira, R. J., Kadaira, A., Mashonganyika, J., Ncube, Q. M., Ngwenya, S., Vinson, G., Wild, R., & Ziwoni, N. (2013). Community intervention during ongoing community violence: What is possible? What works? *American Psychological Association, 19*(2), 196–208. https://doi.org/10.1037/a0032529

Olupona, J. K. (2014). *African religions: A very short introduction.* Oxford University Press.

Rasmus, S., Tricket, T., Charles, B., Simeon, J., & Allen, J. (2019). The qasgiq model as an Indigenous intervention: Using the cultural Logic of contexts to build protective factors for Alaska Native suicide and alcohol misuse prevention. *Cultural Diversity & Ethnic and Minority Psychology, 25*(1) 44–54. https://doi.org/10.1037/cdp0000243

Reeler, T., Chitsike, K., Maizva, F., & Reeler, B. (2009). The Tree of Life: A community approach to empowerment and healing survivors of torture in Zimbabwe. *Torture, 19*(3), 108–193.

Regan, J., & Jennings, P. J. (2005). Airwaves to courage. *Americas, 57*(1), 1–7.

Roland, A. (1988). *In search of self in India and Japan: Toward a cross-cultural psychology.* Princeton University Press.

Royal, T. A. C. (2012). Politics and knowledge: Kaupapa Māori and mātauranga Māori. *New Zealand Journal of Educational Studies, 47*, 30–37.

Swiss, S., & Giller, J. (1993). Rape as a crime of war: A medical perspective. *Journal of the American Medical Association, 270*, 612–615.

Swiss, S, Jennings, P. J., Aryee, G. V., Brown, G. H., Jappah-Samukai, R. M., Kamara, M. S., Schaack, R. D., & Turay-Kanneh, R. S. (1998). Violence against women during the Liberian civil conflict. *Journal of the American Medical Association, 279*(8), 625–629.

Swiss, S., Jennings, P., Weerananthe, K. G. K., & Heise, L. (2019). *Documenting the impact of conflict on women living in internally displaced persons camps in Sri Lanka: Some ethical considerations.* Women's Rights International.

Thornton, R. J. (2017). *Healing the exposed being; A South African Ngoma tradition.* Wits University Press. http://witspress.co.za/catalogue/healing-the-exposed-being/

Waitangi Tribunal (2011). *Ko Aotearoa tēnei: A report into claims concerning New Zealand law and policy affecting Māori culture and identity. Te taumata tuatahi Wai 262*: Waitangi tribunal report. Wellington, New Zealand: Waitangi Tribunal.

Waitoki, W. (2016). The baskets of knowledge: A curriculum for an indigenous psychology. In W. Waitoki, & M. Levy (Eds.), *Te manu kai i te mātauranga: Indigenous psychology in Aotearoa/New Zealand* (pp. 283–299). The New Zealand Psychological Society.

Wallerstein, N., & Duran, B. (2006). Using community-based participatory research to address health disparities. *Health Promotion Practice, 7*(3), 312–323.

Women's Rights International, USA, and the Women's Health and Development Program at Mother Patern College of Health Sciences, Liberia (1998). *Violence against women in war. Workshop I: Raising awareness of violence against women—A manual for training midwives in Liberia* (2nd ed.). Women's Rights International, 1–30.

World Population Review (2020). https://worldpopulationreview.com/country-rankings/countries-in-africa

Collaborative/ Therapeutic Assessment Models

Chapter 3

Assessment, Training, and Social Justice in Community Psychology

Heather Macdonald, Barbara L. Mercer, and Caroline Purves

A change in county government public funding of mental health services brought our psychology clinic (staffed by psychologists, clinical social workers, child and family therapists, and treatment specialists) into the "shoes" of social service child protection workers. Through the funding source called Early and Periodic Screening, Diagnostic, and Treatment (EPSDT), we were tasked to carry our services to people in the community who might not have easy access to clinic treatment. Our clinic had moved from a small, predominantly White, working/middle-class community in the north part of the San Francisco East Bay Area to the Fruitvale neighborhood (once a land of fruit trees) in East Oakland, a vibrant, multi-ethnic community with the city's largest Hispanic population with a preserved culture (formerly the home of the Chicano movement, including the Brown Berets). Although our therapy staff was somewhat diverse, it took nearly 30 years for the diversity on our staff to reflect the diversity of the people we served and to offer the types of programs, in addition to an individual therapy model, that reflected a collective perspective. These services included mental health screening of first-time foster care children, transitional-age youth including sexually exploited minors, case management, and a youth advocacy program staffed by former foster youth. These expansions led to advocacy regarding social policy for foster care, sexual exploitation, and national task forces. We brought into organisational focus our work with each other and our differences, and could no longer ignore cross-discipline collaboration. Our approach to mental health, while attuned to each individual, aspired to a holistic purpose of public, social, community, political, and environmental health. From our clinic's inception in 1979, as both a community and training non-profit psychology clinic, we approached our work systemically and collaboratively, but as our work became linked to a particular community we were pushed to grow to go beyond this as more than an *idea* or *theory* of community. Caroline Purves explores how academically oriented graduate students were challenged but eventually became enthusiastic, in translating their

DOI: 10.4324/9781003124061-6

classroom training into everyday language attuned to their clients. Heather Macdonald shares assessment feedback with an Athabascan Native adolescent; she will then describe a mobile therapy assessment in a climate of social tension and community pain.

Learning and Teaching a New Paradigm of Assessment (by Caroline)

The graduate students' assessment seminar meets weekly to discuss cases and issues of assessment in general. This weeks' meeting is underway. Halley is giving her follow-up report on the testing of the child we talked about in our previous meeting. He is an 8-year-old boy who comes from a family in which domestic abuse (father towards mother) has resulted in authorities stepping in. The boy has been a holy terror in school; he is aggressive towards other students, rude to his teacher, and refuses to do his work. The group suggested ways Halley could talk to the boy about the assessment, explaining what was involved. At first, she seemed to accept the ideas. However, as she described his opposition towards her and refusal to cooperate during this first meeting together, it seemed as if the group's suggestions had flown out the window. She was downcast and dejected. Even though we had talked about these ideas the previous week, once she was in the presence of the boy's difficult behavior, she had lost her grounding.

Again, we explained that she needed to be upfront about the referral. The boy was in a lot of trouble at school; thus, we suggested that she tell him that she knew what a hard time he was having. Further, she had learned that the teachers and his mom wanted some help with understanding why he was always so angry and hitting other children. They wanted some ideas to share with him so that he could have a more successful time at school, both in class and on the playground. The various tests that she was going to use would help him to learn ways he could be in better control of his anger. They would also give him and his mom a better understanding of why he was so mad so much of the time. Furthermore, Halley should tell the boy that she would answer any questions he had all along the way. We all felt that being forthright with this young boy was the most honest, and helpful way to develop a relationship with him. This approach would encourage his ability to understand his behavior and offer new ways of being in the world.

She took these suggestions to heart. With this encouragement from the group in mind, Halley regained her balance; she spoke to the child directly, and while he was not the easiest of children to work with, his attitude was positive and he was as cooperative as he was able.

Wondering how I could be so confident in a tricky situation as well as bring the group along, I began to think about the path that had brought me to this collaborative approach. My first exposure to assessment began in the late 1950s with the classic model of the psychologist as the expert, ideally a neutral presence, and the client to be understood through the use of rather mysterious "tests" or "instruments." Questions asked by the client were either deferred to the end of testing or answered as briefly and neutrally as possible. Children were told only that the psychologist would be playing some games with them.

Over the years, I practiced assessment in a variety of settings and three countries. As I become ever more familiar with the tests and procedures, I relaxed and became more forthcoming with clients. Assessment, as I came to realise, was a two-person enterprise rather than the examiner holding all the cards and the client being kept in the dark.

I also started to recognise some traditional elements in reports that seemed downright weird, if not offensive. For example, the first time I read a report that constantly referred to "the examiner" I became confused. Who was this person? Were there three folks in the room—the psychologist and the "examiner" and the client? It's as if the psychologist wanted to keep a distance from the client while at the same time making their relative relationship clear; the psychologist, that is, the examiner, was in charge while the "examinee," that is, the client, was there to be observed.

Paragraphs organised by test or instrument rather than by aspects of the client's dilemma were another "distancer." IQ results or MMPI scores, for example, were tacked on to the test taker (which is what the client often seemed to have become). What was missing in these reports was how these scores illuminated the understanding of the problems that had brought the client for testing. What was mainly missing in these kinds of reports was the person. Many of the people who would read these reports, including the client, were not psychologists. When the focus is on the test results rather than the meaning of these results, it feels as if the report is directed at another psychologist rather than the client. In fact, this all-too-common type of report leaves that actual work to the reader!

Reports written in "psychologese" rather than standard English can be daunting for both the client and non-psychologist referring agents. It's understandable that after years of studying and learning psychologists are comfortable with "professional" language (when I said to my graduate students that their reports should be understandable to the workman next door, there was surprising—to me, at least—resistance to that idea). However, being able to talk and write about the test findings in an ordinary language requires a deeper understanding of what we have learned about the clients. We are then able to talk with them about the conflicts and pain that have sent them for the referral in the first place. Using technical jargon reinforces a "one-up" stance that makes the psychologist seem to be in a different dimension from the client.

These were elements of an assessment world to which I was only gradually becoming conscious. What actually woke me up was a psychology writers' group that I was part of. The other members were planning on becoming psychoanalysts (which was not my goal, much as I liked the theories). When it was my turn to present, I wrote two pages about my interactions during the testing of a youth in juvenile hall. The family had not followed through on past referrals for counseling. The youth started off surly and reluctant, refusing to talk other than to give brief answers. I had told him the reason for our meeting—the judge wanted to know if he should be in foster care—but the youth was unresponsive. Gradually, however, he warmed up, and then he suddenly blurted out, "I don't want to go to foster care!" He told me that his big brother said he was stupid and wondered if he should go to a foster home. We explored his questions openly and talked about what he wanted. At the end, I asked him how he liked our work together, which he said he did. I suggested that he could have someone to talk with as we did every week and perhaps he should give it a try. He seemed okay with that suggestion, and we parted ways.

The writers' group was positive about the summary, suggesting that I write it up for a presentation. A colleague suggested I read a paper by Constance Fischer—"The Testee as Co-Evaluator" (Fischer, 1970)—which was an eye-opener! My paper, "Feedback in the Psychological Assessment, or What Do I Get Out of It" (1994), was accepted for presentation by both the California State Psychological Association Conference and the Society for Psychological Assessment (SPA). (Interestingly, after these talks a couple of people confessed to me that they used many of these ideas but made sure not to tell their supervisors!)

At the SPA conference, as I was leaving the room where I had just finished my talk, a couple who were sitting in the corridor reached out and caught my arm. "Who *are* you?" they asked. It turned out to be Connie Fischer and Leonard Handler, who had been told about the presentation by Steve Finn. They brought me into the fold of collaborative assessment, which developed into Therapeutic Assessment—thus, C/TA. These three were formidable, nonstop creators and teachers. They were also generous with their time and commitment to changing how psychology evaluations were conducted.

At that time, I was working at an agency that focused on children in the foster care system, which offered plenty of opportunities for me to explore the collaborative approach. I found, far from my early introduction to assessment, that usually, if not initially, during the testing the kids became open to knowing why they were there, what they were being asked to do, and ultimately to coming up with their own questions. "Why can't I remember what I read?" asked a 13-year-old. "I wish my mom and dad wouldn't fight so much," stated a 10-year-old. Sometimes, before we even launched into the testing instruments, a child might tell me what was going on at home that was causing so much distress for them. A report was typically sent to the referring party, often the social worker, but we began having sessions with the foster parents if they wanted to learn more about the child. Ultimately, a co-worker and I created a one-day workshop for foster parents to help them understand more about the assessment process. Their observations on the children's responses to the testing was instructive—behaviors following testing varied from much improved to some negative behaviors (which wore off quickly, apparently). By directly including the foster parents and demystifying the process, the compliance by both the foster parents and the children improved.

One day, Barbara Mercer, a colleague from our graduate student days, asked if I would like to supervise at the WestCoast Children's Clinic in Oakland. Such a great opportunity! The interns were committed to the work, and the staff was excellent. Barbara's assessment program was one of the most respected in the country. Of course, I said "Yes"!

The newly arrived interns in my first group were open to trying these new "radical" ideas, although their graduate training had been the usual "traditional" academic approach to psychological testing. Somewhat methodically, we took on each aspect of an evaluation as it came up. We explored the following: The initial referral, who should be included and how, the reasons for the assessment, how to conduct the assessment, the final results, and how to discuss them and with whom.

Thus, the first focus was the referral: Who was being referred and why? Who were the players in the client's life? Who would benefit from being included, and how would that facilitate change in the child's life? These referrals typically came from social workers, teachers, or other adults in the child's life. How or when to invite foster parents was, again, a new idea that elicited discussion in our group.

An innovative addition to the reasons for the referral involved asking the children and teens to pose their own questions; again, this was a radical move from the clinicians' graduate training. Adolescents were given the choice to pose their questions alone or with their parents. Most of our kids were in foster care, with the referrals coming from the social worker. Often the youngsters were taken aback by the idea, but teens were initially more interested. Once the assessment was underway, they were invited again to ask if there was anything about themselves they were curious about, and they often did ask. There can be an un-stated element of shame for a child who is too scared to ask publicly "Am I crazy?" or "Am I dumb?" When their worst fear is out in the open and the assessor can discuss it without alarm, there is a sense of relief and a different emotional climate in the room.

How and when to include the parents or foster parents in the actual testing took some discussion. The most useful solution was to have them watch from another soundproof room with the child being aware of their presence. Ideally, another psychologist would sit with the adults to help them understand how the testing was unfolding. (Of course, this added considerably to the expense, though the model was great when the funding was available.) The interns found that after some self-consciousness most children settled down to the tasks in front of them. Of course, the interns had to learn to adapt as well!

Writing the report was the next "radical" task. Rather than listing the results from the testing, the interns were charged with thinking about the questions being asked, then arranging the findings by elements in the client's psychological make-up and how these elements were impacting the client's life. Thus, for instance, if there were school problems the test results were related to the underlying causes while offering some ideas for remediation. This person-friendly rather than test-oriented approach was, indeed, a challenge that the interns had to grapple with. As Steve Finn (2007) puts it, it is the assessor's task to put themselves "in our clients' shoes." With a child in foster care, the client can, indeed, be many. Thus, the reports had to be understandable to all the various parties involved.

Then, the real challenge: How to report the findings to the child or adolescent. One can hardly tell a 6-year-old what her scores on the IQ test are or what the Rorschach summary means. The important information has to come in a language that makes sense to her. The most effective way of relating the findings turns out to be using metaphors. This can be in the form of a story, a song, a fable, a graphic mini-novel, or whatever other means seems useful. Sometimes a letter directed to the child answering their questions directly is a helpful option. The group members, after some hesitation, rose to the occasion. Once they put themselves into the mind of the "subject," their creative juices really flowed. Audrey Rosenberg, a member of that first seminar, writes,

> I don't have many memories from that time, but the thing that most struck me was the memory of writing fairy tales for the children I tested. It was such a radical and powerful idea! I especially remember the faces of the children when I read a fairy tale about parental addiction to the children in the grandparents' support group. The otherwise chaotic group was silent and rapt with attention. I remember, too, the experience of writing a fairy tale for a girl with a psychotic process and trying to convey what it felt like to be her and to understand her level of confusion. (personal communication, 2021)

An obstacle that got in the way of the feedback to the child was the impact the actual traumatic experiences had on the child, which was often revealed during the testing process. One path, a very sensitive clinician chose was a soothing, fairytale-like story that made no mention of the "real lived" experience of the child. As we explored the clinician's discomfort with bringing up the trauma in the child's life, she realised that part of our job as psychologists is to help bear these painful burdens in order to help the child learn to manage them (see Purves [2016] for my article on vicarious trauma in supervision). Her final story, while still a "fairy tale," took on the traumatic material in a manageable fashion, which allowed some relief from the early "secrets" the child had been left to bear alone.

Group discussions then became more about feedback in general—who to include in discussing the results and the most helpful way to go about it. The group discussions centered around the relevant parties and the child or adolescent who was the center of the process and concerned who should be involved and how. With an adolescent who was in foster care, this was a particularly sensitive issue as the consequences were often unpredictable. However, with all the adults in their life brought into the assessment process and the adolescent having some say, the chances of a positive outcome with useful recommendations in which the teen had some say were improved. This was very different from the old model of sending a report to the social worker and that being the end of it. With a younger child, the reading of the feedback story was often instrumental in helping the parents or parent figure develop a better understanding of the child's dilemmas than the official report.

It was not long before the Collaborative Therapeutic model was adopted throughout the assessment arm of the clinic. As Barbara Mercer mentions in her introduction to this book, we had several workshops with Stephen Finn, which included live testing sessions with his supervision, making the staff and interns increasingly comfortable with this approach.

One major aspect of the work that we did not discuss directly for a long time was the disparity between the clinicians and the clients. This was a glaring oversight. Initially, the majority of our child clients were African American, Latinx (Hispanic), or bi-racial and bi-cultural. For the most part, the clinicians were White. As the years rolled on, the client base included families from all over the world. Our staff and intern groups became increasingly diverse as well. Issues of culture and race differences became directly addressed throughout the clinic, not always easily and not always resolved. Nevertheless, the ongoing discussions added to the sensitivity and awareness of the clinical staff.

Thinking back to Halley and her initial discomfort and final better outcome, I believe that an unspoken thread that runs through the practice and teaching of assessment is that of rigour and bravery. Clients, both the children or adolescents and the adult figures in their lives—are looking for help; the dilemmas that initiate the referrals can only be resolved when the difficult, often painful issues are faced openly.

The ultimate challenge is for the assessor to find the pathway to make this new understanding accessible. The adults in the child's life are looking for understanding and guidance. The children can, and indeed ultimately do, want to understand and learn to manage both the positive and negative aspects of their life. This is what Halley ultimately chose—to be direct both with the child and the parent. The result was a cooperative child who could complete the assessment demands and find the needed support from parent and teacher. How does rigour and bravery factor into an assessment? The assessor cannot fall back on the carefully structured organisation, clearly defined rolls of tester and patient, and vague answers to questions that have characterised the traditional approach to "psych testing." Rather, this collaborative approach demands both creativity and care yet at the same time rigour in terms of following the structure of the testing instruments. While not particularly easy, it provides the scaffolding to help clinicians share the findings in a way that facilitates both understanding and change. Furthermore, it prepares all the parties to be more open to receive and act upon the test findings, beginning the move towards behavioral changes and improved family dynamics.

"I Don't Trust a Person Who Knows Everything" (by Heather)

The practice of psychological assessment has a long history dating back to the 19th century, when researchers began exploring the various ways in which the categorical differences of biology and behavior could be measured. It is a history intimately intertwined with the late 19th-century and early 20th-century imperial projects of White supremacy and the struggle against colonialism. Yet, as noted in other chapters in this book, traditional testing practices have been slow to combat more inherently oppressive models of psychology that are linked to an older history and slow to integrate cultural, religious, and social contexts into the practice of psychological assessment.

What the three of us aim to suggest in this book is that cultural and community-based models offer a way to shift and transform older paradigms of assessment where the idea is to gain *a final* knowledge about psychological functioning and apply this "knowing" to a person's life. After years of clinical practice, I am less certain that we can truly "know" the data and a person, and I have searched for ways to engage the mysteries or paradoxes that the assessment process often evokes.

Is it possible to open up the space of assessment so that different contexts can come alive as the encounter between people unfolds? In other words: Can psychological assessment be a site of ethics, invitation, transformation, or promise? Psychological assessment is a relational endeavor where we are often witness to suffering that goes beyond language. Can these assessments be a place of listening in depth to someone where the discussion at the end of the process is not a *final* knowing but can begin to reflect some true aspect of their life experience?

In previous published articles, I have explored these questions through numerous clinical events: the young man who began to masturbate during the administration of a thematic apperception test (TAT; Murray, 1943); the blood smear on my face from an unrealised wound that announced itself upon my first meeting with a pregnant client; or the young girl who stood on her chair and screamed until veins bulged from her neck after the first three Rorschach cards were administered (Exner et al., 2005; Macdonald, 2016a/b). All of these scenes contained encounters or events that were unpredictable and that unsettled the typical roles of "assessor" and "client." These encounters unseated the typical arrangements of the known world where the assessor is able to "witness" the client from a distance and apply some kind of data in order to readily interpret, in a straightforward manner, their behaviors. In these moments, the assessor is already more deeply engaged in a relational and social context than they usually realise.

For example, I recently worked with a 15-year-old Athabascan Native woman and her father (her parents were divorced, and the mother attended only a few of the meetings). They had come to see me because the young woman had refused to go to school and her father wanted to know what to do about it. On the first day we met in person, her father handed me a 25-page in-depth psychological and neuropsychological evaluation that was extremely well written. I was shocked; why had they come to me when they already had had a full assessment completed? I posed this question to the father: "What else can I possibly do here when you have a full report?" Without hesitation, he turned to me and said, "The man we saw who wrote this report knew everything, and I do not trust a person who knows everything."

Upon reviewing the report more closely, I noticed that aside from the identification of the client, there was not a single mention of the family's cultural context and their recent move from their Native lands, where they had left behind their tribal homeland. There was nothing left to "know" in psychological terms about the case; it was rather about being in deep relationship with this young woman so that we could engage the unknowable, travel through the labyrinth together, and learn about some of the geography she was navigating.

In our second interview, the daughter revealed a recurring dream. Since she had left Native lands, she had had a dream that there were bright red fish chasing her as she swam in the ocean. She often reported that she woke up from these dreams feeling scared. She then talked more about both her tribe and her clan and how important fish were to her people, but she could not understand why they were chasing her. Through a number of further conversations with the father and the young woman, it started to become clear that there were tremendous collective historical and cultural forces at play in this woman's refusal to go to school. In one session, her father told his daughter stories about how many people in his family had been forced to go to Indian residential schools that required the children to give up their language and culture. This young woman's dilemma was bound up in layers of family history and social traumas and how these had impacted her life.

At the end of our meetings, I still had no idea what the father needed to do about his daughter's schooling moving forward. However, I wrote the young woman a feedback letter that summarised our time together and the conversations we had with her father. In addition, through my research I had found an artist from her Native community who had drawn a mural on the side of a school. The mural was a picture of the ocean with large red fish swimming in it, just like her dream. The difference in the mural was that the artist had also painted a large eagle flying above the fish and the ocean. I included this drawing in the feedback letter. The young woman read the letter silently in my office during our last session together but did not say too much. After she read the letter, she simply said "Yes" and nodded her head.

The best assessment has to offer is a true heart connection with another person that comes from that hidden ethical place in relationship where we lean in and are "listened into the world" (August, 2010)—where we are in relationship with one another in the direction of not knowing, where the map becomes murky and runs off in stained ink.

As another case example (Macdonald, 2016), I once worked with a young African American woman who was eager to be emancipated from the foster care system. At the time of our encounter, she was pregnant and living with her mother. The county worker who had made the referral explained to me that she had concerns about "Dedra" (a pseudonym) leaving the system and losing access to mental health resources. The case manager further suggested that she was worried about the presence of a possible mood disorder since Dedra had exhibited symptoms of extreme irritability, depression, and "impulsive" behaviors that had started prior to her pregnancy. Dedra had returned home to her mother after over a year in foster care, and since that time she had become "obsessed with death." However, the caseworker could not explain to me over the phone exactly what she meant by Dedra's "obsession."

It was fortunate that when I met with Dedra I was working for an agency that prioritised community engagement and often encouraged clinicians to have meetings in the home of the client in order to gather background and experience in the context of the client's world. In other words, there was an assumption that neither the therapist nor the client could be separate from the world in some "objective" manner and that working together in community privileges the spatial and geographic environments as the major factors that shape identity, narrative, and relationship.

When I first met Dedra, she sat down on a kitchen stool in her home and looked at me from across the table. I noticed for the first time the features of her face. Her eyes were a deep brown color with eyelashes that curled perfectly above them. Her belly was enormous beneath a bright yellow cotton T-shirt. She said, "I am having a boy." She picked up her phone and sent a text while appearing to ignore me. A knot formed in the middle of my chest as I pulled out the Minnesota Multiphasic Personality Inventory-Adolescent (MMPI-A; Butcher et al., 1992) and a battery of cognitive tests. A text came back to her with a ring tone I recognised, and I asked her about other songs I thought she might like. She gave me a brief upward glance, and with several keystrokes on her phone, the whole song played.

We talked for some time about her love of music. Although we shared ideas about music, I felt like an intruder. I felt like she knew something that I did not—that I could give her those tests and it would not matter since I would still be the one who did not know or could not know. During this initial testing session, she refused to complete the MMPI-A. She stated, "These are the tests that will put me in jail. You are trying to make me look crazy!" She was not wrong about the problematic nature of perceptual misattributions towards her personhood as a result of culturally biased tests. She had mentioned to me before that she had wanted "White people" out of her business and that this assessment would finally get the White people "off my back." I was confused about what to do next. Dedra paused before asking me the next question: "Do you know about the death of Oscar Grant?" I replied, "Yes. He was shot a week ago by a police officer just outside the office where I work."

Dedra nodded and then looked away in a manner that told me I had missed the point. The fact of the matter was that I did not know her experience at all, nor could I ever really understand it. Then Dedra took me into her bedroom because she wanted me to see her dresser mirror. It became apparent that this related to the original referral question regarding her "obsession with death." On the left side of the mirror was a column of five newspaper obituaries she had cut out and shoved into the edge of the wood. I leaned in close to read each one. All five people who died were African American and male. Oscar Grant was the last in line;

a policeman had shot Grant while he was face down on the ground with his hands cuffed behind his back.

When I looked up, I observed Dedra's reflection in the mirror, with her swollen belly and her baby boy about to come into the world. I felt my body flush with emotion. She wanted me to know the odds. This was not about pity, sentimentality, helplessness, or liberalism. Dedra existed in the quickly disappearing space right between birth and death, and she knew it. Dedra wanted me to get the message: there is an inequitable distribution of power in our culture, a loaded dice game wagered with human lives. I said, "Dedra—this is so cold." She nodded and said, "You better be cold. Because that's how it is."

It seemed that Dedra was working to integrate the violence and death that had been prevalent in her community through the numerous obituaries up on her mirror, the images that represented the pain and/or the losses in her life and in her community. At times, there is simply no language for the trauma, no way to express the unsayable or unspeakable. Her "obsession" with death had nothing to do with some kind of mood disorder or psychopathology but was related directly to her life as it related to social and political events.

I wrote a long a feedback letter to Dedra in which I attempted to stay true to her personhood and true to the issues of justice in her community. In the final paragraphs, I wrote:

> In the opening statement of his autobiography *Blues All Around Me* B. B. King (1996) states, "When it comes to my own life, others may know the cold facts better than me. Truth is, cold facts don't tell the whole story. I'm not writing a cold-blooded history. I'm writing a memory of my heart. That's the truth I'm after—following my feelings no matter where they lead. I want to try to understand myself, hoping that you … will understand me as well" (p. 2). Your baby boy will be learning about his heart through yours. He will want to know how to live in this world, not just to survive, but how to really share himself and his dreams with others. He will want to know how to become his full potential by following his own truth, and you can teach him.

As soon as we finished the final feedback session, I gathered up my things and prepared to leave. She walked me to the door and waited for me to exit with her hands on her hips. It was an awkward farewell and an extremely intimate moment across an abyss of distance, across the unknowable. Once outside, I looked back at her through the closed screen door reinforced with steel bars. She smiled and waved goodbye.

From that point forward, I realised that in order to heal or even to conceptualise psychological wounds, their political and social counterparts would also need to be taken into account. As I write psychological reports, I continue to wonder how to explore psychological, social, and political themes as they relate to an individual within their own developmental trajectory. How could the test data give one a greater understanding of how social, political, and cultural systems interface with the psychological trauma of oppression and of how, in turn, this understanding impacts a notion of human identity, cultural memory, suffering, and freedom? These are tricky questions because one may conclude that their answers imply that a more reflective and sensitive kind of psychology is required or that there needs to be an increase in connection to political realms and an increase in community engagement. However, what some of the authors suggest in this volume is that we need different methodologies in psychological interventions so that we can become more aware of how psychology enters into *what is already social, cultural, and political.*

References

August, P. (2010). Is there a language to Logo's? The end of metaphor and the beginning of time. Unpublished paper.

Butcher, J. N., Dahlstrom, W. G., Graham, J. R., Tellegan, A., & Kaemmer, B. (1992). *MMPI-A: Minnesota Multiphasic Personality Inventory-A—Manual for administration and scoring.* University of Minnesota Press.

Exner, J. E., Jr., Colligan, S. C., Hillman, L. B., Metts, A. S., Ritzler, B. A., Rogers, K.T., Sciara, A. D., & Viglione, D. J. (2005). *A Rorschach workbook for the comprehensive system* (5th ed.). Rorschach Workshops.

Finn, S. E. (2007). *In our clients' shoes: Theory and techniques of therapeutic assessment.* Routledge.

Fischer, C. T. (1970). The testee as co-evaluator. *Journal of Counseling Psychology, 17,* 70–76.

King, B. B. (1996). *Blues all around me.* Avon Books.

Macdonald, H. (2016a). Assessment and social justice (pp. 71–74). In Mercer, B, Fong, T, & Rosenblatt, E. (Eds.), *Assessing children in the urban community.* Routledge

Macdonald, H. (2016b). The foot fetish: Events, reversals, and language in the collaborative assessment process. In L. Laubscher, C. Fischer, & R. Brooke (Eds.), *The qualitative vision for psychology: An invitation to the human science approach* (pp. 290–305). Duquesne University Press.

Murray, H. (1943). *The thematic apperception test: Manual.* Harvard University Press.

Purves, C. (2016). Why are you crying? It didn't happen to you? Vicarious trauma, assessment and supervision In B. Mercer, T. Fong, & E. Rosenblatt (Eds.), *Assessing children in the urban community* (pp. 114–119). Routledge.

Chapter 4

Assessment of Japanese Children: *Hikikomori*

Noriko Nakamura

Although it is difficult to identify the causes of a high degree of social withdrawal and disconnectedness from the outside world, known in Japanese as *hikikomori* (this word is used to describe both the person and the behaviour), I would like to demonstrate that inner disconnectedness is the key to understanding this social withdrawal phenomenon as it results in disconnection within the most intimate relationships (self, parents, spouse) and creates social disconnection from other groups such as school or places of employment. Clients are often asked why they do not attend school, but they themselves do not understand why they cannot feel safe and happy in the outside world. In this case, psychological assessment data play an important role as an "empathy magnifier" (Finn, 2007) to understand the client's disconnectedness.

Hikikomori: Definitions and Etymological History

The case study used in this chapter is of an 11-year-old girl who refused to go to school for three years. At the time of the case, 1993, the word *hikikomori* was not yet in common usage and I was not conscious of the term; instead, I used "school refusal." However, given the same case today, I would use *hikikomori* because the girl's school absence exceeded six months, which is in accordance with the definition given by the Ministry of Health Japan (2010).

The definitions of the terms "school refusal" and *hikikomori* have evolved over time as the phenomena have become better understood. The first term used in relation to truancy in Japan was *gakkou kyoufushou*, which is a translation of "school phobia," a term that appeared in a 1941 article in the *American Journal of Orthopsychiatry* (Johnson et al., 1941). Japanese psychiatrists adopted the term in the late 1950s. The expression conveyed the thinking of the time that students who did not want to attend school were suffering from separation anxiety from their mother.

In 1947, when the Japanese government created the junior high school system we have today, 99% of appropriate-aged children attended school.

DOI: 10.4324/9781003124061-7

However, a survey two years later revealed that 400,000 children of elementary age and 740,000 children of junior high school age were shown to be absent for 30 or more days, and the government set out to identify the reasons. Four main factors were identified: Post-war economic poverty, the desire of some Japanese families for their children to learn the trade of the father along with the perceived irrelevance of school education to the child's future, sickliness due to poor diet and living conditions, and *gakkougirai* (dislike of school). Two government surveys of Tokyo students absent for 50 days or more carried out in 1952 and 1965 showed that absence because of dislike of the school rose from 11% to 41% between those dates. As a result, in 1966, the Ministry of Education began to use the term "dislike of school" for all students absent from school. This term was more easily accepted than "school phobia" as it matched the cultural preference for softer language and did not carry the nuance of being a symptom of anxiety or other type of disorder (Maejima, 2016).

In 1970, a new term, *toukou-kyohi* ("school refusal") came into use, and it remains in use today. However, the introduction of this term led to much negative thinking about the causes of school refusal. Traditionally, the division of responsibilities between father and mother is clearly delineated, and the parent in charge of the education of children is the mother. Over time, the belief developed that if a child refused to go to school, the mother must be too indulgent or the child must be mentally ill, and the term carried a considerable social stigma. So, when the Japanese Ministry of Education made the statement in 1992 that "any student can suffer from school refusal," it was received with huge relief; the student's family or background was no longer automatically considered the cause of the problem.

The first academic reference to *hikikomori* came in an article in the journal *Kyouiku to Igaku* (Education and Medicine; Kitao, 1986), but public awareness of the phenomenon only increased after the publication of the book *Shakaiteki Hikikomori* (Social Withdrawal; Saitoh, 1998; Rosenthal, 2014). The author referred to individuals, predominantly male adolescents, who withdrew from social activity or were not earning a living for months or even years at a time. The term includes school refusers, but they account for only approximately 30% of all hikikomori cases. The remaining 70% consist of those beyond the compulsory school attendance age of 15 and those who first begin to exhibit social withdrawal from the time of further advanced education or after entering employment.

Although the use of the term *hikikomori* is now widespread, I consider "social disconnectedness" (*shakai shadan*) to be a more accurate term as the individuals exhibit a chain of disconnection, first from themselves and then from their families, school, and society.

Hikikomori Rorschach Assessment Data

Between 1989 and 1993, I dealt with the school refusal cases of 30 children (15 boys and 15 girls) aged 10–18 (average 15.7) while I was working at Chiba City Education Center. Although it has not been statistically analysed, comparison of the resulting data from the Rorschach tests I administered to those children reveals that there were two distinct groups of individuals, identifiable by one of the key scores on the Rorschach test, Lambda (L), which indicates the degree of openness vs. defensiveness and disconnection from the outside world. I have continued to find the same division in the multiple cases I have dealt with since then (Nakamura, 2011).

Those in the first group (73% of cases) had a high Lambda score, and I call them "wrapped-up" people, a reference to the transparent film used to wrap up food sold in a supermarket or used at home to preserve leftovers to be put in the refrigerator. I have found these people to be intellectually smart but often academically unsuccessful; they can look out and see the world but are psychologically limited and cannot interact face-to-face with people or meet and fulfil the expectations of others. Typically, they spend their time compulsively playing computer games or chatting over the computer until late at night and are unable to wake up in time for school. During therapy, I explain that the Lambda score is like a wall around the individual and compare it with the individual's physical height in meters. A Lambda of less than 1.0 is expected, but their Lambda scores exceed 1.5.

The second group of hikikomori individuals (27% of cases) had a lambda lower than 1.0 and were more hypervigilant. Hypervigilance (HVI) indicates a psychological state of cautiousness and distrust of the outside world and avoidance of intimate relationships. Again, using the wall analogy, their "wall" is rather low in that they have little defence against what the world throws at them. They are supersensitive and have a higher percentage of HVI positive than the high Lambda individuals. Based on the data, 88% of low Lambda cases were hypervigilant compared with 24% of high Lambda cases.

Case Study: Hypervigilance

Background and Process

The girl in this case study, whom I will call Junko,[1] was born in the western area of Japan and lived there without any difficulty until her family moved to Tokyo because of her father's business when she was nine years old. Before moving, the family lived next to her paternal grandparents, and Junko was close to her paternal grandmother.

Both parents were in their 40s and university graduates; her brother was three years her senior.

The therapy took place over a period of 17 months, beginning in late 1993 and ending in 1995. There were 48 therapy sessions of 50 minutes each, plus four 90-minute sessions of family therapy which the father also attended, including the first session. The other three family sessions were held at approximately six-month intervals. The mother accompanied Junko each time she came until session 42, after which Junko attended alone. When Junko felt too sick to attend, the mother came alone.

I administered the Rorschach to Junko in the fourth session, and on seeing the results I knew that this would be a difficult case requiring at least a year of therapy. I discussed the results with Junko and her mother in the fifth session. Although Junko stayed at home all day reading or drawing, the Rorschach stress indicator score of 5 (m = 5) alerted me as the usually expected score is 1. I pointed out that even though Junko suffered several physical symptoms of stress, such as stomachaches, headaches, eye pain, stiff shoulders, and constipation for days at a time, she was not physically sick, so the source of the stress needed to be identified. The mother responded, "I am the one who is sick from Junko not going to school." I offered the mother a Rorschach test, which took place in the sixth session, and it played an important role in understanding the entire family dynamics.

Junko was resistant to taking any intelligence test because she felt ashamed and inferior in regard to anything connected with academic work. For this reason, I suggested a Draw a Tree Test, which took place in the eighth session, and also suggested that the parents employ a private home tutor, which they did with positive results. Junko finally felt able to take the Wechsler Intelligence Scales for Children-Revised (WISC-R; Wechsler, 1974) intelligence test in session 14.

Phases of Therapy

First Phase: The First 15 Sessions

Presenting Issues. The initial appointment call was from the mother, who explained that her daughter, then 11, had not attended school for over a year. The referral was made on the advice of a famous university hospital psychiatrist in Tokyo. The mother was apologetic and embarrassed for me to know that the father had pushed her into making the appointment and that the daughter was so anxious and nervous that she refused to visit anywhere new. For the benefit of the daughter, I asked the parents to visit me alone first and then tell the girl later at home about their experience.

Initial Session with Parents. During the initial session, the father was very quiet while the mother spoke easily and cheerfully. The mother handed me a referral letter from the psychiatrist that stated: "... not attending school for about a year. For the last two months, school attendance stimulation did not work and it may be better to take time to treat her inner psychological issues." The father explained that "school attendance stimulation" meant that the psychiatrist had asked the father to verbally push the girl to go to school, which had not been successful. Next, the psychiatrist had advised the father to physically catch hold of her, put her into the car, and take her to the school together with her mother. After one failed attempt, the girl had started to hide and had fought back with all her strength against her parents. The father said he was not at all happy to act this way but had done it as he believed he should obey the person in authority. The mother felt she had no choice but to follow the husband's instructions. This unsuccessful maneuver made the parents disappointed that their daughter was not cooperating and that the specialist's advice had not worked. An atmosphere of tiredness and failure enveloped the entire family, and the disconnectedness between the parents and daughter increased. This led Junko to be seen as the black sheep of the family because everybody else was busy working frantically hard, whereas Junko spent her time at home reading books and writing her own manga or other stories.

This session also revealed that the father spent more than half the year away on business trips and that Junko's brother was out from early morning to late at night due to football team practice before and after school, sometimes falling asleep exhausted in the entrance hall on his return home. The mother, who still seemed unaccustomed to life in Tokyo and had few friends and no community network, stayed at home and was in charge of juggling their schedules and dealing with all household matters. Junko also spent all day in the house.

Second Session. Beginning with the second session, Junko was able to attend, accompanied by her mother. Junko said she did not feel safe coming to appointments during school hours because she did not want to be seen by anyone and felt guilty for doing something else during school hours. The small, private consultation room where she would not meet anybody else made her feel safe and motivated to come to see me. Over time, she became able to talk about her experiences. She said that moving had been a bolt out of the blue and that separation from her close friends and grandparents living in the neighborhood was a harrowing experience. While waiting to enter a private school, she had to attend a public school for the first time. She felt out of place at her new school, and one lunchtime, she was eating slowly and became the last person in the classroom; a boy came in and said, "Why don't you eat quickly? I will punch you if you stay here longer; we need to clean the room!" She felt threatened, and the words the boy used, spoken in a different dialect from the one she was used to, shocked her. However, her unhappiness and hesitancy to attend school was met with irritation by her parents, who could not understand why she was not trying to participate in her new school.

Third Session. In the third session, she described "sadache," a word she created to describe her feeling of sadness when she prepared to go to school. When this sadache became serious, she started to cry, and either her mind became blank or she felt her heart had turned to stone. Junko not only suffered sadache but also tremendous irritation, so strong that she almost wanted to destroy the whole house. Instead of destroying it, she found that a way to get rid of this strong irritation was by pinching her mother. The mother did not want to be pinched but did not know an alternative way for Junko to handle her irritation. Junko, her mother, and myself as therapist, together made a team to find out what irritated Junko so much and how could we shift the pattern. I proposed some tests, such as the Rorschach, to find out. She was very cautious but at the same time curious about the cause of her problem and how she could deal with it.

Rorschach Test Details. At the very start of the Rorschach, when I handed her the first card, she did not pick it up. Card 1 was soon put on the table, and she responded that she saw a jack-o'-lantern. Following the procedure, when only one response is given, I encouraged her to take time and look more closely. From the second card onwards, she spontaneously and quickly reported what she saw and gave a total of 41 responses; 22–25 responses are considered the expected range.

Assets and Strengths. It is valuable to recognize and emphasize the strengths of the person from the Rorschach data before starting a course of therapy. Although Junko was complex and easily frightened, she was a girl who (1) was up for anything and was looking for some fun (Afr = 0.58 not lower than 0.45 indicating an openness to emotion); (2) was open to the outside world (L = 0.64); (3) was relatively realistic, as long as she was not overwhelmed by threat or confusion (WDA = 68%); (4) was clearly a hard worker, as shown in the number of responses she gave (R = 41); and (5) accepted the social conventional interpretation of things (four popular responses).

Understanding Junko from the Rorschach

Junko's Rorschach results evidenced low Lambda (L = 0.63) and hypervigilance. From these results, I understood the two main factors that had led to Junko's school refusal and hikikomori behavior. First, she was tired. Having an overactive brain, the 11-year-old girl had to protect herself psychologically as she was easily overwhelmed. (M = 17, M −= 10, HV, low Egocentricity Index, M-passive, m, Dd). Second, she was disconnected from her own decision-making processes and how she saw the world. An example of this was that the order in which she gave her responses was confused on 9 of the 10 cards, and this made her difficult to understand. Other professionals might have mistakenly interpreted this result to mean that Junko was psychotic or schizophrenic. The harder she tried, the more difficulty she had communicating (X −= 46%, Dd = 19). She was also disconnected from herself and denied the emotions she was feeling (FC = 2, CF = 1). What I understood from the Rorschach data was how stressed out Junko was but also how good she was at hiding her stress so that neither her parents nor the consulting psychiatrist could recognize it or sympathize with her.

Junko and I talked about the goal of the therapy, the purpose of our work together, and I asked what would be her ideal self if I could help her achieve it. After I gave the Rorschach test and explained her complexity and how difficult it was for outside people, even her parents and close friends, to understand her, she was happy to hear this result and seemed to trust me to find the key to "fix" her. After that, we became closer but I was always cautious, keeping my physical distance, as I knew Junko was hypervigilant. Junko and I came to a consensus that the goal of the therapy would be "Make Junko's 'sadache' disappear". This was an ideal goal as her sadache consisted of many painful physical and emotional feelings. Junko explained in detail her severe backache, shoulder ache, tension in her neck, and pain in her eyes. She said she had experienced constant headaches all her life, but nobody in her family believed her (a medical report showed no dysfunction). She was constantly constipated for about four to five days at a time. All these physical symptoms were rather vividly explained, and I suggested she receive physical therapy or massage, which was successful as the physical therapist took her physical complaints seriously and explained she would need rather long-term therapy. This led her to have someone outside of her immediate family who was close to her to support her on a weekly basis.

The assessment process proceeded slowly. I invited Junko to do the intelligence test in the eighth session, but she refused to do it. Then, I asked her to do the Draw a Tree Test, as I knew Junko was good at drawing. However, she refused again, but this time the mother interfered and instantly said in a sharp tone of voice, "It is not difficult at all, I can show you how to draw a tree," and she drew an 'apple tree' in a minute (Figure 4.1).

Looking at her mother's drawing, Junko snapped, "It's embarrassing! That can't be a tree!" Junko got a pencil and drew "a tree of mystery" with an unknown type of fruit that nobody had ever seen (Figure 4.2).

The differences between the Mother's and Junko's trees were similar to the differences in their Rorschach results, reflecting the simplicity of the mother's approach and the complexity of the child. This could be seen in the mother's Rorschach data, which appeared at first glance to be

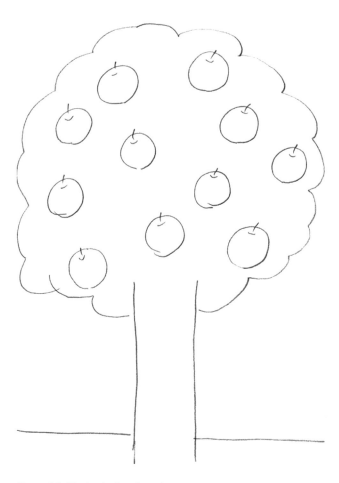

Figure 4.1 Mother's drawing of a tree.

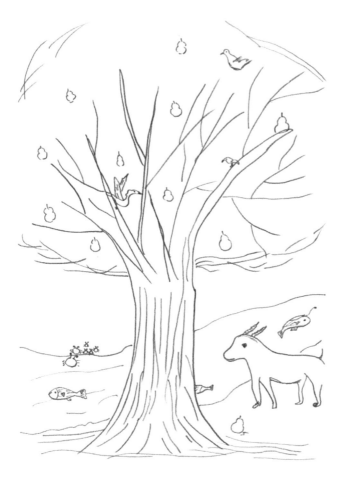

Figure 4.2 Junko's drawing of a tree.

normal although it was a short record ($R = 15$). The mother appeared to be functioning well enough with no apparent problems ($COP = 2$, $X+ = 53\%$, $WDA = 83\%$, $EA = 7$, $D = 0$, $FM = 3$, good processing, self-value with objectivity, and capacity to connect with people: $T = 1$). The source of the "sickness" or stress she referred to may have been in relation to her emotions. The Mother could modulate her emotions under usual circumstances, but under emotional stress, she became overwhelmed (4 blended/M.FC'.m.FD, and 5 blended/M.FC'.m.CF.FD responses on cards III and IX, respectively, both with human content) and lost her focus (5 DR in I-II-IX-X). Most importantly, the Mother was trying to avoid loaded emotional situations (low Afr = 0.36) and to hold back and tolerate uncomfortable feelings in herself (C' = 3), resulting in her feeling severe frustration.

Fortunately, Junko became interested in taking the intelligence test (WISC-R) and did it in the 14th session. She did it because she wanted to complete all the tests that I had prepared for her. Although she refused to do the vocabulary subtest, she rather enjoyed all the performance tests. Her PIQ was 126 (very high average). The subtest scores were Picture Completion (17), perfect for her age; Picture Arrangement (11), Block Design (12), Object Assembly (17), and Coding (10). Her verbal subtests results were Arithmetic (18), perfect for her age; Similarities (13), Comprehension (10), and Information (8). Her assumed verbal IQ was 111 and her assumed full IQ was 118. This was a big relief for not only Junko but also for all of us, including the parents and myself. What was more, Junko was eager to catch up with her studies even though she was not able to attend school. That led us to think about hiring a tutor to help her prepare for her return to school and to be a communication partner from outside her family. This succeeded as Junko very much liked the tutor, who was a pretty, gentle-natured university student in her early 20s. Junko asked her parents to increase the number of tutoring visits, and gradually the two become closer, not only through catching up on her studies but also through chatting about her drawings and sharing other interests.

By the end of 15 sessions, all the assessment data for Junko and her mother were ready, and I scheduled a feedback session with Junko and both her parents. At that session, the father revealed he had similar tendencies to Junko, explaining that he was shy, quiet, and obedient and had difficulty making friends and dealing with new situations. He added he was also as stubborn as Junko when he needed to be. The mother added that her husband's mother was the "queen" of the family that everybody had to obey. The mother sympathized with the father because he was so under his mother's control that he had lost his own intuition or natural desires. The father seemed to have repressed them all to try to meet external expectations. He did not talk much during the session, but he seemed to understand the similar nature he shared with his daughter. He commented that his family could be grouped into two: One being himself and Junko and the other being his wife and son. He even added that that might be the reason why it was easier for him to understand Junko than it was to understand his wife. Junko said in a later session that she felt closer to her father for the first time and understood why she could not make her mother understand her.

Second Phase: The Middle Block of 22 Sessions—Trial and Error

Key persons who played an important role in the middle part of the therapy were the tutor, physical therapist, and Junko's paternal grandmother. Junko accepted rather attentive physical and mental support well. The fact that Junko accepted support from the outside was a bonus of the feedback session. Sharing the data with the parents and discussing Junko's Rorschach, WISC-R, and Draw a Tree results enabled the parents to understand her for the first time. Furthermore, Junko felt encouraged by hearing an episode revealing her father's difficulties when he was young. His sharing about his character enabled her to release the deep shame that she had felt about being "the bad one in the family" and feeling that "nobody likes me and nobody will accept me."

The new topic that became significant during the middle section of therapy was the paternal grandmother. It became apparent that Junko was attached to her before the family moved to Tokyo and used to visit her house after school. One day, when talking over the phone, Junko was surprised to know that not only herself but also her grandmother had become sick after Junko's family moved away. The grandmother felt sad and lonely, resulting in physical heart pain, especially at dusk, which was very surprising as her grandmother used to be tough and strong. The grandmother told Junko that when her heart hurt, medication was helpful, and she recommended Junko to get some for herself. Junko had found someone who could share her sadache. This led Junko to visit a psychiatrist and ask for medication. She was prescribed low dosages of three medications (a tricyclic anti-depressant, an anticonvulsant, and a sedative) for the purpose of minimizing the ups and downs of her emotions. This was a dramatic change as before her grandmother's recommendation Junko had never wanted to visit a psychiatrist or take medicine. The medications were efficacious, and she appreciated the effect of feeling lighter and less bothered by headaches and sadache.

Junko was not able to attend the graduation ceremony at her elementary school; her parents attended the ceremony instead and obtained the elementary school graduation certificate for her. She could not attend as she was afraid of meeting people who knew her. This led her to think she might join a summer camp where everyone was new to her. However, in less than a week she returned home from the countryside after her parents went to pick her up. Junko reported it was too soon for her to try to join the group and it was very tiring because of the tension she felt all the time all day long, and her lack of sleep and constipation had caused her to start feeling sick again.

One positive outcome of Junko's time away from school was that she wrote a series of fantasy novels based on an adventure story of the struggle of an alien who wants to be a human being. Junko was shy about letting me know about her writing but looked happy when she reported it.

Third Phase: Last 15 Sessions: Junko by Herself

At one session, I had the opportunity to listen to the mother's story because Junko was absent and the mother came alone. When Junko was three or four years old, the mother had had a slight fever for a whole year and did not feel well. It seems that was the hardest time for her after her marriage because she found out that she had to obey her mother-in-law absolutely and nobody could go against the mother-in-law. Finally, the mother's answer to this situation was to "not think for herself" and switch her mind off. After moving, the mother was alone in Tokyo, not knowing what to do or how to make herself feel at home in the new environment without her mother-in-law nearby. We talked about doing something she was interested in by taking some courses for adults. She chose some activities that released her stress. I encouraged the mother not to feel responsible for her daughter staying at home but rather to go out and find some activities outside the home that would make her happy, which proved to be an effective tactic. After losing the mother-in-law's direction, she was at a loss and needed my permission to enjoy some activities by herself. I added that the mother's feeling happy would be the best medicine for Junko.

Because of the mother's new activities, Junko had to come to see me by herself for the last 10 sessions. It was interesting to hear her report about wandering around the streets and the small local area she explored before and after the sessions with me. This showed her emerging independent spirit. Junko made the significant decision to quit the mission school and transfer to a public junior high school in order to put herself in a very new place.

For the first time, Junko came to the session with her father and discussed her new school, which her father thought was a promising idea. Junko bought a new school uniform and started to think about focusing on attending school and quitting the therapy.

Post-therapy

Junko was 13-years-old when she left therapy, and five years later, when she was 18, I had an opportunity to talk to her over the phone. According to her report, her public junior high school had not been as suitable as she initially had thought, but she had been able to graduate. After graduation, she had chosen to go to a "support school," which provided special support for attaining certified graduation from senior high school. Junko said this support school had suited her and was easy to attend. As she was one of the best students there, she had been admitted to a junior college on a recommendation, and she was majoring in education. Junko stated that at last she was happy and busy, enjoying her college life with friends. She explained her experiences at the support school had brought back some of her confidence in herself. She was able to keep up with the work, she met teachers she liked and could trust, and she felt respected and protected there. By listening to her story, I recognized how much she had recovered her self-esteem and self-acceptance. Her journey to find connectedness to herself had taken time.

Cultural Context

The Role of the Expert and Others in Authority

Japan is a hierarchically structured society, and respect and obedience are expected from lower ranks toward higher ranks. The rank depends on a person's age or on their position of authority. In the case of Junko, there were three areas where this factor impacted the situation. The first was the mission elementary school that wanted to have Junko graduate successfully and enter junior high school, otherwise they would lose face; the school's reputation was at stake. The school recommended the psychiatrist to the parents, who felt they could not go against the school's wishes.

The second area of rank was the psychiatrist. Doctors, teachers, and experts are addressed by the title *sensei*, and it is considered improper to question a sensei's opinion. From the time of their school education, Japanese people are trained to not ask questions but to just accept what they are told. Even though the father felt uncomfortable following the psychiatrist's questionable instructions, he could not question them or seek a second opinion.

Third, the grandmother ruled over the household because of her age and status as the husband's mother. Wives are expected to follow their mother-in-law's directions without question, and husbands expect their wives to do so. As husbands are frequently away from home or may even live without their family in another city, if transferred there by their company, they have little power or interest in controlling the far-away relationship between their mother and wife.

Shame Culture

In this case, all of the family members had graduated from a distinguished private mission school except Junko, and this was a source of shame and disruption for the family; they considered her going to a public school uncouth. Also, the parents constantly praised and fussed over Junko's brother, sending an unspoken message of disapproval to Junko. In turn, Junko was ashamed of disappointing her parents. Her feelings of shame were released after the Rorschach results were explained.

Absent Fathers/Workaholism

In Japan, devotion to one's company comes before responsibility to the family. In this case, Junko's father worked for the family company that had been founded by his father, and as he was the first son, he was under tremendous pressure to succeed. His being absent from the home for half of the year is a typical scenario for Japanese businessmen.

With the Benefit of Hindsight

A Reinterpretation of the Results

This case, which is now 28 years old, is still vivid in my memory and resonates within me. I was a fledgling clinical psychologist at that time and was trying to use assessment in a collaborative way. Fortunately, my private practice allowed me to communicate closely and freely and to use the test results directly in communicating with clients. This was how I created the Rorschach feedback session. I was excited to try discussing the meaning of the data and understanding the actual experience behind the background that clients explained. This was one of my cases during that period. I learned from a workshop led by John Exner, the Rorschach expert and creator of the Comprehensive Rorschach Scoring System (1993), how useful it is to identify not only the child's but also the mother's Rorschach data. I learned how Rorschach could be used in understanding relational issues between a couple or among family members.

This case with Junko was one of my first experiences of grasping the meaning of relational issues. The mother was trying to feel nothing, while Junko was trying to feel everything. Loneliness connected the two of them from different directions. The mother was lonely after her marriage, which was under the obligatory control of her mother-in-law. She stated that she was almost married to her mother-in-law, not to her husband; she was at the mother-in-law's disposal and her husband was totally out of the picture. Only now can I understand the mother's way of drawing an apple tree, her saying "It's not at all difficult, I can show you, this is how." This was her way of solving the task, doing whatever she was asked to do, and not hesitating or being troubled.

Now I understand why the mother showed her opinions and emotions only in an indirect way (5 DR out of 15 responses). She forced herself to keep calm and not to be involved in feelings (low Afr.), and she tried to keep her distance and was defensive (4 PER). She was in between trying not to be involved and becoming too complex, exactly as shown in the Rorschach blends. I was too naive at the time to understand all these underlying conflicts and hardships that were causing the mother's irritation.

Family Changes

At the time of the therapy, I did not consider seriously the implications of the family's move to Tokyo or that it had impacted not only Junko but all the family members. As Junko explained, it was 'a bolt out of the blue'; there were many losses of intimacy at the same time, and the whole family had to adjust to a new nuclear family system. The father and son were able to adjust by working hard outside the home, but it was difficult for the mother and Junko to adjust to the new situation without the presence of the paternal grandmother, who had been the most important figure for them. My interpretations of the mother's Rorschach and Draw a Tree Test were too simplistic. I did not recognize that the mother, like Junko, had no self-image and that her self-effacing approach was her survival tactic.

Therapeutic Assessment vs. Collaborative Assessment

In 1993, I had not even heard the expression *Collaborative Assessment* (CA) yet, nor *Therapeutic Assessment* (TA). If I took this case now, what would I do differently, I asked myself. Although I knew that the presence of the father and getting him involved was an important factor, especially when dealing with young people, I only gradually came to understand the importance of the family dynamics in this case. If I were to take the case now, following TA training and with the help of the TA structure (Finn, 2007), I could ask more clearly for the father's commitment and help him understand the importance of his voice. The TA procedure has the advantage of gathering the experience and history of the couple. In this case, the couple's dynamic and the family system affected Junko's psychological development a great deal.

Conclusion

This 1993 case of an 11-year-old girl took place when school refusal was beginning to be recognized as a social problem in Japan. Now we use the term *hikikomori*, the official term for a person who stays at home more than six months without involvement in any social activity, to cover these cases. Each of these individuals has their own reasons for being stuck at home. One way to untangle their invisible struggles is to use visible psychological assessment data, such as I described in Junko's case; her psychological assessment revealed that she was neither psychotic nor schizophrenic but had reasons for not being able to express herself or interact with society. The therapeutic process took time, and the family's involvement was one of the keys to the success of the process. Projective methods and collaborative family assessment feedback played important roles in accessing the narratives of the family members in the context of Japanese cultural traits.

Just as the Japanese word *umami* has been adopted in the culinary world in recent years to describe a fifth taste that had existed all along but had not been recognized outside Japan until it was identified and given a name, so the word *hikikomori* is now being adopted around the world to describe cases of social withdrawal. However, the prevalence of cases in Japan suggests that the culture of not speaking one's thoughts or opinions, obedience to authority, and shame based on saving face, which form the bedrock of Japanese society at home, in schools, in the workplace, and in social interactions in general, is the root cause of the disconnectedness that has resulted in the *hikikomori* phenomenon.

Note

1 Identifying information discussed in this chapter has been changed to protect clients' privacy.

References

Exner, J. E., Jr. (1993). *The Rorschach: A comprehensive system, Vol I: Basic foundations* (3rd ed.). John Wiley & Sons.

Finn, S. E. (2007). *In our clients' shoes: Theory and techniques of therapeutic assessment*. Routledge.

Kitao, T. (1986). Dropout apathy, Hikikomori. *Kyoiku to Igaku, 34*(5), 439–443.

Johnson, A. M., Falstein, E. I., Szurek, S. A., & Svendsen, M. D. (1941). School phobia. *American Journal of Orthopsychiatry, 11*(4), 702–711.

Maejima, Y. (2016). History and theory of school refusal and school nonattendance – A discourse history of children who don't or can't go to school. *Arts and Sciences* (Tokyo Denki University), *14*, 23–47.

Ministry of Health (Japan). (2010). New guideline for the evaluation and support of hikikomori. https://www.mhlw.go.jp/file/06-Seisakujouhou-12000000-Shakaiengokyoku-Shakai/0000147789.pdf

Nakamura, N. (2011). Bringing tests to life in collaborative/therapeutic assessment wrapped-up people. International Society of the Rorschach & Projective Methods 2011. Tokyo Symposium presentation paper. Tokyo, Japan.

Rosenthal, B. (2014). *Is it safe to come out yet? Analysis: Japan's policy for hikikomori*. Scholar's Press.

Saito, T. (1998). *Social withdrawal revised*. PHP Institute.

Wechsler, D. (1974). *Wechsler intelligence scale for children—Revised*. Psychological Corporation.

Chapter 5

Growing Empathy with Complex Clients in Developing Countries: Collaborative/Therapeutic Assessment in Latinoamérica

Ernesto Pais and Daniela Escobedo-Belloc

Common to both Mexican and Argentinian psychologies and their cultural contexts are the influence of psychoanalytically oriented theories that have served as the foundations of graduate programs. These theoretical academic programs have shaped mental health service delivery in Latinoamérica and have served as a basis for the Collaborative/ Therapeutic model that we present in this chapter through descriptive case material of two clients with complex experiences in life.

Argentinian and Mexican Demographics

The first country that we present is Argentina. It has a current population of more than 44 million people, and its distribution is similar to other countries in the region that have higher population densities in the big cities. Ethnicity is different from other countries in Latinoamérica: 95% of Argentina's citizens are White, and less than 1% have Native American origin (INDEC, 2010) this is mainly due to the wave of European immigration in the late 19th and early 20th centuries and the very early freeing of Black slaves in 1813. As in other countries in the region, poverty has increased from 5% to 45% in the last 50 years (1970–2020). Also, young people represent a significant group in that more than 25% of the population is under 14 years old (INDEC, 2020).

The second country, Mexico, stands out for its great cultural and ethnic diversity as well as the economic inequality among its 126 million people. Today, the majority of Mexicans are genetically admixed; most have a pre-Columbian Indigenous and European genetic substructure, with African represented to a lesser extent (5%; Moreno-Estrada et al., 2014). However, less than 7% of the population speak a native language (INEGI, 2020). Some cities towards the center and north of the country have a 4% poverty rate compared to the cities in the south, where it reaches 70%, including 30% living in extreme poverty. Regarding the

DOI: 10.4324/9781003124061-8

distribution of wealth, 34.1% of the wealth is in the hands of the richest 1% of the population and 64.4% belongs to the richest 10% (Castañeda, 2020).

Psychological Underpinnings

As described by Ponza (2011), psychology was born in Argentina not only as a therapeutic theory of Freudian inspiration but also as a critical expression and an attempt to investigate the constitutive assumptions of modern thought in the search for human emancipation. This approach also allowed Lacanian psychoanalytic methods to be introduced in the early 1970s in a society that became immersed in a process of political crisis and cultural modernization in the 1970s and 1980s after many military coups, dictatorships, and social, cultural, and thought repression. Sigmund Freud was introduced in the 1910s and Melanie Klein in the 1950s to Argentinian psychology; Jacques Lacan even today is one of the most-cited authors in university psychology programs. The Lacanian approach was introduced in the 1970s, reaching its peak influence in the 1980s. Some authors relate these events to political and intellectual developments.

Psychological Studies in Latinoamérica

Mexico and Argentina have the universities with the largest number of students in Latinoamérica. However, in Latinoamérica the dropout rate at the middle and higher levels has been reported to be around 50% (Didou Aupetit & Jokivirta, 2015). These countries also have in common a strong influence of Catholicism, although less so in their capitals.

Psychology as a discipline has been studied and researched since the 1890s in both countries. In this context, Ezequiel Chávez offered the first psychology course in México, and Rodolfo Rivarola and Ernesto Weigel did the same in Argentina. Nevertheless, the first bachelor's programs in psychology in either country were not founded until the 1950s (Klappenbach & Pavesi, 1994). Around 1916, Aragón combined the German experimental and the French psychoanalytic influences and founded the first experimental psychological laboratory in Mexico (Escobar, 2016). In 1950, the psychoanalytic theoretical presence established itself and was consolidated through the Sociedad Psicoanalítica Mexicana A.C, promoted by Erich Fromm. This was a significant step toward the foundation in 1962 of the International Federation of Psychoanalytic Societies (IFPS). Today, diverse evidence-based training is available in Latinoamérica. including psychodynamic, cognitive-behavioral, and systemic disciplines. Attachment- and trauma-informed courses, as well as dialectical-behavioral and mentalization (Bateman & Fonagy, 2013) treatments, have arrived in the last two decades and they show a gradual but steady advance.

Argentinian Theoretical Framework

Theoretical frameworks for psychological research in Argentina changed from 1900 to 1950, when psychology programs were introduced. Such research was initially inspired by the empirical work of William Wundt's Leipzig Laboratory, which was founded in 1879. But since 1920, philosophical approaches criticizing experimental and empirical research have been well received in Argentina, leading to the situation of psychology in Argentina from 1940 up today (Fierro and Freitas Araujo, 2021): Argentina has an underrepresentation of non-psychoanalytic theories and psychotherapies, the absence of solid epistemological and methodological discussions, and an attitude oriented more to philosophical backgrounds than empirical studies.

Currently, Argentina has one of the highest numbers of psychologists in the world, with a ratio of one psychologist per 500 inhabitants (World Health Organization, 2014). As stated above, psychoanalytic approaches derived from the European analytic and object-relational models of Freudian, Kleinian, and Lacanian theories are the most common in the country. These approaches influence psychological assessment as well (Klappenbach, 2007).

Some Argentinian diagnostic techniques have been developed, such as the Cuestionario Desiderativo (Celener de Nijamkin & Guinzbourg de Braude, 2000; Sneiderman, 2014) and the Sistema Argentino para la interpretación del Rorschach for Rorschach inkblots (Passalacqua & de Colombo, 2000). A relevant characteristic of psychological assessment in Argentina is that since the 1950s it has been strongly process-oriented (Frank de Verthelyi, 1999), even though test adaptation has also been very important. Some Argentinian authors have worked on psychological assessment as a process and on "psychodiagnosis" and have introduced collaborative techniques (Lunazzi, 2018).

Mexican Theoretical Framework

Regarding the history of psychological assessment in Mexico, Santamarina in the 1920s and Boder, and Diaz Guerrero in the 1960s are significant because of their efforts to adapt psychological instruments. Diaz Guerrero emphasized the need to understand Mexican identity and pursued a transcultural psychology. He published several self-reporting scales to measure attitudes and beliefs of the Mexican population, such as the level of "machismo" (Alarcón, 2010; Galindo, 2004).

By 1926, personality assessment was being practiced in the legal context, such as the juvenile court, and in infant health and psychiatric services. Since 1950, the Sociedad Mexicana de Psicología A.C., and since 1999 the Sociedad Mexicana de Rorschach y Métodos Proyectivos A.C., have promoted training, research, and development of tests. Among Mexican test standardizations, the Wechsler Scales and the Minnesota Multiphasic Personality Inventory-2 (MMPI-2) and the MMPI-2-RF (Ben-Porath & Tellegen et al., 2008/2011), stand out, similar to the situation in Argentina.

Clinical Services in Latinoamérica

It is a long journey to achieving a generalized level of opportunities for professionalization in the field of psychological assessment, both in Mexico and Argentina, due to economic inequality and insufficient postgraduate programs with an emphasis on psychological assessment. In Argentina, 78% of the students have access to undergraduate programs in public and free universities, which are ranked higher than private and other Latin American universities. For instance, the Universidad de Buenos Aires, a public and free university, is the highest-ranked university in Ibero-América. The lack of postgraduate courses on psychological assessment may be related to the absence of free education at this level.

Therapeutic Assessment

Therapeutic Assessment (TA) proposals have been introduced in different places around Latinoamérica and are described in articles and presentations (see, e.g., Escobedo, 2018; Espinoza-Reyes, 2020; Pais, 2019; Sanz & Pais, 2013). As stated in Smith (2016), the TA model is itself culturally responsive, so the introduction of TA in Mexico and Argentina allows in particular for working with clients of diverse cultures. Collaborative/Therapeutic Assessment's evidence-based theoretical frameworks, including attachment theory, Fonagy's concept of mentalization (Bateman & Fonagy, 2013), and intersubjectivity, are relevant for the comprehensive assessment and treatment for complex cases involving trauma in adverse contexts such as poverty and political and societal crises.

In Argentina, TA is addressed in graduate and postgraduate programs. This is also the case for bachelor's degrees in psychology at the Universidad Abierta Interamericana and Universidad del Salvador and the specialist course on psychological assessment of the College of Psychologists of the Province of Buenos Aires as well as the International Postgraduate Course on Collaborative and Therapeutic Assessment at the Universidad Abierta Interamericana. In Mexico, TA is taught in the north of the country, in a master's degree in psychotherapy at the School of Medicine in the Universidad Autónoma de Nuevo León and in a systemic track specialization at the Universidad de Monterrey.

Our Clinical Background

We come from different contexts and clinical pathways. In Mexico, Daniela works mostly with adult and child populations within a university hospital in its psychiatric department and in private practice. In Argentina, Ernesto began to notice the therapeutic effects of assessment feedback in 2007 while doing psychological assessment in a state institution for adolescents convicted of crimes, and he started introducing some collaborative techniques in his work. Both of us assess and treat patients with severe personality disorders and complex trauma who are from different cultural and socioeconomic backgrounds. Also, we strive to work within a relational approach with an empathic and humanistic perspective. Our backgrounds have allowed us to appreciate the value of the model proposed by Finn (2007). Thus, we started our training in TA more than 10 years ago. In Mexico, a colleague had contact with TA at the Society for Personality Assessment's annual convention. This connection generated a very well-received set of TA conferences, a formal study group, and supervision opportunities. In Argentina, TA was introduced in studies related to multi-method assessment. It was very well received, both for being process oriented as well as for its dynamic theoretical framework. Currently, Ernesto is running the University Center for Collaborative and Therapeutic Assessment in Buenos Aires, where clients from disadvantaged social contexts receive pro bono services.

Casework in Argentina and Mexico

In order to share our clinical work with TA from different cultural backgrounds, we introduce two cases. Both cases are clients from upper socioeconomic backgrounds in a private practice setting, although we do have experience applying the therapeutic/collaborative model in public health and academic settings based on both public and private funding. These cases describe the step-by-step process of a therapeutic/collaborative assessment. They show a nontraditional type of psychological assessment that uses standardized measures in a collaborative way to create a therapeutic intervention and result. These two complex cases reveal a core precept of TA: The use of psychological tests as *empathy magnifiers* (Finn & Tonsager, 1997) to bring empathy to what each client has experienced and allow the clinician to be "in their client's shoes"

(Finn, 2007) so they can understand from their client's perspective and assist the client in making links from their symptoms and questions about themselves to their life experiences and create new ways forward. These cases illustrate how the Therapeutic/Collaborative model is ideally suited to clients from varied backgrounds in our two countries.

The Case of Porcia in Argentina: "Why do I have this ritual?" (by Ernesto)

The first case that we would like to introduce concerns a 31-year-old White woman, who was dealing with a variety of family tragedies. She had been in therapy previously but couldn't resolve her current symptoms, nor could she deal with these issues from an early age despite her ability to maintain what she termed a "positive attitude." This TA helped both the client and the therapist to get in touch with emotions that were cut off from her awareness and the now costly dilemma of always "trying to be positive." Both test measures and a more in-depth (or "extended") inquiry into her responses on test measures enabled me to get into the client's shoes and understand why it was particularly painful for her to experience any negative emotions.

Background and Referral

Porcia is a 31-year-old woman who was referred to me by a colleague after receiving treatment for 7 months from a therapist with a psycho-analytic framework. Porcia said it was not helpful, so she started looking for other types of therapy in order to resolve a particular disruptive ritual she was dealing with as well as "old problems that are related to that ritual."

Porcia expressed in her first interview that she was very happy with her partner, to whom she had been married for 5 years after living together for a few years. She had studied business management and received her degree in the usual time and manner. Currently, she was working as a teacher. She had worked in the field of e-commerce for the past 10 years. In the last 5 years, she was the commercial manager for two big global e-commerce companies. Today, she co-owned a successful e-commerce business.

To help understand her background, Porcia describes the following as significant:

- Her parents were physicians.
- When she was 2 years old, her parents divorced, and her father died when she was 3 years old.

- After her father's death and until she was 6 years old, her mother had a partner. Porcia shared that she used to call him "Dad."
- When Porcia was between 10 and 15 years of age, her mother became addicted to drugs, mainly cocaine, and developed what Porcia described as promiscuous sexual conduct.
- When Porcia was between the ages of 11 and 13, her mother made two suicide attempts.
- Porcia moved several times from Buenos Aires to other cities in the suburbs. Sometimes she stayed with her maternal grandparents. She had a hard time due to being separated from her friends and relocated to another school.
- When she was 17, she was very depressed and stopped going to school. After 2 months of therapy, she was able to rejoin her regular activities.
- In the last 10 years, she has gone through different medical interventions. Among the most relevant, she required surgery to remove a breast implant that had become encysted. Also, she was hospitalized due to constipation and other physical problems.

Initial Session Based on the Therapeutic/Collaborative Model

The goals of the initial session are to enlist the client as collaborator, lower their anxiety about the results and the process, and let them introduce their own narrative about their self and worldview. Another important goal is to build upon questions that the client wants to have answered through the assessment and to explore the context where these questions arose.

Regarding my first impressions when I met Porcia, I was surprised by how extremely fast she talked (reflecting both her anxiety and for her amazing processing speed). She also seemed very nervous and overwhelmed, expressing her daily problems in an anguished way as if they were impossible challenges. Porcia came across as a smart person, frequently using psychological jargon while talking about herself. However, as introduced before, this is relatively common in Buenos Aires because of Freudian theory being widespread in Buenos Aires. Other things that clearly stand out are that she is very talkative, expressive, and somewhat impressionistic. Nevertheless, I was very comfortable with this initial session and felt quite attuned to her emotions as they came through.

I proposed that Porcia and I work together on questions to guide the assessment. She said she had to solve a specific problem. However, she said she did not want to solve it in a "linear" manner because she had many other issues that surely were related to it.

She told me that her problem was a ritual. Every morning she used a rectal suppository that she had not needed since she had first used it

10 years ago, and she had to wait between 1 and 2 hours before going to the toilet. She had been doing this for the last 10 years with a medical prescription for the suppository for a diagnosis of gastritis that the treatment was supposed to remit in a few days. With a sad look and great frustration, she expressed that only after waiting these 2 hours could she start her day. She quickly related this to a series of problems that this ritual had brought about, such as not being able to go on trips without inconvenience or to leave home early. Also, it had affected her sexuality since her sexual desire had diminished. While she was talking about this, she looked at the floor for the first time and shared that she thought that she had lost sensitivity in her erogenous zones after arousing these parts of the body with the suppository, a conclusion she had arrived at with her previous therapist.

Questions Developed with Porcia

Porcia had three main questions. (1) *Why do I have this ritual? What unsolved things from my life am I putting into this ritual?* Every time she tried to stop doing the ritual, she felt very sad and anxious, had stomachaches for several days, and was not able to defecate. She has tried several medical methods, but none of them have worked.[1] She highlighted that the ritual began 10 years ago after she recovered from gastritis thanks to the suppository. She says that, because of the suppository, she does not have stomachaches or problems with her diet. She also shared that even though she knows the suppository is not needed now, she thinks that if she stops using it she won't be able to defecate, as happened before. (2) *What is my emotional maturity age?* She stated she felt very emotionally immature. She added that her friends used to tell her this, and she recognizes that she experiences every problem as if it is a crisis. (3) *Why is it that I get so defensive with people?*

After we met, I thought about how smart and resilient she had to be in order to cope with the complex and adverse events in her life. It also seemed to me that we were achieving a good connection and that she had begun to share issues that were not easy for her. I also had the feeling that she needed to talk about all these things superficially so she could maintain a sense of comfort, strength, and integration. I respected this way of bonding throughout the entire session.

Standardized Testing Sessions and Standardized Results

The initial session is followed by one or more sessions in which standardized tests are administered according to standardized procedures (Finn, 2007). The Therapeutic/Collaborative Assessment differs from the traditional psychological assessment in that (1) tests are used that are closest—in their face validity—to the client's central questions about herself; (2) each test is introduced to the client according to its relevance to her assessment questions; and (3) a special method is used here, the *extended inquiry*, that consists in engaging clients in targeted, collaborative discussions of their experience of a test or personally significant responses. As well, Porcia was asked about her experience through the tasks, paying special attention to addressing events that seemed related to her questions for the assessment.

We spent four sessions working on this step of the process. Initially, we used two tests. Her question about her ritualized suppository behavior led us to administer a measure of obsessive-compulsive disorder (OCD) (Sánchez-Meca et al., 2011), and the second measure we used evaluates different dimensions of emotional awareness. Her scores on the OCD measure showed a diagnosis of obsessive-compulsive was unlikely, and in the second measure, "emotional hiding" was above average (Samper-García et al., 2016), suggesting that she kept her emotions under wraps and hid them from others.

Next, we used the Rorschach Inkblots (R-PAS; Meyer et al., 2011), and in the following session, she completed the MMPI-2 (Butcher et al., 1989), a self-report personality profile. Finally, we used the Early Memories Procedure (Bruhn, 1992), in which the client is asked to recall earliest memories or events, describe these events, and then rate them regarding how positive or negative they were and how clear vs. fuzzy they are now.

All the tests were followed by an extended inquiry (Finn, 2007) that allowed the client to make associations to her responses. For instance, it was a very important moment in the process to realize that none of the six memories included in the Early Memories Procedure, (considered to be a metaphor for the client's core unresolved issues) had a negative feeling of any kind for Porcia. In the extended inquiry, she asserted that those memories were significant to her. After that, I invited her to talk more about the fact that all her memories were associated with only positive feelings. She was surprised when she realized this, for the first time in the whole process, and she was silent for a while. We were able to build a new narrative about how important it was for her to be vigilant and to keep in mind only positive experiences. We began to talk about how she needed to banish those emotions that were too upsetting for her.

Utilizing Standardized Test Results as an Intervention. A common way to help clients implement more adaptive solutions to their problems in daily life is to share with them hypotheses derived from the assessment findings. We accomplish this in an intervention session once testing is completed by bringing into our conversation problems in the client's life that are the focus of the assessment (Finn, 2007). In this manner, sharing our findings elicits different emotional reactions in clients that are related to their problems in daily life and helps them to be receptive to findings that would otherwise be rejected. In order to proceed with the assessment intervention session (Finn, 2007), the assessor must conceptualize integrating background information, testing, and the clinical experience of the client. Accordingly, I next share some meaningful test results and some possible interpretations. These results assisted us in transitioning to a therapeutic intervention.

MMPI-2. I administered the MMPI-2, a self-report personality profile, to look at Porcia's clinically significant symptoms specifically related to her questions about her physical problems. Porcia was open and non-defensive on this measure although she showed some level of rigidity in her processing and a relatively conventional way of being. To summarize, she perceives herself as someone with few problems in general but with health concerns related to her ritual, and she manifested some defensive strategies of denial (Silin & Sanz, 2019). Thus, the defensiveness she noted about herself did not seem to be a reluctance to be open but a defense to protect her emotional vulnerabilities.

Porcia's profile elevations on MMPI Scale 1 (a scale of physical complaints) and Scale 3 (a measure of [an almost cheerful?] denial of pain or depression) suggests that her emotions constellate in physical problems combined with an opposite desire to minimize her pain. Caldwell's (2001) interpretation of the origin of this personality profile proposes that due to a lack of physical soothing or solace when anxious, the infant or child develops physical symptoms instead of a connection to their own emotions. Also, they may show avoidance of anger and have difficulties recognizing conflicts in their life and relationships. This fits with Porcia's painful childhood history—her extreme and overwhelming emotional experiences, particularly early parental death as a toddler, closely following parental divorce; her mother's depression, suicide attempts, addiction, and unavailability for parenting. Yet, her profile on this measure reinforces how she keeps painful emotions at bay in order to maintain an overly positive outlook. This MMPI-2 profile supplemented the history that Porcia and I had shared about her life and gave us a clue about how to answer her worries about her problems in her life.

Rorschach. Results from the Rorschach and standardized R-PAS scoring helped to further understand Porcia's adult successes and how she dealt with her early trauma and loss. The Rorschach confirmed her strengths and coping strategies with well-preserved processes of perception and judgment. However, she tended to perceive her world in a rigidly conventional way at the cost of her self-expression. Rorschach scores reflecting stress and distress levels that she felt day to day were below average, confirming that she did not allow herself any thread of vulnerability.

After Rorschach administration and coding, I was impressed by some other findings. Mainly, there were two aspects. On the one hand, since her history had many traumatic experiences, I was surprised by her low scores in the Rorschach critical content scales associated with trauma. She was a successful and intelligent person; however, her testing showed a lack of complexity—she gave bare-bones answers with few thematic flourishes. This constricted presentation paired with such a painful history has been noted as a type of cognitive constriction found in traumatized populations (Viglione Towns & Lindshield, 2012). At the same time, her protocol had no signs of anger, giving credence to the notion that she wanted to stay clear of her instinctive feelings.

Early Memories Procedure. Results so far were consistent with her Early Memories Procedure and the overabundance of positive memories, such as," I remember dancing with my mom the day I finished preschool. I remember that she had on a polka-dot dress and a red cap and I was feeling very well," or hardly relevant memories such as, "I remember being in the movies with my cousin. I had just learned to read and he took me to see the premiere of *Batman*. I remember that the subtitles were very fast and I asked questions all the time." She finished answering the final question—"Why do you remember these memories?"—by saying, "Because in most of my memories, there are very important people in my life."

All of this allowed me to conceptualize that a relevant aspect in this case was precisely that the client had so far managed to keep out of her awareness the negative events and emotions that she had undergone throughout her life. By doing this, she cut off negative memories like grief and shame. She was aware that these early losses were relevant for answering her assessment questions and were most likely related to her health and physical symptoms.

I hypothesized that Porcia had suffered anguish, associated with the unresolved early loss of a parent and later childhood traumatic experiences of an unavailable, severely depressed mother with addiction problems, yet on her own, she had been able to cope and take control of her life in a very positive manner, with great accomplishments in academic, work, and social environments. Somehow, her success in keeping negative emotions dissociated to the point of not even recognizing embarrassing or sad situations from her past or current life allowed her to keep those feelings under control. This protected her from reliving the distress and anguish of a painful past. However, this over-control had become "out of control" in relation to her presenting symptom: A daily suppository ritual with its both soothing and disruptive effects that functioned as a way to keep her "messier" emotions in check.

My goal for Porcia's intervention session was to bring into the room and her awareness her concerted effort to banish the negative emotions that life events may have caused her. Through this process, with her considerable strengths, we could create together a new narrative, placing her in a more accurate, compassionate, and active role when unpleasant feelings and difficulties arose.

Tell-Me-A-Story (TEMAS). The Tell-Me-A-Story assessment (TEMAS) is a narrative test that presents a series of ethnically relevant contemporary pictures that embody chromatically attractive, structured stimuli to pull for specific cognitive, emotional, and personality functions. In this case, the TEMAS (Costantino et al., 1993) was selected for several reasons. First, an Argentinian adaptation is available (Costantino et al., 2014; Dupertuis & Pais, in press); the Argentinian adaptation includes some changes to the cards in order to make them more culturally sensitive (e.g., a soccer field instead of a football field) as well as administration and scoring adaptations and different validation studies. Second, it arose from the administered techniques because Porcia presented a level of immaturity in her modulation of emotions related to her second assessment question. The TEMAS (both for the type of contexts it proposes and for the inclusion of color) might help elicit these emotions to a greater extent. On the other hand, the test presents antithetical scenarios (e.g., a child studying or doing their homework to get good grades vs. playing or dancing with siblings and/or friends) in a very explicit manner, which evokes simultaneous positive and negative emotions, one of the test's most important objectives. I hypothesized that Porcia would probably not delve into the most unpleasant part of the antithetical situations. Finally, in the TEMAS card, the bottom of one side of each picture is strongly associated with a playful situation, and from this patient's history we know that she dedicated very little of her childhood to playing due to what she went through in her life. However, these times of playing were very important to her since she cherished some of those early memories.

Porcia was given a card showing a situation that was very simple to resolve: A mother giving a command to her daughter (run errands). A father is in the background. Friends are urging the girl to jump rope with them. Porcia tells a common story that she resolves in a peaceful manner: The child stops playing and obeys her mother in order to be able to do her homework. She recognizes aspects of tension and conflict, but they are shallow and quickly solved by being obedient.

A second card shows a youngster sleeping in bed dreaming of a picnic with a woman. A figure enters through the bedroom window at night. In this case, Porcia has a very long reaction time, 33 seconds, unlike the first card (3 seconds). Then, Porcia narrates the following story: "She went to bed because she was feeling ill and she's dreaming ... [It takes her a long time to continue with the story] It's like she's dreaming in the same situation, and a friend comes to pick her up, and she goes on a picnic with her friend. When she wakes up, she feels fine." She left out the intruding figure altogether.

At this time, I invited her to try to tell an alternative story, which was difficult for her. She began explaining why she came up with the first story, and then she took some more time thinking of an alternative. Then, she stated: "The other option is that she's sleeping and a burglar breaks in.... In that case, the story would not be so good.... Okay, she's dreaming that a burglar broke in or that she went on a picnic with a friend..."

In the face of this situation, as it is usually done in therapeutic assessment, we invite the client to the "observation deck," where they are asked to review their production. When she was faced with this, Porcia said: "I can't believe I didn't recognize this part as someone breaking in to steal—it's so obvious! It's something that really surprises me.... I've thought about it several times. It's like I can't, I can't come up with negative things in my mind.... It's like what we did with the memory test; they were all positive memories. It's really incredible, even I find it incredible that it can't be—I can't stop it, I can't even think." Her stories helped me to deeply understand how far she had to go in order to keep negative emotions out of her experience.

Porcia reported feeling ashamed of what she wasn't able to do. After holding her emotions, we continued investigating, and she was able to share her fear of losing control and of bringing up emotions that she could not face.

We discussed how she had been dealing with very hard situations in her life and the adaptive coping mechanism she was using as I shared with her the meaning of her scores on the personality profile (the MMPI-2) and some of the scores on the Rorschach. After that, I proposed that we look at situations on the TEMAS cards that could help her rework this old narrative of hers based on her fear of losing control and find a way to begin facing negative emotions.

One card shows a girl studying and daydreaming about becoming an actress, a doctor, or conversely, a bag lady; a second card shows a boy and a girl dressed up in grown-up clothes in the attic while looking nostalgically at a crib and some baby toys. With these cards, we could talk together about how she might use her strengths to face the anguish that could arise in these situations. Porcia was able to tell stories that included the negative aspects of the cards and the fears elicited by them ("She's afraid that if she gets in touch with negative emotions she won't succeed, and so she'll become a bag lady").

Using these cards, we worked on creating a new narrative, a story where Porcia allowed the passage of a girl who has gone down a long, sinuous road and yet managed to be successful but at a cost—because she made such an effort to forget her intense losses and difficulties—and has become a young adult who has managed to be successful because she does have skills to begin to face difficult situations, including the negative ones.

At the end of this session, Porcia expressed that she would like to delve into these unpleasant emotions from which she has been running for a long time. Even though she felt she could move forward in that direction on her own, she expressed that she would appreciate having a shoulder nearby to rest on or to cry on in those moments in case she needed to do so. Here, she was able to talk about how much her friends and her husband helped her to feel secure and comfortable, but she also mentioned how hard it was for her to move forward expressing her emotions and how different it was for her when talking to me. After that, we were able to discuss how important it was for her to keep working on this with a therapist who could help her feel secure and comfortable enough to talk about going deeper into this kind of emotions.

Summary and Discussion Sessions

In the summary and discussion sessions, assessors verbally present test results, their case conceptualization, and recommendations to clients and then involve clients in answering their assessment questions developed at the beginning of the assessment. In order to achieve this and to optimize the therapeutic uses of test results, information is discussed initially with level 1 findings, then level 2 findings, and finally level 3 information, moving from the information closest to how the client perceives herself (level 1) to those aspects that are most dissonant with her self-perception (level 3).

During the session with Porcia, she was invited to confirm, modify, or reject possible interpretations of her test scores and give examples of how such findings showed up in her life. Porcia and I each shared how moved we felt with these test results that seemed so close to her life and to her problems in life. She also expressed that she was somewhat impressed by the idea that she was making a huge effort in order to suppress the extremely difficult events in her life but noted that the test had helped her to understand that these were also a significant part of her life as well as showed her resources to move through them. We also worked on building a new narrative that connected her initial assessment question of

"Why do I have this ritual?" with these new findings about her emotional connection. In this sense, we worked on how the way she controlled emotions was similar to controlling her anxiety through the suppository. If she could tolerate some negative emotions it might translate to helping her with her difficult rituals. Some months after the TA, she stopped using the suppository, and she shared that she was very happy to find the way out using her own resources: "I noticed that there was not such a big deal with that; it was just based on how I could manage the anxiety of not using the suppository."

As is generally done in TA, I prepared written feedback in the form of a letter to Porcia answering her assessment questions and test results in language that was comprehensible and accessible to her. The letter summarized the collaborative understandings that had emerged during the process, as well as offered suggestions, for example, to start therapy in order to be able to swim not only on the surface but also to go deeper through those situations that had become difficult for her.

Even though this is a single case, there are some key cultural axes that allow us to think about some of the rationales for the uses of TA in Argentina. Just to emphasize one, Argentinian clients are accustomed to asking questions that, even though they sometimes seem very intellectualized (see the Conclusions section for more on this), need a dynamic and intersubjectivity-based approach. For example, Porcia's assessment question of "Why do I have this ritual?" introduced the background and context of a symptom that allowed me to introduce the TA model as well as a systemic view of the symptom. Also, the use of a stimulus adapted to the Argentinian population is very important since it results in a familiar and culturally relevant situation that evokes the client's dilemma in the relationship with the assessor.

Case of Alba in Mexico: "Why Can't I Get Over It?" (by Daniela)

In Mexico, access to private medical treatment, psychotherapy, and psychological assessment, remains confined to the upper socioeconomic levels. However, educational institutions are able to provide specialized psychological and psychiatric services at low costs. In this context, social public health care covers a low percentage of the mental health demand due to the limitations of the health system in general and the need to improve governmental awareness of mental health needs. However, the collaborative and therapeutic model has been implemented within the public health system, with good acceptance. This has been done as part of an established program of interdisciplinary assessments at the Psychiatry Department of the Universidad Autónoma de Nuevo León in Monterrey, Mexico.

Background and Referral

Alba was a young, single Mexican Latin woman with Spanish ancestry, in her late 20 s, who came to my private practice. Her height was above average, and she had long brown, loose hair that wandered around her face. My attention was drawn to her puzzled gaze. She had an edgy facial bone structure and big eyes that tended to stay fixed and open wide. Despite her sophisticated vocabulary, she had significant difficulty maintaining an orderly discourse. Thus, Alba went from detailed descriptions of episodes of intense anguish in her life to silences and gaps in her narrative. She had a previous history of multiple treatments since her adolescence and reported being diagnosed with anxiety, depression, and attention-deficit disorder. At that time, she manifested depressive symptoms and severe anxiety, which included intrusive images. Sometimes, she visualized her knee being smashed by a hammer; other times, she had the impression that trucks or buses were going to run over her in the street.

We started an assessment while I referred her for consultation with a psychiatry colleague. Meanwhile, she managed to get the authorization of her parents to undertake professional studies in the country's capital. She had long waited for this opportunity to gain independence and put some distance between herself and her family, with whom she had a history of conflict.

She continued pharmacological treatment in the capital, along with psychotherapy. Eventually, she completed professional studies in the field of foreign relations and politics and managed to keep working in her profession for about a year until she was fired. This event was the last in a series of stressful events, including the end of a romantic relationship, all of which made her feel dubious about her ability to be independent. Therefore, at the end of 2019, still in her 20 s, she returned to the north of the country, where she had been raised, and decided to take up counseling with me. I offered her and her family a collaborative assessment. Her parents accepted since they were concerned about their daughter's long evolution of symptoms of anxiety and depression as well as her difficulties in socializing and being autonomous. At that time, Alba's interaction with her family was minimal, and they constantly got into heated discussions about the family's conservative culture. Alba had plans to apply to a foreign master's degree program and decided to stay at her parent's home throughout the process. I thought that it could be useful if her parents started a family assessment with a therapist within my consultation team, and every member of the family agreed to the proposal. The family therapist helped me assess the strengths and vulnerabilities of the family system and was available throughout the evaluation in order to contain Alba's anxious parents.

She also promoted the construction of a shared narrative regarding the feedback sessions.

Alba came from a high socioeconomic stratum and grew up within a conservative family. Her father owned a business, and her mother worked at home. Alba was the youngest of three siblings who were in their 30 s, and, from her perspective, they lived according to the family's expectations. This implied a stereotyped social agenda where being socially active, marrying before their 30 s, and having children are achievements required for having a "normal" life.

Initial Sessions

Alba stated that her problems arose from long periods of punishment imposed by her parents in which she was asked to stay in her room if she questioned any of her family's rules or ideas. She stated that since her puberty, and especially throughout her adolescence, socializing with her peers was almost impossible due to these punishments, and she would spend several days at a time isolated and caught up in reading fantasy novels such as the Harry Potter series. She expressed these events with resentment and a sense of helplessness and blamed herself, wondering why she could not overcome them.

As the main objectives of her assessment, she elaborated on questions about the impact on her life of her childhood experiences. In her words:

> Why can't I get over what happened to me throughout my child-hood? I feel guilty because it was not physical abuse. However, I recall it every single day with a sense of burden, not being able to move forward. How can I feel less guilt and better use my potential for the future, if I have it? How can I explain to others what happened to me?

Nevertheless, she had also a question related to our previous work to-gether: "How can we assess the things that happened to me if I am not even able to talk about them?" Her question was challenging, but I felt reassured considering that the therapeutic and collaborative approach emphasizes maintaining a rhythm of compassion and firmness and pro-motes listening carefully to the person in front of us while searching for positive changes (Finn, 2005, 2007). Also, I managed to explain to her openly how versatile and useful the tests are and how they allow us to approach from different modalities and perspectives what hurts or scares us (Aschieri et al., 2010). Throughout the assessment, I noticed her gra-dual experience of trust since she questioned less often whether I believed what she was saying about her life. The feeling that she was being taken as someone who exaggerated or even lied always haunted her.

Standardized Testing and Extended Inquiry

Based on the chronicity of her symptoms and the face validity of the test regarding her childhood experiences, I decided to use the Minnesota Multiphasic Personality Inventory-2-Restructured Form (MMPI-2-RF, 2008/2011) to assess her symptom experience and to help me get in her shoes by amplifying her self-perception. Also, I selected the Rorschach Inkblot Test administered and scored with the R-PAS Performance Assessment (Meyer et al., 2011), the Dissociative Experiences Scale (DES; Carlson & Putnam, 1993), and the Adult Attachment Projective Picture System (George et al., 1999), in that order, focusing on a relational trauma and attachment perspective. Finally, I used the Tell-Me-A-Story Test (TEMAS); (Constantino et al., 1993) to elicit the potential for change.

We started with the MMPI-2-RF and the DES. Her protocol showed intense discomfort and severe symptoms. Thus, it had elevations in the scale of Infrequency (atypical responding) that in a clinical setting can be related to high distress. Similarly, scores associated with thought alteration, anxiety, depression, and hopelessness were high on the scales of Hopelessness, Dysfunctional Negative Emotions, and Suicide. Her DES also showed a significant level of depersonalization, derealization, and flashbacks.

At this point, I paused to discuss with her some of the findings of both tests as a collaborative resource (Engelman & Allyn, 2012). I was concerned by the intense discomfort she was experiencing and especially about her elevated Suicidality Index. Regarding this, Alba explained she did not consider hurting herself. Instead, she recalled difficulties in staying motivated and focused on school and work. We wondered if her dissociative symptoms worsened her attention deficit. The current hopelessness and lack of meaning in her life were evident, but her attitude remained cooperative and she was interested in gaining understanding.

Subsequently, Alba was enthusiastic about taking the Rorschach Test for a second time. We had used it years earlier on our first contact. I used the R-Pas System and then an extended inquiry. In her protocol, the Ego Interference and Perception and Thought Indexes stood out at the 98th percentile, showing interference in her thought and perception processes as well as the Suicidality Index in the 84th percentile. Thus, her performance was consistent with the MMPI-2-RF personality profile.

Alba's protocol made me think of profiles common in patients with trauma and vulnerability to mood dysregulation (Viglione et al., 2012). When taking the Rorschach, she had intense emotional reactions. Her R-PAS Critical Content Index, often used as a measure of traumatic content, fell into the 97th percentile. Throughout all her sessions, we had a difficult time staying focused. Several stimuli triggered memories from the past, and she got caught in emotional downward spirals which required pausing and containment. Accordingly, her answers to the Rorschach were complex and diverse; it was no surprise that Harry Potter was among them. On the other hand, a lot of her responses managed to convey her experience of anguish and long journey of traumatic experiences. As an example, this is her response to Card IV:

> I think this was the original Rorschach monster response [smiling]. A giant monster with super heavy strides and stomping and spitting lava. Is it wrong what I'm saying?... These are his feet, they are gigantic, you are looking at them too close or he is deformed.... The fire in the closest part looks more intense.

In the extended inquiry, she added: "I could associate the monster with my parents, feeling overpowered by this thing... for example, in discussions with them."

When working with the Adult Attachment Projective Picture System, a developmental measure of adult attachment that identifies attachment-related content (e.g., agency, connectedness to others in relationships), defensive processing, and attachment trauma, responses such as the following to the Bench Card (a sketch of a child alone on a bench with her head on her knees) told of haunting experiences from Alba's past that were still present:

> I imagine the bricks or so … I imagine like a rare medieval dungeon, it may have a window of this size where you cannot see a lot, and it is at night. I don't know, I feel how easy I could be this person.... Not because she did something wrong but because … for the same reason, because they can't understand her. They punished her and sent her to the dungeon and she felt helpless. What happens after … Well, what happens after, well, nothing … I mean no … Like, there is no end to this. You just have to deal with it, and this is going to happen again … and you have to learn to deal with it or how to moderate your actions to avoid this as much as possible.

In the extended inquiry, Alba remembered a past where her "truth" was never admitted, like the time when her mother accused her of mocking her while they were at a beauty salon. Alba tried to clarify that she was not laughing at her mother. However, her mother left her at the salon and threatened to ground her a couple of hours before her high school prom. The above projective story and the memory of her mother showed the sense of helplessness and paralysis in her life that, in conjunction with her attachment fraught with confusion and restriction, implied her need to find new strategies to move forward in her life.

At this moment, she shared how, in recent years, she had joined a social network group with a trauma agenda. Also, she recalled concepts she reviewed at graduate school, such as an undermined sense of agency. We were able to talk about the impotence and confusion that comes along with experiences of invalidation. She felt satisfied with her being able to reach out to this group on her own and having the opportunity to collaborate in the assessment with input from her professional knowledge.

So far, her testing results made me think of a pattern of dysregulation and avoidance common in complex trauma (Armstrong, 2012; Tarocchi et al., 2013). At times, Alba had emotional, anxious, and rage-filled crises, especially while arguing with her parents. The rest of the time, she manifested avoidance and dissociated and put her life on standby, a strategy that helped her while she was isolated and grounded. It was of great help to me to have a parental interview in which I focused on Alba's development. To my surprise, her parents were able to describe how Alba had been a very complex and sensitive infant, with a long history of difficulty sleeping. They recalled her inquisitiveness and intolerance of several stimuli, such as particular types of visual images. Her discomfort seemed funny to the family and was made the occasion for siblings' teasing and shaming her by exposing her to these kinds of pictures. Also, they reported remembering little about her being grounded and punished and had a hard time trying to understand why they were so significant to Alba.

Alba was worried about what her parents had said about her. However, she felt reassured by my efforts to integrate both perspectives and was satisfied with her parents' participation. I was committed to preserving the assessment as a safe place, and she managed to collaborate and stay curious about her inner life, sometimes even with a playful approach (Handler, 1999, 2008). As a relevant sequence in her Rorschach, I noted the symbolism in Cards V and VI:

Card V. R12, W: Like a worm, a snail.

Card VI, R13, D1: Like a spaceship that is taking off, but kind of NASA.... The thrusters pushing each other with all this fire! It seems like lava with different intensities of heat or temperature.

Card VI, R14, D3: A Star of David, but half, not as it should be: half deformed.

When I asked her to elaborate on these responses Alba was very interested. In the extended inquiry, we discussed whether there could be a symbolic element of the slow pace in her snail-like response. I shared with her how she transmitted a feeling of spending a huge amount of time and effort trying to process and contain the cognitive and affective elements of her everyday experience mixed with her memories of the past. At the time of the assessment, Alba had been unemployed for almost a year and had spent several days without stepping out of her room, just sleeping or watching TV. Thus, she dreaded the consequences of trying to move forward. At the end of this inquiry, she added: "In my life, plans are convictions, you have to defend them to death from family scrutiny, but then there is no way you can change them." The possibility of planning and talking with her family about job options or academic programs paralyzed her.

Around her spaceship response, she commented:

> An astronaut goes to space and defies gravity and the absolute universal truth.... It requires a lot of courage to get out into space. It is difficult even for those with training; six humans in a small room can get violent.... It implies a huge sacrifice and a lot of fear. It is more probable that everything goes wrong. You need discipline, dedication, passion, and love of what you are doing.

Her elaboration was revealing. Her early experiences implied a world full of absolute truths, without a space for intersubjectivity. Defying this world was terrifying, almost a life-or-death task, even if you had some treatment or training. I asked her what could be her outer space. She replied: "I think politics, philosophy, and cooking, but everything is kind of paused right now." Also, by that time the family was considering applying for Spanish or Portuguese citizenship through Spanish and Jewish ancestry connections. Alba wondered whether the Star of David related to nationality issues and the possibility of accessing European academic programs.

At this time, we had discussed some aspects of complex trauma since Alba was familiar with a trauma perspective. It made sense to both of us how her past experiences and current manifestations interfered with her cognition and sense of agency. We were able to go through her Rorschach scores and think about examples where her perception was interfered with. We associated these manifestations mainly with a hyper-alert stance as a common response to trauma. Patients with a traumatic background benefit from this thorough process of recognition and validation. Only after this was Alba able to look at her parents from a different perspective. Accordingly, she identified possible traumatic experiences in their early development, such as a harsh and rigid family context. This made it a little easier for her to empathize with them. However, she seemed stuck in the past and very ambivalent about moving forward. I thought about using Constantino's TEMAS cards, as they emphasize decision making, in order to explore her dilemmas regarding change.

Intervention

This session was quite complicated because Alba's life narratives were so intertwined with traumatic content. Nevertheless, we were able to work with a card that shows a girl with outstretched arms standing at the junction of two roads in a forest with friends calling to her to join them for a walk on the right-hand road. She stated:

> It is within the path that my parents want, the known path and [this is] the one that I want, which looks quite lonely. But I know that at least in this one [she points to the independent path] there may be a chance of happiness if I do it right. Sometimes I laugh, I think, what if I don't handle it well, I lose my judgment, I forget what I have relied on, I forget everything. And I am nowhere. And I am in a pit. Because it has happened to me. That which lightened my load I forget, and I come to think that I will never understand. I forgot the part that clicked with me, and another thing that helped me feel better, and I forgot what it was.

I worked on containing her affect, which was complicated since she expressed a sense of hopelessness. Finally, she added that even though she was trying to do her best, meditating and practicing yoga, she wondered what was still blocking her.

Feedback

In her feedback session, she kept asking if there would be a time when she might be able to find a meaning and purpose in what had happened to her. It was important for me to help her integrate different factors around her trauma. We talked especially about her intellectual capacity, which was evident in her professional knowledge. We also spoke of her sensitivity, which made her very aware of her environment despite her parents' policy of no questions being allowed at home. I reassured her that her knowledge of psychological and social concepts was a remarkable strength for overcoming trauma. She also was able to state that there had been no way that she could have controlled what had happened to her and to acknowledge the impact of her childhood experience. We reflected upon her long history of treatments that apparently never included a trauma and systemic perspective. However, she felt very ashamed and resentful of not being able to accomplish more and of all the time she thought she had lost.

At the same time, I had a feedback session with her parents in conjunction with the family therapist. I reviewed with Alba the information I would use in a presentation to her parents. With her permission, I showed the parents some of Alba's answers that conveyed her experience of trauma, among them the narratives from the Attachment Projective Picture System, such as the one of the girl in the Bench Card being punished and helpless in a medieval dungeon. It was important for us to help the parents understand her perspective as well as to keep their perspective in mind. The parents had several doubts around complex trauma, so we emphasized the emotional impact of the sense of relational disconnection, conflictual interactions without the ability to repair her relationships, and how this affected Alba's trusting within her attachment system. They came closer to empathizing with her perspective. Alba accepted a second opinion about her psychiatry practitioner and stayed in twice-weekly therapy with me. Her parents accepted further family sessions.

Update

Alba started the assessment with a psychiatric consultation from my professional team. Her anxiety and dissociation improved significantly, to the point that, together, we were able to discriminate between dissociative manifestations and the possibility of epileptic seizures. Eventually, she was diagnosed with complex partial left lobe epilepsy and also received treatment from a neurologist. I was able to supervise her case in a Collaborative/ Therapeutic Assessment supervision group for Latinoamérica coordinated by Dr. Filippo Aschieri and my coauthor Ernesto Pais. They helped me identify the importance of dissociation as a manifestation of Alba's conflict around or reluctance to leave the past behind because of the risk of having to invalidate it. This was obviously related to her dilemma regarding change and the complex dynamics within her question of "Why can't I get over what happened to me?"

Nowadays, Alba has been more open to social interactions and expresses the joy of spending time with friends and her nephews. She planned and was able to move to Mexico's capital city. The family therapist helped contain her parents' anxiety and their fantasy that Alba might even get involved in illicit ways of earning money. At Mexico City, she has been able to reconnect with her mentor and professional activities. She updated her resume and has had three important job interviews in her professional field. However, it has been difficult for her to pursue a job during the COVID-19 pandemic, which worries her, while she waits for a job offer that will meet her financial needs. Her relationship with her parents is still stressful, as were the few family sessions held throughout the previous year. However, she feels less guilty about taking her own path. After 4 months in Mexico City, she was able to ask her mom to spend a weekend with her. She was upset because her father joined them for a couple of days of what she had thought was going to be a girls' experience. However, they were able to spend a lot of time together without arguing, and Alba said she couldn't remember a previous time when she missed being close to her mother, as she had recently. Alba had proposed a path with her parents and their control, but it was a lonely path. Nowadays, it occurs to me the possibility of a third path, one where she feels sufficiently independent and still connected with them.

Alba's assessment is an example of the benefits of Collaborative/ Therapeutic Assessment procedures such as extended inquiries, family interventions for young adults, using the testing as empathy magnifiers, and using the assessment to impact a family system positively (Finn, 2007; Tharinger et al., 2008).

Conclusions

Although there is much evidence regarding the effectiveness of Therapeutic Assessment around the world, so far, we are not aware of studies of this approach in Latinoamérica. In this chapter, we have intended to show how the collaborative model and Finn's therapeutic assessment model can be carried out in diverse cultures through sharing cases in Argentina and Mexico. Likewise, we include the use of standardized tests in our contexts, particularly the use of the multicultural technique TEMAS.

We believe that in this chapter we have managed to explain how the Collaborative/ Therapeutic Assessment model enhances the work with complex clients who have had traumatic experiences. In this sense, the use of techniques within a collaborative context as empathy magnifiers allowed us, as clinicians, to understand our clients' problems in life and their dilemmas related to change in a much more precise and compassionate way.

Each cultural context has its own specific requirements. In this sense, Ernesto has found on many occasions that, perhaps due to the culture in Buenos Aires where there is a high proportion of people in therapy or who have previously been in therapy as well as a widespread understanding of Freud's theory, clients usually give somewhat intellectualized responses to assessment questions, stripped of connection with emotions, related to some extent to what Fonagy and Target (1996) called a pretend mode mental state. Questions like "Why?" are very common in Argentina, and Ernesto usually intervenes to build questions that are more change-oriented and include emotional states, such as "How is it to ..." or "How can I do ..."

In Daniela's Mexican context, the adaptation of the model to an academic and institutional setting has proven the viability of working collaboratively in a psychiatry department, where master's program students train in psychotherapy and psychological assessment. Recently, we have implemented with good results at least one summary and discussion session with a client in which the student's supervisor participates if the client thinks they might benefit.

Also, both authors have shared their experience of emphasizing family participation in the assessment of young adults, in a similar way to conducting TA with adolescents. This can be done with the client's consent as a way to work on a systemic path in the healing process.

As stated before, TA is itself culturally responsive. This model, combined with culturally sensitive therapists who communicate with clients in their native language and use standardized tests in their countries, allows the therapists to get into clients' shoes and collaborate with them to build a more coherent, compassionate view of themselves.

Finally, we know that much work still needs to be done in relation to therapeutic assessment in Latinoamérica and in other Spanish-speaking countries, but we believe that the results achieved with our clients, exemplified by these two cases, are promising in relation to the challenges of therapeutic assessment in our region.

Note

1 I contacted Porcia's medical doctor, who shared that physical causes had been ruled out and that Porcia's symptoms were related to her emotional life.

References

Alarcón, R. (2010). El legado psicológico de Rogelio Díaz-Guerrero [The psychological legacy of Rogelio Diaz-Guerrero]. *Estudos e Pesquisas em Psicologia*, *10*(2), 553–571. Recuperado em 08 de feveiro de 2021, de. http://pepsic.bvsalud.org/scielo.php?script=sci_arttext&pid=S1808-42812010000200016&lng=pt&tlng=es

Armstrong, J. (2012). Therapeutic assessment of a dissociating client: Learning internal navigation. In S. E. Finn, C. T. Fischer, & L. Handler, L. (Eds.), *Collaborative/therapeutic assessment: A casebook and guide* (pp. 27–46). John Wiley & Sons.

Aschieri, F., Finn, S. E., & Bevilacqua, P. (2010). Therapeutic assessment and epistemological triangulation. In V. Cigoli & M. Gennari (Eds.), *Close relationships and community psychology: An international perspective* (pp. 241–253). Milan: Franco Angeli.

Bateman, A., & Fonagy, P. (2013). Mentalization-based treatment. *Psychoanalytic Inquiry*, *33*(6), 595–613.

Ben-Porath, Y. S., & Tellegen, A. (2008/2011). *Minnesota Multiphasic Personality Inventory-2- Restructured Form (MMPI-2-RF): Manual for administration, scoring, and interpretation*. University of Minnesota Press.

Bruhn, A. R. (1992). The early memories procedure: A projective test of autobiographical memory, part 1. *Journal of Personality Assessment*, *58*(1), 1–15.

Butcher, J. N., Dahlstrom, W. G., Graham, J. R., Tellegen, A., & Kaemmer, B. (1989). *Minnesota Multiphasic Personality Inventory-2 (MMPI-2): Manual for administration and scoring.* University of Minnesota Press.

Caldwell, A. M. (2001). What do the MMPI scales fundamentally measure? Some hypotheses. *Journal of Personality Assessment, 76,* 1–17.

Carlson, E. B., & Putnam, F. W. (1993). An update on the Dissociative Experiences Scale. *Dissociation: Progress in the Dissociative Disorders, 6*(1), 16–27.

Castañeda, D. (2020, July 30). *La Riqueza en México y su Medición [Wealth in Mexico and its Measurement].* Economía y Sociedad. https://economia.nexos.com.mx/?p=3213

Celener de Nijamkin, G., & Guinzbourg de Braude, M. (2000). El Cuestionario desiderativo. (The Wishful Questionnaire). Editorial Lugar.

Costantino, G., Litman, L., Waxman, R., Dupertuis, D., Pais, E., Rosenzweig, C., Forti, G., Paronik, J. & Canales, M. M. (2014). Tell-Me-A-Story (TEMAS) assessment for culturally diverse children and adolescents. *Rorschachiana, 35*(2), 154.

Costantino, G., Malgady, R., & Rogler, L. (1993). Tell-Me-A-Story (TEMAS). Western Psychological Services.

Didou Aupetit, S., & Jokivirta, L. (2015). Higher education crossing borders in Latin America and the Caribbean. *International Higher Education, 49,* 17–18. https://doi.org/10.6017/ihe.2007.49.7979

Dupertuis, D. P., & Pais, E. F. (in press). El Test TEMAS (Tell-Me-A-Story). *Evaluación Clínica en Sociedades Multiculturales [Clinical Evalution in Multicultural Societies].*

Engelman, D. H., & Allyn, J. B. (2012). Collaboration in neuropsychological assessment: Metaphor and intervention with a suicidal adult. In S. E. Finn, C. T. Fischer, & L. Handler (Eds.), *Collaborative/therapeutic assessment: A casebook and guide* (pp. 1–24). John Wiley & Sons.

Escobar, R. (2016). El primer laboratorio de psicología experimental en México [The instruments in the first psychological laboratory in Mexico]. *Revista Mexicana de Análisis de la Conducta, 42*(2), 116–144.

Escobedo, D. (2018). Peter, an adolescent who didn't want to grow or grow up. *The TA Connection: Resources for Therapeutic Assessment Professionals, 6*(2), 9–15.

Espinoza-Reyes, M. D. C. (2020). The use of collaborative/therapeutic assessment with oppositional defiant disorder: A longitudinal case study. *Rorschachiana, 41*(2), 200–222.

Fierro, C., & Araujo, S. D. F. (2021). Psychology qua psychoanalysis in Argentina: Some historical origins of a philosophical problem (1942–1964). *Journal of the History of the Behavioral Sciences, 57*(2), 149–171. https://doi.org/10.1002/jhbs.22070

Finn, S. E. (2005). How psychological assessment taught me compassion and firmness. *Journal of Personality Assessment, 84*(1), 29–32.

Finn, S. E. (2007). *In our clients' shoes: Theory and techniques of therapeutic assessment.* Lawrence Erlbaum Associates.

Finn, S. E., & Tonsager, M. E. (1997). Information-gathering and therapeutic models of assessment: Complementary paradigms. *Psychological Assessment*, *9*(4), 374.

Fonagy, P., & Target, M. (1996). Playing with reality: I. Theory of mind and the normal development of psychic reality. *The International Journal of Psychoanalysis*, *77*(2), 217–233.

Frank de Verthelyi, R. (1999). *Temas en evaluación psicológica [Subjects in psychological evauation]*. Lugar Editorial.

Galindo, E. (2004). Análisis del desarrollo de la psicología en México hasta 1990: Con una bibliografía in extenso [Analysis of the development of psychology in Mexico until 1990: With an extensive bibliography]. *Psicologia para América Latina*, *2*. http://pepsic.bvsalud.org/scielo.php?script=sci_arttext&pid=S1870-350X2004000200004&lng=pt&tlng=es

George, C., West, M., & Pettem, O. (1999). The Adult Attachment Projective: Disorganization of adult attachment at the level of representation. In J. Solomon & C. George (Eds.), *Attachment disorganization* (pp. 462–507). Guilford.

Handler, L. (1999). Assessment of playfulness: Hermann Rorschach meets D. W. Winnicott. *Journal of Personality Assessment*, *72*(2), 208–217.

Handler, L. (2008). A Rorschach journey with Bruno Klopfer: Clinical application and teaching. *Journal of Personality Assessment*, *90*(6), 528–535. 10.1080/00223890802388301

INDEC. (2010). Censo Poblacional Nacional 2010 [National population census 2010]. Instituto Nacional de Estadística y Censos. http://www.indec.gov.ar

INDEC. (2020). *Encuesta permanente de hogares [Permanent household survey]*. Ministerio de Economía de la República Argentina.

INEGI. (2020). *Censo de Población y Vivienda 2020 [Census of population and housing]*. Instituto Nacional de Estadística, Geografía e Informatica. https://www.inegi.org.mx/programas/ccpv/2020/#Documentacion

Klappenbach, H. (2007). Professional psychologist degree in Argentina: From the beginnings to nowadays. In A. Columbus (Ed.), *Advances in psychology research* (Vol. 38, pp. 1–32). Nova Science Publishers.

Klappenbach, H. A., & Pavesi, P. (1994). Una historia de la psicología en Latinoamérica [A history of psychology in Latinoamérica]. *Revista Latinoamericana de Psicología*, *26*(3), 445–481. https://www.redalyc.org/articulo.oa?id=805/80526305

Lunazzi, H. (2018). *La evaluación terapéutica y la clínica de la pantalla: Relectura del psicodiagnóstico [Therapeutic assessment and the screen clinic. Re-reading the psychodiagnosis]*. Lugar Editorial.

Meyer, G. J., Viglione, D. J., Mihura, J. L., Erard, R. E., & Erdberg, P. (2011). Rorschach Performance Assessment System: Administration, coding, interpretation, and technical manual. Rorschach Performance Assessment System.

Moreno-Estrada, A., Gignoux, C. R., Fernández-López, J. C., Zakharia, F., Sikora, M., Contreras, A. V., Acuña-Alonzo, V., Sandoval, K., Eng, C., Romero-Hidalgo, S., Ortiz-Tello, P., Robles, V., Kenny, E. E., Nuño-Arana, I., Barquera-Lozano, R., Macín-Pérez, G., Granados-Arriola, J.,

Huntsman, S., Galanter, J. M., Via, M., ... & Bustamante, C. D. (2014). Human genetics: The genetics of Mexico recapitulates Native American substructure and affects biomedical traits. *Science, 344*(6189), 1280–1285. https://doi.org/10.1126/science.1251688

Pais, E. F. (2019). TEMAS as therapeutic intervention with adolescents and adults. In Y. P. Zinchenko (Ed.), *XVI European Congress of Psychology: TEMAS (TELL-ME-A-STORY), a multicultural test and treatment modality for the 21st century* (pp. 426–428). European Congress of Psychology.

Passalacqua, A. M., & de Colombo, M. A. (2000). *El psicodiagnóstico de Rorschach: Sistematización y nuevos aportes [Rorshcach's diagnostic: Systematiztion and new contributions].* Ediciones Klex.

Ponza, P. (2011, March 31). Psicoanálisis, política y cultura en la Argentina de los sesenta[Psychoanalysis, politics and culture in Argentina of the sixties. *Nuevo Mundo Mundos Nuevos.* https://doi.org/10.4000/nuevomundo.61036

Samper-García, P., Mesurado, B., Richaud, M. C., & Llorca, A. (2016). Validación del cuestionario de conciencia emocional en adolescentes españoles [Validation of the emotional awareness questionnaire in Spanish adolescents]. *Interdisciplinaria, 33*(1), 163–176.

Sánchez-Meca, J., López-Pina, J. A., López-López, J. A., Marín-Martínez, F., Rosa-Alcázar, A. I., & Gómez-Conesa, A. (2011).The Maudsley Obsessive-Compulsive Inventory: A reliability generalization meta-analysis. *International Journal of Clinical and Health Psychology, 11*(3), 473–493.

Sanz, I. A. E., & Pais, E. F. (2013). Organización multi-nivel de resultados en psicodiagnóstico. Pautas para aplicación en técnicas de auto-atribución y de atribución al estímulo [Multi-level organization of results in psychodiagnosis. Guidelines for application in techniques of self-attribution and of attribution to the stimulus]. In E. Benito (Ed.), *1° Congreso Latinoamericano para el Avance de la Ciencia Psicológica, La evaluación y diagnóstico psicológico en contexto: investigación y práctica.* Asociación para el Avance de la Ciencia Psicológica.

Silin, P., & Sanz, I. A. E. (2019). *Evaluación de la personalidad e interpretaciones clínicas con el MMPI-2 [Evaluation of the personalized clinical interpretation with the MMPI-2]* Pedro Silin.

Smith, J. D. (2016). Introduction to the special section on cultural considerations in collaborative and therapeutic assessment. *Journal of Personality Assessment, 98*(6), 563–566. 10.1080/00223891.2016.119645

Tarocchi, A., Aschieri, F., Fantini, F., & Smith, J. D. (2013). Therapeutic assessment of complex trauma: A single-case time-series study. *Clinical Case Studies, 12*(3), 228–245. https://doi.org/10.1177/1534650113479442

Sneiderman, S. B. (2014). *El Cuestionario Desiderativo. Aportes para una actualización de la interpretación [The Desiderative questionnaire. Contributions for an interpretive update].* Editorial Paidós.

Tharinger, D. J., Finn, S. E., Austin, C. A., Gentry, L. B., Bailey, K. E., Parton, V. T., & Fisher, M. E. (2008). Family sessions as part of child psychological assessment: Goals, techniques, clinical utility, and therapeutic value. *Journal of*

Personality Assessment, 90(6), 547–558. https://doi.org/10.1080/002238908023 88400

Viglione, D. J., Towns, B., & Lindshield, D. (2012). Understanding and using the Rorschach Inkblot Test to assess post-traumatic conditions. *Psychological Injury and Law, 5*(2), 135–144. https://doi.org/10.1007/s12207-012-9128-5

World Health Organization. (2014). *Mental Health Atlas*. WHO.

Chapter 6

Culture and Psychological Assessment in India

Kakli Gupta

Historical View of Indian Mental Health

The mental health profession, in the scientifically advanced form that it currently exists in the Western world, is only about four to five decades old in India. While the first psychiatric hospital was set up as early as 1745 in Bombay (now Mumbai), most centers in India from 1745 to 1912 functioned more as "lunatic asylums" (Nizamie & Goyal, 2010). In 1912, in colonial India, one of the first treatment centers (Central Institute of Psychiatry; CIP) was set up at Ranchi, Bihar. The first psychiatric out-patient service was set up in Calcutta (now Kolkata) in 1933 at Carmichael Medical College. After India gained independence in 1947, the number of psychiatric hospitals in India surged. The range of services offered started increasing and included child and adolescent clinics and neuropsychiatric services. The first clinical psychology laboratory in the country was set up in 1949 at CIP, Ranchi. In 1954, the Department of Psychology and Human Relations was created through the All Indian Institute of Mental Health (presently the National Institute of Mental Health and Neurological Sciences, or NIMHANS) in Bangalore (Nizamie & Goyal, 2010). In the late 1950s and early 1960s, many other hospitals with outpatient mental health services were set up in big cities such as Delhi and smaller cities such as Lucknow, Amritsar, Rohtak, and Chandigarh.

However, one of the most impactful impetuses to the evolution of the mental health profession in India came in August 1982 when the National Mental Health Programme (NMHP) was adopted by the Government of India. This programme was formulated to offer mental health services in the country to ensure availability and accessibility of minimum mental health care for all, to encourage the application of mental health knowledge in general health care, to promote community participation in the mental health services development, and to stimulate efforts towards self-help in the community. While focusing on these goals, there has been a gradual shift from mental illness to mental health, recognizing the

DOI: 10.4324/9781003124061-9

preventive aspects of mental and neurological disorders. (Prasadarao & Sudhir, 2001, p. 36)

Since then, many programmes and policies have been put in place by the government to address mental health care in India. The last 20 years have seen a significant evolution in the quality, variety, and availability of mental health services in the nation. In a parallel way, the need for mental health services has increased exponentially in the country. A comprehensive study done on the prevalence of mental health issues in India in 2019 revealed that "in 2017, one among every seven people in India had a mental disorder, ranging from mild to severe. The proportional contribution of mental disorders to the total disease burden in India almost doubled from 1990 to 2017" (World Health Organization, 2019, p. 157).

The challenges of the stigma around seeking mental health services (Gaiha et al., 2020), lack of mental health awareness, and tendency to rely more on families than trained professionals for emotional support continue to deter a large percentage of the population from seeking mental health services. And while the last two decades have seen some reduction in this stigma, at least in the urban population, there are not enough mental health professionals to meet the need.

According to the World Mental Health Atlas (2019), there were 0.3 psychiatrists per lakh [3 psychiatrists per 1 million] of population in India. Psychologists and psychiatric social workers were even fewer. The median number of psychiatrists in India is only 0.2/100,000 population compared to a global median of 3 per 100,000 population. Similarly, the figures for psychologists, social workers, and nurses working for mental health are 0.03, 0.03, and 0.05/100,000 population.... We currently have 9000 psychiatrists, 2000 psychiatric nurses, 1000 clinical psychologists, and 1000 psychiatric social workers. We would need an additional 30,000 psychiatrists, 37,000 psychiatric nurses, 38,000 psychiatric social workers, and 38,000 clinical psychologists. As per the calculations, it will take 42 years to meet the requirement for psychiatrists, 74 years for psychiatric nurses, 76 years for the psychiatric social workers, and 76 years for clinical psychologists, for providing care for 130 crore [1.3 billion] population, provided the population (assuming both general population and mental health human resources) remains constant. (Bada Math et al., 2019, pp. S652–S653)

Thus, India is at an interesting juncture—on the one hand there has been a huge expansion with more well-trained professionals available, many more training programs, and many more clients reaching out to professionals proactively. On the other hand, we still need much more. Even with only a minority of the population reaching out for help, we struggle with a shortage of quality professionals.

My Journey to Becoming a Psychologist

Beginnings in India

Twenty-five years ago, when I chose to study psychology, I was completely oblivious of the above reality of the state of mental health in India. Growing up in a nuclear family in India but staying in close proximity to my extended family (grandparents, cousins, uncles, and aunts) had shown me different flavors of human relationships—affection, bonding, politics, hurt, competition, envy, support, love, pain, and complexity! I was impacted by all of it, in healthy and unhealthy ways, and it somehow led me to want to become a mental health professional.

My parents were understandably anxious about my decision—25 years ago, a bright young woman wanting to become a clinical psychologist was not exactly a reason for pride in Indian families. Not only did the profession not seem lucrative there was also a worry—"What if working with mentally unwell people makes our daughter mentally unwell?" Things are different now. Psychology is in high demand in India, and it is quite competitive to get into reputable colleges offering psychology. But back then, it wasn't as challenging. I got into one of India's most reputable colleges for psychology and started my education in 1996.

When I imagined what I would do as a clinical psychologist, I imagined myself as a therapist—talking to people and helping them feel better. I didn't know much about psychological assessments. We had a basic introduction to "psychological testing" during our undergraduate training, but it seemed more of a "fun" thing to do with people rather than a "credible" way of getting to know about their psyche.

During my master's program in clinical psychology, I received a strong theoretical exposure to different schools of psychology—psychoanalysis, cognitive behaviour therapy, social psychology, etc. Psychological assessments were also introduced, but the training and material used were far from adequate. For instance, the Rorschach Inkblot Test was taught in a vague manner; we learnt some versions of the psychoanalytically oriented Klopfer system, but it was not systematic. During our internship at a hospital, psychological tests were sometimes requested by the psychiatrists, but the prescription usually mentioned one particular test, such as "TAT" or "Rorschach." We didn't use a "battery" of tests. "Patients" were not always given feedback about the "test results." The psychiatric consultants sometimes used these to diagnose the patients. I didn't feel experienced in interpreting the data, nor did I have any close assessment supervision. Consequently, psychological "testing" was something toward which I developed a "nonenthusiastic" attitude. I didn't learn what it could do, it didn't feel credible enough, the test material felt obsolete, and I did not feel adequately trained for it.

Doctoral Training in the United States

My feelings about psychological assessment did not change until my second year of the PsyD program at a professional college in the US. For the first time, I saw test material that was well organized and up-to-date and had a clear method and rationale. "Cognitive assessments" and "personality assessments" were taught separately over a period of 2 years. We spent months learning how to interpret Thematic Apperception Test (TAT; Murray, 1943) stories, how to administer the Rorschach using the Exner Comprehensive System (Exner & Weiner, 1995) using standardized norms, and, eventually, how to use data from a variety of tests and put it all together to help understand an individual. It all made more sense, and I started to see how it could help the real lives of real people.

While these 2 years had definitely helped me feel differently about psychological assessments, it was only during my third year of the doctoral program that I learned about the process of Therapeutic Assessment enabling me to broaden my view of psychological assessments. At WestCoast Children's Clinic in the San Francisco Bay Area, I saw how 8-year-old kids were given feedback from the psychological assessment process. They could take something from their own assessment that was not just for their caregivers or social workers. My trainers, in contrast to my master's program assessment teachers, were excited about assessments, and their enthusiasm was infectious. How could someone love assessments so much? I understood that once I did a few of them myself. For the first time, I wrote stories for children addressing their own questions from the assessment, and even though not every child would respond verbally to the feedback, seeing how they felt understood by the story (A rabbit named "Hoppy" whose mother got sick) or how it made them feel "seen" and how it "touched" them was heart-warming.

One of my favorite moments was getting a warm smile from an African-American adolescent who was very disengaged throughout the assessment process. The assessment showed that not only did he have a lot of psychological trauma, he could also hardly read or write due to severe learning difficulties and several gaps in his education. He would often listen to music on his CD player during our breaks. At the beginning of the assessment, I asked him what he wanted to know from this assessment. He asked, "How does the mind work?," which I thought was his way of asking, "How does my mind work?" Given his difficulty with reading and his interest in music, I thought his question was best answered in the form of a song, which I wrote and sang for him. He was surprised that what he perceived as a "boring assessment process" could culminate in a song about his life.

The Therapeutic Assessment approach made it possible for me to integrate assessments meaningfully with the therapeutic process. It no longer felt like I had to wear two different hats as a psychologist. It was also a time of personal growth for me—psychology and creativity came together in an attempt to make a difference in the lives of my child and adolescent clients.

Return to India

While I was in the thick of this learning process, a medical emergency at home required me to move back to India. I had grown up in Delhi, one of the biggest cities in India, but now I was moving to Chandigarh, a smaller city about a 4-hour drive from Delhi. Chandigarh is one of the first planned cities in India and boasts of its beautiful architecture and well-organized infrastructure. People mostly speak Punjabi, Hindi, and English. There is a large population of Sikhs in the city.

I had no idea how willing and open people in this city would be to come to a psychologist. While bigger cities in India were beginning to open up to the idea of visiting a psychotherapist, there was still a lot of stigma attached to "needing an outside person" in smaller cities and towns in India.

> **What will people say?** In India, this singular age-old social precept is relevant for everyone. It cuts across the lines of gender, caste, religion, socio-economic class, and region. It reigns supreme in regulating people's decisions, because should people's vulnerabilities become public knowledge, they will invite judgement, gossip and drama. It also suppresses much-needed psychological care.... The social pressure to be "normal" manifests in unhealthy stigma and pressure against getting help. Stigma to appear normal. Stigma to keep the family drama invisible. Stigma to protect the family honor. Stigma to force yourself out of the need for help.
>
> (Taniparti, 2018)

I was skeptical that my clinical training would be utilized in this small city in India, but a big part of me was also looking forward to offering something back to my own people. While training in the United States, I had felt privileged. I dreamt of coming back and sharing my services in my own country and training more people so we could have a bigger community of well-trained clinical psychologists. The timing of my return to India felt premature and driven by external circumstances, but I felt a step closer to my dream.

At first, I explored the option of joining some hospitals or practices of local psychiatrists/psychologists in the city. But, I was disappointed to see that psychological services were offered very differently from the psychodynamic, client-centered, and relational training I had received. The medical model dominated. Patients waited to see psychiatrists and psychotherapists (sometimes for hours), and the session duration was not standardized. The prevalent approach seemed largely cognitive behavioural.

While in the United States, I still saw myself as a fresh graduate, but in India, I had to step up and set up my own practice. That seemed like the only way in which I could work more professionally and relationally. Because I specialized in working with children, adolescents, and families, it seemed appropriate to approach the local pediatricians to let them know about the services I could offer. Most of them were happy to hear about what I did as they felt that a lot of kids they saw for "health concerns" had underlying psychological struggles.

> In India, mental health and seeking help remain shrouded in shame. One of the most acceptable forms of expression of suffering is through the medium of the body. The hospitals here are full of people walking in with unexplainable symptoms and diseases. Research on the psychosomatic disorders, where thinking and feeling are evacuated into the body, is bare. Psychosomatic disorders are the most radical and extreme form of psychic reduction that not only affects the emotional well-being of the individual but his physical well-being as well.
>
> (Agarwal, 2018, p. 53)

Within a month, I started getting referrals. Parents would typically call for concerns about enuresis, school refusal, behavioral problems at school, lack of interest in studies, sexually inappropriate behaviours, and sometimes more directly for symptoms of depression or anxiety.

Tests and Costs in India

While setting up my practice, I also thought of establishing a library of psychological tests. I definitely wanted to put my Therapeutic Assessment skills and knowledge to good use. But I didn't realize what this would mean financially until I visited one of the few stores in Old Delhi where test materials were sold. The catalogue had a list of tests made in India or adapted in India and tests that were imported from the United States or the United Kingdom. The Indian tests were quite affordable. The imported ones were not, definitely not for a new practitioner like me, but they seemed exorbitantly priced even for the more experienced version I imagined myself to be in 5–6 more years. I realized that even if I invested in the material by taking out a loan, it would take me years to recover this investment given that the fee for assessments in India would work out to be much lower.

For instance, in 2006 the WISC-IV (Wechsler, 2004) in India cost 55,000 INR (approximately 1,250 USD) and the Minnesota Multiphasic Personality Inventory (MMPI) (Butcher et al., 1993) cost 42,000 INR (950 USD), while an hour of therapy in 2006 in the city I lived in cost around 300 INR (6 USD). Even now, the average fee charged by seasoned therapists in India for one session is 30–35 USD per session. Potential clients would have to be told why their child or adolescent could benefit from the assessment, and they would definitely not be willing to pay anything more than 3,000 INR (68 USD) for a psychological assessment in 2006. They only knew about blood tests or X-rays, and those would cost much less than that. Why would they be willing to pay any more for a service they did not have any familiarity with? Also, health insurance does not cover outpatient services in India, and mental health services are even more unlikely to be covered. The cost has to be borne by the family themselves. I had the option of using the "Indian tests," but many of them were standardized in the 1960s and seemed fairly obsolete. We did have an Indian adaptation of WISC-IV (published in 2004), but the price was comparable to the price of the WISC-IV in the United States.

The clinic in the United States charged 1,500 USD for a full psychological assessment done by a predoctoral intern like myself back in 2006, which was the fee paid for by *public* funding for low-income families. It would take me 20–30 hours from start to finish, including writing a feedback story or song or letter. In India in 2006, for the same work, I would get paid a maximum of 5,000 INR (114 USD) by the more well-to-do families. However, I would have had to pay the USD equivalent price to buy the basic test material: the Wechsler Intelligence Scales for Children-IV (WISC-IV) (Wechsler, 2004) , and the Wechsler Individual Achievement Test (WIAT) (Wechsler, 2009), personality profiles like the MMPI (Butcher et al., 1993), the Rorschach Plates (Exner & Weiner, 1995), and projective stories like the TAT. The finances did not make much sense, so I decided to go slow on procuring the test material and used the older editions of test material that my clinic in the United States had given to me. Due to financial considerations, I could not always spend 20–30 hours on each assessment. So, I used these more as tools to get to know the child and build a connection.

Clinical Work with Indian Families

My next few months were full of observation and learning. I went through a process of reorienting myself to my culture, finding a way to make my training in "Western psychology" work with the nuances of

Indian culture. In Chandigarh, I spoke to most of the clients using a mixture of Hindi and English. Some clients spoke in Punjabi, which I understood but couldn't speak. A majority of the Punjabi-speaking clients could still understand Hindi.

As I sat through many "first initial consults," I began to see a few patterns.

"Why Should I Believe You?" Pattern

Many times, as I heard the parents describe the child's symptoms, I could see very clearly how the symptoms seemed connected with recent stressors the family had been experiencing. For example, Grace was 10 years old when her father brought her to me with complaints that she refused to go to school. Grace's parents had recently separated, and her mother had left the house. It was clear to me that this child needed therapy right away as, most likely, she was dealing with loss, grief, and anger which needed containment. But the father was not sure what her school refusal had to do with the parental separation. I did not really feel the need for an assessment with this child as I believed that a lot of her emotions would begin to unfold in the play therapy itself.

Sensing ambivalence in the father, I suggested a "psychological assessment" for the child. The father seemed more willing to invest in a 4–5-session assessment process rather than a vague process of counseling based on a vague hypothesis. After the assessment, I found that for this father (and for many more parents), my tentative, subjective working hypothesis was not as powerful as "data" from the assessment. Creating an assessment was the way I was able to link Grace's refusal to go to school to a family issue. Once the data confirmed that their child's behavior had an emotional basis, he was more willing to accept therapeutic help.

This was a bit confusing for me in the beginning because, in Indian culture, "doctors" tend to be trusted and respected. Patients see doctors as authority figures and tend to not question their views. Why was I not being seen the same way? Perhaps because I didn't have a white coat and a stethoscope dangling over my neck! I had to work harder to make myself sound credible. Assessment data gave me that credibility. Also, doctors often rely on blood tests and X-rays to arrive at a diagnostic picture. Themes from the assessment, especially "numbers" from the Rorschach or MMPI, made me sound more convincing to some of the parents.

As a rule, then, I started every new child or adolescent referral with an assessment—play observation, sand play, Projective Stories (TAT/CAT), Rorschach Inkblot Test, Early Memories Procedure (Bruhn, 1992), etc.

I used these tools just to get to know the child and to use my "observations based on data" as a powerful way of helping the parents see what was going on with their child:

"Things are fine in the family" Pattern

Over time, I also began to notice that parents would not always reveal everything that was going on in the family in the initial consultation. Either some important things would not be mentioned at all or significant details would be left out. While this also happens in other countries and cultures, Indian culture is particularly prone to creating this pattern. Being a collectivistic culture, "family" is a very sacred unit in India. Sharing/discussing/revealing family secrets outside the family creates a much larger sense of betrayal and shame than in more individualistic cultures.

> The Indian family: large and noisy, with parents and children, uncles, aunts and sometimes cousins, presided over by benevolent grandparents, all of them living together under a single roof. There are intrigues and secret liaisons, fierce loving and jealous rages. Its members often squabble among themselves but remain, in most cases, intensely loyal to each other and always present a united front to the outside world.
>
> (Kakar & Kakar, 2007, p. 8)

In contrast to the modern West, the Indian experience of the self is not that of a bounded, unique individuality. The Indian person is not a self-contained center of awareness interacting with other, similar such individuals. Instead, the traditional Indian, in the dominant image of his culture, and in much of his personal experience of the self, is constituted of relationships. He is not a monad but derives his personal nature interpersonally. All affects, needs, and motives are relational and his distresses are disorders of relationships—not only with his human but also with his natural and cosmic orders.... This emphasis on the "dividual" (rather than the individual), transpersonal nature of man is not limited to traditional, rural India. Even with the urbanized and highly literate persons who form the bulk of patients for psychotherapy, the "relational" orientation is still the "natural" way of viewing the self and the world.... In practice, a frequent problem arose when I thought the psychotherapy was going well and the client was well on the road to a modicum of psychological autonomy, and then family members would come to me and complain, "What are you doing to my son/daughter? S/he is becoming independent of us.

S/he wants to make her/his own choices now, thinks s/he knows
what is best for her/him and doesn't listen to us."

(Kakar, 2018, pp. 168–169).

While I wanted to understand the context of the child and their family
thoroughly in the beginning, I started to appreciate how I could potentially be treading in delicate territories. Once again, starting with "assessment" helped as the data gave me some clues and direction about
what needed to be explored in the family. It was interesting to see how
data-driven exploration allowed much more detailed narratives of the
family situation to emerge. It seemed that seeing some "spill of family
dynamics in the data" took away the sense of betrayal/shame of sharing
"family secrets" for the parent. I guess it was as if the "data" had already
shared the secret with me; now it was just a matter of confirming it.
Krishiv and Sanya are examples.

Krishiv

A mother called to consult for her 14-year-old son, who she said was
struggling with depression and "not trying to come out of it." Only the
mother came for the first session. She said the father was busy. Very well
put together, extremely well dressed, the mother seemed concerned but not
helpless. When I asked about the family stressors, she said there were
the usual ones like any family would have—some business problems, but
nothing unusual. She said they had moved into a new house recently, and
she had been busy organizing things in the new house. She and her son lived
with her husband and mother-in-law. I suggested we do some assessment
sessions. Krishiv came for the first session (and, unfortunately, the only
session). He hardly spoke to me but seemed very willing when I invited him
to do a sand tray. He covered the sand tray with trees, and next to each tree
he placed little people carrying weapons, and it appeared as if the trees were
going to be cut by these people. When I asked him to tell me about the tray,
he replied with just one sentence: "This is devastation." The boy couldn't
tell me anything more, and our session was rather short.

I followed up with his mother, letting her know that Krishiv seemed
quite angry to me and that it seemed that something had been making him
feel very hurt and upset. I wondered if there was something in the family
that could explain why he might be feeling this way. The mother told me
that the family was struggling with having lost the family business and
the familial home due to the father's drug addiction. The mother had no
choice but to continue in the marriage because her own parents refused to
support her and she had no college education herself to find a job. From her
outward demeanor, she had come across as a very sophisticated, well-put-
together woman who spoke excellent English. I would never have guessed

that this was someone who had gotten married right after school (at the age of 19 years) and did not have any college education or career. She came from a wealthy business family and was married into another wealthy business family. But now, with her husband's drug addiction, everything was falling apart. She told me that her own parents' message was very clear—she did not have their support if she even thought of stepping out of this marriage.

This was the state of many women in the families I got to know through my work with their children. Traditional Indian families (and even many urbanized ones)

> tend to treat their daughters, explicitly or implicitly, as *"paraya dhan"*, meaning members of the family they will marry into. Thus, the daughter is socialized to become a good wife, a good daughter-in-law and a good mother through the "reinforcement of traits such as self-effacement, self-sacrifice, submission, devotion, chastity, purity, tenderness, fidelity, dependence, tolerance of pain, resilience, and patience"
>
> (Saraswathi & Pai, 1997, as cited in Gupta, 2005, p. 28)

Many women stay and suffer in bad marriages because they don't have the financial independence or the wherewithal to live independently. The children in these families become carriers of symptoms that belong to the family.

Unfortunately, Krishiv did not want to come for any further sessions. I am not sure if that was his decision or if there were other factors operating.

Sanya

A Chandigarh mother called me for help with her 7-year-old daughter Sanya. She had seen a pediatrician, who had referred her to me. Sanya had been masturbating excessively in private and sometimes even in public, had become very *ziddi* (stubborn), and had been crying a lot lately. After the initial phone call, I asked the mother to come without the child for a parent meeting. She came by herself. The child's father did not come. The mother said he was busy. Once again, the mother came across as very well put together. I sensed some resentment in her towards Sanya for embarrassing her with the "shameful" symptom of masturbation. When I asked how long these symptoms had been going on, the mother said that she had been noticing these changes ever since Sanya's *bua* (father's sister) had moved into their home with her two daughters (8 and 3.5 years old), while going through a divorce. Sanya lived with her parents, younger brother, and paternal grandparents, and now her aunt and two kids had also moved in.

The mother reported everything else was okay, really, and she did not understand what was wrong with the child. I told the mother that I would like to see the child for a few sessions and assess what might be going on. While I did have a strong hunch that the child's symptoms had something to do with the aunt and her kids moving into their home, based on my earlier experiences, I decided to not share that with the mother till I had some more evidence from the assessment sessions.

The next week, I decided to start Sanya's assessment with play observation. I showed her the playroom. She chose to play with the dolls and told the following story: (Figure 6.1)

> This is a family consisting of mother, father, seven children (three *didis* [elder sisters] are college going, three are school going, and one is a baby sister). Mother works very hard the whole day doing things for everybody. One day, the power [electricity] goes off and the mother gets hurt by the wall while on her way to get a candle. She cries for a while and then goes and gets the candle. At night, she realizes the candle is still lit, and that's when she hears voices from people outside asking them to leave the home. She says no and goes to sleep. The next morning, the people break in and the family is thrown out, and they are crying.

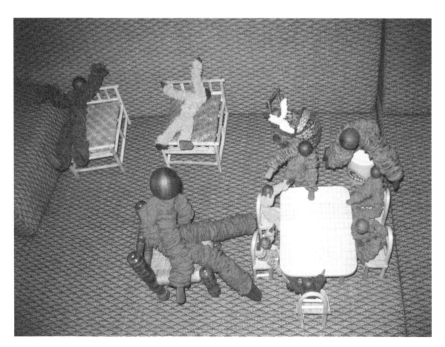

Figure 6.1 Sanya's Play Story.

Sanya's face showed no emotion. I said to Sanya that that must have been awful for the family. She quickly replied, "No, they are okay!"

The themes from Sanya's play were quite powerful and evident: An overburdened mother who is not really taken care of by anyone else (mother gets hurt, cries for a while, and then goes about doing what she needed to do, with no one coming to help her or asking her if she was okay); a family which is "thrown out" of their own home (strong feelings of being displaced from one's own home); loss and sadness.

Respecting the child's confidentiality, I did not want to share the details of the play sequence with the mother. But I called her in, and this is how the conversation unfolded:

Kakli:	I have had only one session with Sanya, but I was struck with some strong themes in her play. Can you help me make sense of it?
Sanya's mother:	Sure
Kakli:	I got an indication that she could be worried about losing her home, and maybe she is worried about you, too? Does that make sense to you? Can you say anything more about it?
Mother:	Well, I told you that my *nanad* [husband's sister] has moved in with her two kids. We had to give them Sanya's room because there is no other large-enough room where the three of them could stay. Sanya had to move into her younger brother's room. Also, my nanad and her kids get a lot of sympathy from my husband and my husband's parents. Everyone feels bad for them because they are going through divorce. If Sanya tells her dad that she misses her room, he gets upset with her, saying she is not kind. Also, my responsibilities at home have increased a lot. My nanad is feeling depressed, so I have to cook for her family and my own family and the in-laws. There are also financial hardships. My husband and mother-in-law have taken my gold jewelry from my wedding and will be selling it to get money to pay for my nanad's court case. My husband also spends time with his sister and her kids much more. He and I have been fighting more [starts to cry].
	In the traditional Indian view, which still exerts a powerful influence on how even most modern Indians view marriage, parent-sons and filial bonds among the sons override the importance of the couple as the foundation of the family.

Cultural ideals demand that the universal dream of love, that constitutes and seeks to find its culmination in the couple, be muted. They enjoin the family to remain vigilant lest the couple becomes a fortress that shuts out all other relationships within the extended family.

(Kakar, 2018, p. 168)

Kakli:	Wow! That's an awful lot of changes in a short span of time, and very painful ones. Sanya must be feeling a lot of loss… she has had to give up not only her room but also her time with her father and attention from her grandparents. And you are dealing with so much loss too—your jewelry, your financial resources, your husband's time and attention, and so much added responsibility.
Sanya's mother:	Yes, on top of that, this girl is embarrassing me with masturbation. I can't handle all this.
Kakli:	I can see how this must be so overwhelming for you, and shaming, too. Masturbation is normal in children, and when it is excessive, it could be a sign that it is being used for self-soothing. Do you see why Sanya might need more soothing and comfort right now?
Sanya's mother:	I get it, she is going through a lot of changes. She hates my nanad's kids.
Kakli:	Of course, she hates them. For her, they have taken away so much from her. So, we understand she would be angry. Do you think she might also be anxious? Soothing is usually a way to calm down anxiety. What might she be worried about?
Sanya's mother:	I don't know.
Kakli:	Any chance she could be worried about you?
Sanya's mother:	Me? Why?
Kakli:	You are going through a lot yourself. And children, especially older ones, especially daughters, can be quite attuned to their mother's feelings. Somehow, Sanya's play suggested that she worries about you. She might feel you have to handle all of this by yourself and there is no one to contain your sadness.
Sanya's mother:	[starts to cry again] But I don't show her my feelings. I tell her we just need to go through this and help her aunt and her kids
Kakli:	You may not show it, but she senses it. And maybe she resorts to self-soothing mechanisms like masturbation

	because she doesn't want to burden you with her emotions too much when you are already so overwhelmed.

Sanya's mother: So, how can I help her?

Kakli: I guess the first step is to understand why she might be masturbating so much. How do you feel when I say it could be a way she self-soothes because she is overwhelmed herself with loss and resentment and she also worries about you because she senses your sadness?

Sanya's mother: Makes me feel better. At least, I am not feeling so ashamed.

Kakli: Right now, you are going through a lot yourself, so I don't expect you to be able to hold Sanya's feelings as much as you could have at other times. Maybe I can help her contain those through our sessions. Would you like to try that?

Sanya's mother: Yes

I saw Sanya for few more assessment/therapy sessions. I also tried to rule out any possible sexual abuse that the child might be going through. Sanya's masturbation symptoms reduced significantly after a few sessions.

Unfortunately, the mother stopped the therapy sessions at this time, thinking that now "everything" was better. My advice to continue sessions for a few more months to prevent relapse was not followed.

"Symptom Relief Is Enough" Pattern

As with Sanya, I saw many children where the initial Therapeutic Assessment provided symptom relief. Sadly, some of the parents did not continue with therapy, thinking that the problem had been resolved.

Move to Bangalore

After practicing for 2 years in Chandigarh, I moved to Bangalore—a big, metropolitan city in South India also known as the Silicon Valley of India. It was a pleasant surprise to find a much higher mental health awareness in this city. Bangalore houses one of the biggest and oldest mental health institutes in the country—NIMHANS (National Institute of Mental Health and Neurological Sciences)—and there are many psychiatrists, psychologists, and counselors in the city whose work and contributions have made the residents of this city much more open to seeking mental health services. With regard to psychological assessments, cognitive assessments (IQ, ADHD, learning difficulties, etc.) are quite extensively done in Bangalore, but very few professionals do "emotional assessments."

Bangalore also has a very high population of families where parents have studied/worked in the US/UK/Australia or other developed countries and have returned to India to be closer to their families. These urban Indian families are more Westernized and also usually more open to seeking mental health services.

In Bangalore, I have not felt the need to start seeing every child with an "assessment." My use of assessments is now more need based—when an understanding of what might be happening with the child is not clear based on initial interview(s) with parents or when a child is already in therapy and there seems to be a "stuckness" or when there are clear questions guiding a psychological assessment.

"Open to Assessment But Not to Therapy" Pattern

Over the last 10 years, I have come across situations where an adolescent or an adult client was referred for therapy by family members but the client did not think they needed it. They were not willing to invest in an open-ended therapy process, but they agreed to a shorter, structured engagement of psychological assessments. For some of them, the process of assessment brought about a significant shift. Ragini is one such client I got to work with. Using the therapeutic/collaborative model, the work with Ragini and other clients demonstrates how an assessment can open clients to deeper therapeutic work. Using and sharing assessment tools and data in a transparent way with people becomes similar to short-term therapy and can produce lasting results.

Ragini

Ragini, a 19-year-old young woman, was referred to me by her father. She had dropped out of her architecture course after 3 months and had been staying home for the last 6 months. While it is normative for adolescents and young adults to stay with their parents in India, not attending college is rather unusual. Ragini's parents said that she had become very inactive and seemed "stuck" somewhere. They were beginning to get worried about her. Ragini, on the other hand, told her parents that she just wanted to be "lazy." She was not convinced she needed any help. I recommended that we do an assessment since there was no overt acknowledgement of concerns or symptoms on Ragini's part. I told the parents to tell Ragini that this could be a way for her to get to know herself better. Ragini came, but only on her mother's insistence.

Ragini came across as a quiet person with a pleasant demeanor. She said she had joined the architecture course by her own will. No one had pressured her in any way. She went to college for about 3 months and then stopped going because "she didn't feel like it." She did not seem forthcoming when it came to exploring her feelings. I asked her if she had any questions about herself or her life that this assessment could help address. She replied, "I don't know." I then gave her a list of questions typically asked by young people her age and asked if any of the questions seemed applicable to her for herself. She identified four questions from the list: (1) What kind of a person am I? (2) Why can't I concentrate? (3) Why do I feel so confused? Why can't I make up my mind? (4) Why am I so lazy? On further exploration, she didn't say much about the first, second, and fourth questions, but for the third one, she said she always feels confused, never gives straight answers, and often finds herself saying "I don't know." When I asked her to describe how confusion felt to her, she said she didn't have any feelings and was not an emotional person.

Following this initial interview, I introduced the projective drawings (a series of drawings: House, Tree, Person, Person of the Opposite Gender, and a Person in the Rain), followed by some projective questions. Ragini's response to the Person in the Rain (Verinis et al., 1974) drawing stood out as most meaningful. She said, "There was a lot of rain and so it had flooded. The person was okay with it. He felt that he got stuck in that place but he can go where he needs to go." Her drawing and the description conveyed a mixture of feelings—on the one hand, there seemed to be a minimization of being "flooded." On the other hand, there was a sense of hope and confidence in being able to resolve her "stuckness" (Figure 6.2).

The following session, I administered the Rorschach Inkblot Test using the Exner Comprehensive Scoring System. Ragini gave a valid protocol with a normative 25 responses and a Lambda of 0.67, indicating a responsiveness to the task and an emotionally rich protocol. Ragini's first response as she "signed in on Card I had a similar theme to the Person in the Rain drawing. She said, "Something is flying in the air, reaching for something; it is going up, higher and higher." Once again, her desire to grow, rise, and do well in life came through, quite a contrast to her "lazy" presentation.

One of Ragini's responses on Card II was, "Looks like a volcano, lava all over the place; lava because of red color. Volcano erupted; everything is flying everywhere." This response was of course quite a surprise coming from someone who said she was not emotional and did not feel anything. I wondered if she felt she had to keep a tight lid on a deep sense of anger and helplessness that she felt inside so it would not get out of control. Interestingly, on the same card, she also saw a "bridge," conveying a sense of a hopeful transition.

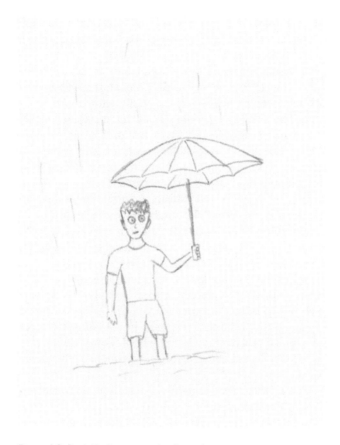

Figure 6.2 Ragini's Person-in-the Rain drawing.

On the next card, which often captures a person's view and experience of relationships, one of the things Ragini saw was "two people screaming," suggesting the possibility that she might have experienced emotional intensity or aggression in her close relationships. She gave a texture response on Card IV—"Monkey's head, Spanish monkeys with lot of hair near the neck (hair because of the pattern [touched card])." This also left me feeling hopeful—she was expressing warm attachment feelings on a card that pulls for relation with masculine/authority figures. In contrast, her response on Card VII, one which pulls for relation with feminine figures, indicated a need for individuation and separation. She said, "Looks like something is falling; this top part is breaking off from the part at the bottom."

Another meaningful response came on Card VIII, where she said, "Looks like two locked-up chains." I wondered if this was a reference to locked-up feelings inside her. On the same card, she gave another response, "Looks like a mossy lake, green parts make it look mossy and contaminated," suggesting a possible experience of contamination and ambivalence in close relationships.

The Exner scoring system revealed that Ragini had an "extratensive pervasive" style of coping (EB = 2:5.5), which meant that her typical problem-solving strategy was to interact emotionally with others to try out various solutions. This seemed surprising as she had described herself as "unemotional" and other scores pointed to her preference to avoid emotions. Ragini also scored a 4 out of 5 aspects on the depression constellation, suggesting that she might not qualify for a diagnosis of depression but she definitely had depressive features. Her egocentricity ratio was 0.12, indicative of very low self-esteem. A form dimension score of 1 was encouraging as it suggested she might have the ability to introspect. A GHR:PHR (Good human to poor human response ratio) of 1:3 suggested that she had a tendency to perceive hostility and anger in interpersonal relationships. An isolation index of 0.44 suggested that she was fairly isolated, which was particularly concerning for a person who had an extratensive style of coping. People with an extratensive style of coping need to reach out to others in order to cope and solve problems. She did not have a single whole human response in the entire protocol, confirming that she avoided others and was left with a skewed perspective about relationships. This reflected her referring symptom of pulling away from life in the world.

Overall, Rorschach suggested that Ragini's natural temperament and coping style was more emotional than cognitive. Her self-esteem was significantly low. Her interpersonal relationships had been confusing—at times loving, at times "contaminated" by conflict and lack of emotional attunement. All of these interpretations were only in my mind at this point. I did not share any of this yet with Ragini.

At our next session, we did the Early Memories Procedure, a task in which the client is asked to describe her earliest memories from childhood, narrating them as a scene and then responding to four questions: Which part of this memory is the clearest, how old were you, what is the feeling about this memory, and if you could change one thing from this memory, what would that be? Ragini shared six memories in total, of which I am sharing the four that seemed most significant.

Memory 1: I am in my parents' house and sitting on my father's legs while he is lying down. I was playing with him, and perhaps the TV is on in the background.

Which part of the memory is clearest to you? Me sitting on his legs and holding his knees.

How old were you? Perhaps 3 years.

What is the feeling about this memory? Happy; nostalgic.

If you could change one thing, what would it be? Nothing.

Ragini seemed very connected with her feelings as she narrated this memory. As I listened, I couldn't help but smile, conveying a sense of enjoying this warm fuzzy feeling with her. I was also happy to see that she was beginning to open another door to her emotional world to me.

Memory 2: I am a little bit older, maybe 3 or 4. My mother had made bitter gourd for dinner. I really hated it. I was forced to eat it. Both Mom and Dad insisted that if I tried it, I might like it. I tried it, and I threw up. Mom got mad at me for first refusing to try something I didn't like and then for throwing up. I began to cry.

Which part of the memory is clearest to you? Me refusing the food. What is the feeling about this memory? Amused.

If you could change one thing, what would it be? Probably, me just eating it and liking it. I think I didn't even try to eat it. I should have.

As I was listening to the description of the memory, I felt bad for that little child. It felt a little too much to be scolded for throwing up. I was struck that Ragini said she felt amused and that she felt she should have just eaten the food. I wondered why she didn't say she felt bad or angry at her mom/parents for forcing her to eat something she hated. I decided to not bring this up yet. We continued.

Memory 3: In the place where we stayed, me and my older sister went out to play. One day, she ran away to play with her friends and I got lost; she would often do that. I was crying. Just walking around the place. She found me later, but after about 1.5 hour or so. She was shouting at me because I made it harder for her to find me as I kept walking instead of staying in one place. We just went home, and I cried the whole way.

Which part of the memory is clearest to you? Me trying to find her; that time felt very long.

What is the feeling about this memory? I probably shouldn't have stuck with her and just played with younger kids.

How old were you? About 4 years.

If you could change one thing, what would it be? I wish I just stayed home and avoided the whole thing.

I nodded my head, conveying a lot of validation for the little child who must have felt so lost and scared. Again, I was struck that what she wanted to change was to not have gone with her sister, instead of feeling let down by her sister and wishing she would have kept her close to her or at least not scolded her for getting lost. While I was itching to say this to her, I decided it would be better to wait till we reached the end of this task so I would not color what she was going to recall next.

> Memory 4: It was my birthday, and there were quite a lot of people in the house, but for some reason I didn't want to go out. I was sitting in the room, and I was crying in the room, and they kept calling me and I wouldn't go out. Later, my aunt came into the room, spoke to me for a while, took me to the hall where everyone was, then I was fine.
>
> Which part of the memory is clearest to you? Me sitting in that room. How old were you? 4 to 5 years.
>
> What is the feeling about this memory? A bit bad. It was my birthday, people wanted to see me, but I was avoiding them.
>
> If you could change one thing, what would it be? I should have just gone; don't know why I did that then.

There was a lot of sadness in the room while Ragini was narrating this memory. It was becoming clear to me that she had a strong tendency to blame herself rather than other people. I was finding myself feeling strong emotions. I asked Ragini how it was for her to tell me some of her childhood memories. She replied that she was surprised with all that had come out. She said she did not know she had these memories and that she had feelings around them. I let her know that I was experiencing a lot of emotionality from her in this session, which was different from how I had experienced her in the previous sessions. We both agreed that this session had been very "powerful."

I asked Ragini if she noticed any pattern to her responses to the "What would you change, if you could?" question following each of the memories. She said she hadn't. I said,

> In many of these memories, you were feeling sad, unhappy, alone, and what you wanted to change was your *own* response to these situations, not the response of others. For example, when you got lost, you wished you had not gone with your sister and had stayed home, but I was wondering if you wished your sister was more sensitive to you, took better care of you, or someone realized the fact that you must have been so scared having been lost for what felt like a long time. When you were narrating this memory, I could not help

but think of that little Ragini feeling so lost and alone. It must have been so scary for her, and instead of getting comforted around her fear, she ended up getting scolded.

Ragini listened attentively. I asked her to see if she noticed this pattern in the other two memories. She nodded. We spoke more about her tendency to self-blame and to not see the role of the other's inability to tune in to her feelings. We also spoke about how her feelings may have gotten lost in the process and that she ended up believing she didn't have feelings, when in fact, she was a very emotional person.

Ragini came back after a week. She said that after the last session, she went back home and asked her mom why no one ever asked her how she felt. Her mom said that whenever they did ask her as a child how she was feeling, she would say, "I don't feel anything." So, over time, they assumed that she was just different and maybe she really didn't have feelings.

Ragini also said that she was doing more things around the house for the last few days. Her mom noticed that her activity level had increased and called it "magical." Ragini added that she was thinking of taking up an internship in film-making, which was something she had been wanting to do for a while. She said she had identified one good place a few months ago but had not pursued it until now. It felt like Ragini had begun to get "unstuck"!

While the Early Memories Procedure session had already felt very powerful, I wanted to complete the assessment with the Thematic Apperception Test. Not surprisingly, Ragini's stories had themes of low self-esteem, lack of attunement from the mother, and self-blame, which matched what was seen on the Rorschach and the Early Memories Procedure.

Ragini's story for a card showing an older man and a younger man was heartening. It was a story of a very good village carpenter who goes to the city to find more work. He gets a good job, does really well, and lives a much better life. One day, his employer, who is stuck in a legal case, asks him to be his witness to help him get out of the case. He wants the carpenter to lie. The carpenter knows it is wrong to lie, but he is worried about losing his job. First, he says okay, but then he refuses at the last minute. He loses everything—his job, his money—and goes back to being the carpenter he was. The carpenter feels relieved, while the boss is surprised that the carpenter stood up for himself. This story conveyed hope in Ragini's ability to let her true self take over in an assertive way.

We followed this session with an individual feedback session in which Ragini and I addressed her assessment questions. The discussion centered around how, contrary to her belief, she was actually a fairly emotional person deep down. We also spoke about the possibility that what she had been calling "laziness" was more likely unexpressed sadness and self-blame.

Even though Ragini was 19 and technically an adult, within the Indian cultural context, it seemed appropriate to offer feedback to her parents from the assessment since they had been so concerned about her. In India, a 19-year-old is still very much a part of the family, and the psychological separation of adolescence may just be starting around this age.

> The hallmark of adolescence as defined by Erikson … is to evolve one's own sense of self and establish one's personal identity. This psychological separation is supported by the normative practice of physical separation from the family, initially in the form of greater time spent by adolescents away from their parents and family and later as an actual moving out of the familial home. However, in most Indian families, children do not leave home unless necessitated by educational and job requirements or marriage for girls. Even the earlier phase of adolescents' spending more time with their peers than with their families is minimized in most traditional families, though it is on the rise in more urban families. Thus, adolescence is not experienced the same way in most Indian families as in the west.
>
> (Gupta, 2005, p. 29)

Ragini wanted to do the feedback as a family session, but only with her parents. She didn't want to include her sister in this session. Ragini sat between her parents. Her father appeared pleasant but was a man of few words. Mother was the most expressive, very open and forthcoming but probably depressed. I started by expressing my pleasure with Ragini for investing so well in the assessment process and for her openness to this journey, despite her initial hesitation. The mother spoke about the changes she had experienced in her in the last few weeks and expressed gratitude.

The mother spoke a little bit more about Ragini's childhood and herself as a mother. She had started working just a year after Ragini was born, and she could not be there for Ragini much. She felt guilty. She said she believed that Ragini was just like her father—she didn't really get emotional easily and maybe she just didn't have feelings the way the mother and her elder daughter tended to. I intervened and said that Ragini was very emotionally sensitive and that in many ways this was her strength. By now, Ragini was looking a bit low. I stopped the discussion and asked her how she was feeling.

She just shook her head, saying, "Nothing."

The mother said, "See, this is how she always responds."

I looked at Ragini and asked her, on a scale of 0 to 10, how angry was she feeling at that moment. She said, "Five." I asked her how sad was she feeling. She said, "Eight" and then burst into tears. This was the first time Ragini's parents had seen her cry in a very long time. We gave space to Ragini to feel all that she was feeling.

I said it was very courageous of her to allow himself this experience and that it was very heartening to see her parents, especially her mother, being able to acknowledge that they might have missed engaging with this part of Ragini and that over the years, a faulty belief about her being unemotional got established.

Ragini had decided to pursue her course in film-making in 3 weeks. She said she would be leaving the city in 2 weeks' time. I let her know that I would be available whenever she felt the need to talk. I did recommend that it would help her to be in psychotherapy. She said she would let me know if she wanted to talk.

What helped Ragini? The specificity of eliciting her early memories, coupled with empathic listening on the assessor's part, lowered her guard significantly. Just like her aunt, who stayed with her and helped her face the guests at the birthday party, the assessor, by remaining attuned to Ragini's emotional process, supported her in being able to face the "collective," the world.

Last, the family session seemed to have really helped Ragini because (1) she got acknowledgment and validation from the mother about her unavailability to her as a young child and (2) she received attunement as well as permission to feel her feelings from the assessor.

Assessment Tools for Therapeutic Intervention

While psychotherapy and counseling services have become in high demand in India in the last 10 years, and even more so since the start of the COVID-19 pandemic, assessments in India are still largely cognitive (to assess for developmental delays, intellectual difficulties, attention problems, and learning issues). The high cost of test materials, the inability of most clients to afford the cost of assessments, and the lack of advanced training in conducting assessments, especially projective tools, are the largest obstacles in the growth of use of psychological, and especially emotional, assessments in India. Also, at a time when the country is facing a serious shortage of mental health professionals who are adequately trained to provide counseling or psychotherapy services, rigorous training in tools such as the Rorschach Inkblot Test, Minnesota Multiphasic Personality Inventory (MMPI), Thematic Apperception Test (TAT), and other projective or actuarial measures seems like a luxury most training programs can't afford.

As an intermediary option, I have found it helpful to use some assessment tools for therapy. For instance, sometimes, when my counseling supervisees have felt stuck while working with a client who finds it hard to share spontaneously in the session, I have shown them how to administer the Early Memories Procedure and try to use that as a way to get to know their client better. Many clients respond well to the safety provided by the structure of a "task." Many of my supervisees have no training or experience in using this tool, but keeping the Therapeutic Assessment model in mind, we make sense of the data in supervision and the supervisee counselor is able to then use this understanding to connect with the client and help them open up and feel understood.

Similarly, many of us use projective drawings as a way to connect with a child in the initial session. This has been especially useful when, during the pandemic, sessions with kids have had to be done online. Sentence Completion is a task we often use with children and adolescents as a "fun game" that can lead to meaningful and deep psychological engagement. The therapist pops up a statement, and the client has to complete it almost as a free association. The therapist can create a sentence at the moment or think of a few beforehand, keeping in mind the context of the client's life. Assessment tools have become powerful therapeutic interventions in many of these situations.

Conclusion

Over the last decade, I have had the opportunity to work with many clients who were helped through Therapeutic Assessments. In some cases, they eventually became convinced to see a therapist. In other cases, they did not go for therapy, but the assessment helped them with insight and healing. There have also been situations in which a family member (typically a parent) of a client who was assessed reached out for therapy after experiencing it vicariously through their son or daughter. The relational focus of Therapeutic Assessments has worked well with the Indian culture—clients' skepticism about the psychological process gets addressed through a transparent process of arriving at an understanding; at the same time, "data" tells part of the family narrative and makes it easier for the client to share the rest without necessarily feeling a heavy sense of betrayal towards the family.

One of the aspects I enjoyed the most when I was learning how to do Therapeutic Assessments two decades ago was the room for creativity in helping clients feel understood. Most mental health professionals in India experience the limitation of resources—training, experienced colleagues, mentors, test materials, financial support, and time. But those of us who have grown up in the Indian culture are also quite adept at *jugaad*—creative ways of problem solving using minimal resources. In my experience, the Therapeutic Assessment model's primary focus on relating with a client while using tools and communication creatively has worked well with this Indian mindset of using the resources available to address the problem at hand.

The pandemic has created an environment of grief and anxiety, and many more people in India are reaching out for psychological help. While this has increased the demands on the limited number of mental health professionals, it has also been heartening to see how psychiatrists, psychologists, counselors, and social workers are trying to come together, helping each other out through peer support, supervision, consultation, and sharing training resources. India still has a long way to go to develop adequate mental health resources, but there is progress at many levels, especially in the use of creative ways of connecting and relating with clients to help them feel seen and understood and to heal.

References

Agarwal, U. (2018). Of mothers and therapists: Dreaming the Indian infant. In M. Kumar, A. Dhar, & A. Mishra (Eds.), *Psychoanalysis from the Indian terroir* (pp. 37–54). Lexington Books.

Bada Math, S., et al. (2019). Cost estimation for the implementation of the Mental Healthcare Act 2017. *Indian Journal of Psychiatry, 61*(4), S650–S659. https://www.ncbi.nlm.nih.gov/pmc/articles/PMC6482705/

Bruhn, A. R. (1992). The Early Memories Procedure: A projective test of autobiographical memory II. *Journal of Personality Assessment, 58*, 326–346.

Butcher, J. N., Dahlstrom, W. G., Graham, J. R., Tellegan, A., & Kaemmer, B. (1993). *MMPI-A: Minnesota Multiphasic Personality Inventory-Adolescents: Manual for administration and scoring.* University of Minnesota Press.

Exner, J. E., Jr., & Weiner, I. B. (1995). *The Rorschach: A comprehensive system—Vol. 3: Assessment of children and adolescents* (2nd ed.). Wiley.

Gaiha, S. M., Salisbury, T. T., Koschorke, M., Raman, U., & Petticrew, M. (2020). Stigma associated with mental health problems among young people in India: A systematic review of magnitude, manifestations and recommendations. *BMC Psychiatry, 20*, 538. https://bmcpsychiatry.biomedcentral.com/track/pdf/10.1186/s12888-020-02937-x.pdf

Gupta, K. (2005). *Intergenerational cultural differences: Learning from the experiences of immigrant families from India* [Unpublished doctoral dissertation]. California School of Professional Psychology.

Kakar, S. (2018). Psychoanalysis, culture, and the cultural unconscious. In M. Kumar, A Dhar & A. Mishra (Eds.), *Psychoanalysis from the Indian terroir: Emerging themes in culture, family, and childhood* (pp. 165–178). Lexington Books.

Kakar, S., & Kakar, K. (2007). *The Indians: Portrait of a people.* Penguin Books.

Murray, H. (1943). *Thematic apperception test manual.* Harvard University Press.

Nizamie, H. S., & Goyal, N. (2010). History of psychiatry in India. *Indian Journal of Psychiatry, 52*(7), 7–12. https://www.indianjpsychiatry.org/text.asp?2010/52/7/7/69195

Prasadarao, P., & Sudhir, P. 2001. Clinical psychology in India. *Journal of Clinical Psychology in Medical Settings, 8*(1), 31–38.

Saraswathi, T. S., & Pai, S. (1997). Socialization in the Indian context. In H. S. R. Kao & D. Sinha (Eds.), *Asian perspectives on psychology* (pp. 74–92). Sage Publications.

Taniparti, N. (2018, May 11). The worries of 'Log Kya Kahenge?' on mental health. *The Wire.* https://thewire.in/health/social-factors-behind-the-stigma-that-surrounds-mental-health-in-india

Verinis, J. S., Lichtenberg, E. F., & Henrich, L. (1974). The draw-a-person in the rain technique: Its relationship to diagnostic category and other personality indicators. *Journal of Clinical Psychology, 30*(3), 407–414.

Wechsler, D. (2004). *The Wechsler Intelligence Scale for children* (4th ed.). Pearson Assessment.

Wechsler, D. (2009). *Wechsler Individual Achievement Test-Third Edition* (WIAT-III). Psychological Corp.

World Health Organization. 2019. The burden of mental disorders across the states of India: The global burden of disease study 1990–2017. *Lancet Psychiatry, 7*(2), 148–161.

Section III

Collaboration and Immigration

Collaborative Assessment From a Transcultural Perspective: Cooperativa Crinali's Experience in Milan, Italy

Marta Breda, Nicole Fratellani,
Francesca Grosso, Ilaria Oltolini,
Benedetta Rubino, and Stefania Sharley

A Brief Introduction to Cooperativa Crinali's Work with Migrants

In the last years of the 20th century, Italy went from being a country of great emigration—as demonstrated by the percentage of Americans with Italian origins—to a country of immigration. The phenomenon of immigration to Italy is in fact fairly recent and is constantly growing; foreigners living in the country increased from 2.3% of the population in 2004 to 8.7% in 2019 (Caritas & Fondazione Migrantes, 2019; Caritas Italiana et al., 2004). Initially, most migrants arriving in Italy were men coming from North Africa or Albania who worked in factories or agriculture and women who travelled alone from the Philippines, Peru, Ecuador, Moldova, or Ukraine and worked as housemaids or carers for children and the elderly. Once their working lives were stabilised, these migrants reunited with their families, where possible, by arranging their move to Italy. Migration thus brought about a new type of client base, who often did not speak Italian and who found that local services (healthcare and also social and psychological care) were poorly prepared to deal with new requests and unequipped to work with migrant families.

The attitude towards migrant people in Italy is ambivalent. On the one hand, in Italy migrants have free access to some important services, such as healthcare and schooling. This is the result of a process of institutionalisation, which has granted everyone access to these services, but could also be rooted in a deep-seated characteristic of Italian culture: A strong sense of generosity and a willingness to share with everyone what the country has to offer. On the other hand, it cannot be denied that Italian legislation regarding welcoming migrants, rescues at sea, citizenship, and asylum seeking has become more stringent and rigorous over

DOI: 10.4324/9781003124061-11

the last few years. As far as public opinion is concerned, a few alarming details have emerged. Firstly, over half (51%) of Italian citizens perceive in a negative way migration flows coming from outside of Europe (European Commission, 2019); this is a result of the stereotypically negative narration on the subject by mainstream media. Another worrying piece of data is the significant growth of hate, intolerance, and racism, both on- and offline, in Italy and in the rest of Europe (Fondazione ISMU, 2021). Racist insults targeting members of minorities, which would once have been considered unacceptable, have acquired social media visibility (ECRI, 2020). The rise of right-wing parties, in Italy and many other European countries, has contributed to the development of this climate of intolerance and hate.

Having witnessed the increasing numbers of foreign women accessing local services and hospitals, in 1996 a group of women with diverse professional backgrounds (psychologists, social workers, midwives, gynaecologists) founded Crinali (an Italian word for the imaginary lines on mountain ridges that form the boundaries between watersheds), an association that later became a social cooperative. Our Transcultural Assessment Group is part of Crinali.[1] The aim of Crinali's work was to facilitate the interaction with these new clients (especially women and children), to welcome them, to understand them from both linguistic and cultural perspectives, and to respond to their health and social needs at important times in their lives, such as pregnancy, the birth of children, and the children's placement in school (Cattaneo & dal Verme, 2005). The first step was the organisation of a training course for migrant women who were competent Italian speakers and wanted to embark on a new professional journey modelled on the experience of other European countries, that of linguistic and cultural mediators. The choice of *female* linguistic-cultural mediators stemmed from the observation that, in all cultures, the helping professions are characterised by a prevalence of female figures, who are more easily accepted than males. The fact that the mediators themselves had experienced and psychologically processed their migration and the struggles relating to moving to Italy would help them identify with clients' troubles while also facilitating communication with clinicians (not just from a linguistic point of view).

This is the short story of how Cooperativa Crinali's work started; subsequently, it extended its areas of intervention while continuing to collaborate with public services. Linguistic-cultural mediators began working in family counselling centres and the "health and help centres for migrant women and their children" which were set up in two Milanese hospitals. A multi-professional team, which linguistic-cultural mediators are permanent members of (Bevilacqua et al., 2001), operates in these centres and enables the implementation of a comprehensive approach to the client that deals not just with health problems but also with psychological, social, and cultural issues. As a logical consequence, the cooperative subsequently began to focus more on the psychological aspects of migrant people's distress. Having witnessed the difficulties migrants encountered in accessing traditional psychological services, Crinali activated a transcultural consultation service (Cattaneo & dal Verme, 2009, 2020) inspired by the theoretical model of ethno-psychiatry and the in-depth and extensive research and clinical practice conducted by Moro (1994, 1998) with migrant children and families.

In recent years there has been an increase in the number of migrant children referred by schools to local services for learning or behavioural problems and of parents reported to the Juvenile Court for inadequacy or abuse (Tribunale per i Minorenni di Milano & Procura della Repubblica presso il Tribunale per i Minorenni di Milano, 2018), and the need for assessment has become pressing. For this reason, Crinali activated a psycho-diagnostic assessment service with a transcultural perspective, which our group is in charge of. In brief, our methodology is supported by the theory on which Moro's aforementioned transcultural consultation is based, by studies on multicultural assessment (Dana, 2005), and by Collaborative Assessment (Finn, 2007). The latter is particularly well suited to work with migrants because it enables the clinician to better understand the client as well as their country and culture. It is important that the clinician becomes acquainted with the individual client's sociocultural etiquette and attends specific training in order to overcome the temptation of an ethnocentric attitude. The clinician should also become competent at using (a) the anthropological register to recognise cultural factors linked to the psychosocial environment of origin; culturally significant interpretations of stress factors; and the role of religion, traditions, and parental and social ties; and (b) the psychological register to identify the levels of individual functioning; resources and impairments; and the destabilising impact of migration and acculturative stress.

In response to requests from local services, we identified an assessment procedure aimed at carefully reducing the risk of pathologizing culturally connoted representations, family models, and behaviours. In addition to the linguistic-cultural mediator's presence and the careful use of diagnostic tools, we believe it is crucial to arrange a preliminary meeting with the referring provider and all the people involved in order to share and explain the assessment procedure and collect the questions needed to set up the assessment. We subsequently organise

- transcultural anamnestic interviews, using genograms to explore the client's personal history;

- the administration and discussion of acculturation scales to understand the strategies used to face migration and entry into Italian society;
- the administration of tests to assess personality and cognitive functioning; and
- a final summary and discussion session with the people involved and the referring provider.

The final reports, containing the responses to the diagnostic questions, are handed to the referring provider and—in the form of a personalised letter in both Italian and the client's native language—to the client.

Collaborative assessment is not widely used in Italy, and diagnostic procedures are often carried out in a much more "traditional" way in which assessor and client have distinct roles and the aim of the test administration is to identify a diagnosis and treatment. A complete mapping of Italian psychological assessment services is not easy to carry out since many providers of this type of services are part of the private and non-profit sectors; this makes it even harder for migrant people who need access to these services to find out about them and get in contact with them (Médecins Sans Frontières, 2016). Within mental health services, migrants may encounter staff not adequately trained to work with migrant clients, poor (or no) use of linguistic-cultural mediation, and little flexibility in the use of Western diagnostic categories. However, as far as Milan and Lombardy are concerned (the geographical reality we work in and thus know best), we have noticed a growing interest in the use of collaborative assessment and a greater openness towards a type of psychological evaluation that considers the client as an active part of the assessment process.

The aim of this chapter is to introduce our way of working, which is constantly evolving. Migration flows change, and the increasingly more frequent and globalised exchange of knowledge influences cultural representations and often destabilises the reference points of migrant people, who have already been subjected to the traumatic experience of migration and to the acculturative stress resulting from it.

The Approach of Crinali's Transcultural Assessment Group and the Essential Role of Linguistic-Cultural Mediation

An assessment can be very stressful and worrying for any client; this is even truer for those who are not familiar with the language and the intricate Italian system. Confusion, fear, bewilderment, and sometimes anger can characterise the first approach to assessment, not least because it can be very difficult for someone coming from a different cultural background to understand the reasons lying behind and the sense in participating in such a process. The assessment setting entails the presence of two assessors and a linguistic-cultural mediator (who should be the same person throughout the assessment process). The latter is an essential figure for two reasons. The first—and more intuitive one—is the necessity of relying on a translation which is as accurate as possible. Secondly, the figure of the linguistic-cultural mediator is a source of reassurance and trust because she belongs to the client's country of origin; she is viewed as an intermediary with White people, as the migrant client never really knows to what extent White people can be trusted (Cattaneo, 2015). It is not enough for the mediator to be a competent translator; thanks to her knowledge and understanding of both worlds, she has the paramount task of enabling the encounter between different cultures. Aballouche (2002) compares linguistic-cultural mediation to a bridge that not only enables communication and mutual understanding between the clinician and the client but also promotes a constructive change in the relationship between culturally diverse people. This valuable presence can inform us of the client's relationship with their country of origin. A refusal to use their native language could signify either the need to exhibit a good command of Italian or the fear of being judged by the mediator, who embodies their home culture, or the need to distance themselves from their cultural roots. In a situation where anxieties, fears, and confusion come into play, ensuring the presence of a figure who can be perceived by the clients as similar—as a bearer of the same culture and language, as somebody who fully understands their values and way of thinking and with whom they can express themselves without the fear of constantly being misunderstood—facilitates the creation of a respectful and welcoming environment and conveys a willingness to collaborate and to understand different points of view.

For those conducting the assessment, mediation is also essential because it aids the operation of cultural decentering[2] by providing the context required to interpret clients' answers and behaviours without mistakes and preconceptions.

For instance, Said is a Moroccan father who has spent 30 years in Italy and has never gone back to Morocco since the day he migrated. He explicitly refuses the presence of the Arabic mediator by stating he does not need it and by choosing to carry out the whole assessment in Italian. However, when he encounters linguistic issues and difficulties relating to culturally determined mental schemas, he appeals to the mediator in an attempt to reduce the intense sensation of shame he is feeling. While in Italian Said's thoughts are vague and indefinite, in Arabic they acquire a clearer form and content. Mentally returning to Morocco places him in a safe haven that enables him to regulate his emotions and become an active protagonist of the assessment.

Diagnostic Tools

Acculturation Scales

Acculturation scales are usually the first tool we use when we begin an assessment. Administering an acculturation scale can be very useful in building a therapeutic alliance and selecting the best diagnostic tools to use; moreover, exploring the clients' acculturation strategies[3] is essential to be able to interpret their test results. We normally use at least one of the following scales: A modified version of the Brief Acculturation Scale (BAS; Paniagua, 1998), the Multigroup Ethnic Identity Measure (MEIM; Phinney, 1992), and the Acculturative Stress Inventory for Children (ASIC; Suarez-Morales et al., 2007). All three measures are easy and quick to administer and, like almost all acculturation scales, they were created and validated in North America. Despite not being validated in Italy and hence not useable by us in a quantitative way, after being translated and adapted to the Italian context, these scales can be used in a qualitative way and additional questions can be asked in order to identify responses that may have been influenced by social desirability since clients may provide socially desirable answers to appear more integrated into the host culture and more competent speakers of Italian than they actually are.

Karim is an Egyptian man in his 60s who has been living in Italy for almost 20 years. During the administration of the acculturation scales, he states that he speaks Arabic only at home with his wife, who moved to Italy from Egypt just over a year ago; by contrast, he says he mainly talks in Italian with his friends and work colleagues. He declares himself proud of his culture and especially of being Muslim. But it only takes a little delving into Karim's daily life to understand that his integration into the host culture and interaction with Italian people are actually quite limited. In addition, it emerges that he has a strong attachment to his cultural roots and that his future plans are completely oriented towards returning to his country of origin. Karim states that he rarely goes out, mostly to attend important religious gatherings in which he participates as the community's spiritual guide. He adds that his main wish is to return to Egypt and start a business there.

Despite his answers matching an assimilative style, after asking Karim a few more questions regarding his habits, we soon find out that behind an apparently assimilative strategy hides a separation style and a lack of openness towards interacting with the host society, which he sees as a temporary home despite the many years he has spent in Italy. It is understandable that, while facing an unknown assessment situation, Karim wants to provide answers he thinks are "right" in order to appear integrated into Italian society and to protect himself from the intrusiveness of the tests.

With adults and adolescents, we use a version of the BAS, modified by Noseda and Bevilacqua (2002), which explores a few essential areas of cultural belonging (language, sociality, and food), and the MEIM (which mainly investigates ethnic identity search and the feelings linked to belonging to a specific ethnic group). With children, however, we administer the ASIC,[4] which focuses on migration-related stress and potentially discriminatory experiences.

Mei is an 8-year-old girl; she has Chinese origins but has spent almost her entire life in Italy. She is fluent in Italian (which she prefers to Chinese), and she talks to her parents in both their native language and Italian. When asked if she misses her country of origin, she says she does not and she explains that, on the contrary, she misses Italy when she is on holiday in China.

Mei's acculturation strategy is assimilative, from her responses to the ASIC's items emerge a very strong identification with Italian culture, which she perceives as her own, a detachment from Chinese culture, and an absence of immigration-related stress. The questions relating to perceived discrimination, however, reveal the presence of discriminatory experiences. Despite Mei feeling Italian, she is well aware that she does not look Italian to her peers; she explains that it bothers her a lot when her schoolmates exclude her from games and activities because of her ethnicity.

The Rorschach Test with Migrant Populations

The transcultural use of the Rorschach test[5] (Rorschach, 1942) is a real challenge. Rorschach himself was concerned with issues in the transcultural use of his test and described the cultural differences relating to the frequency of psychopathologies and symptoms among the inhabitants of the Canton of Bern and those of the Canton Appenzell Innerrhoden in his native Switzerland (Rorschach, 1942). Subsequently, Exner (1986) noticed that, when comparing data relating to White and non-White Americans, his Comprehensive System was not totally suitable for transcultural use. The issues relating to the Rorschach's transcultural use are diverse, and close attention needs to be paid during both its administration and the interpretation of the data.

As far as the answers to the cards are concerned, people see different images according to their culture of origin; the content is the variable that is most influenced by the home culture (Nakamura et al., 2007). As in a case that we assessed, a client coming from Morocco is likely to say they see "ostriches" in Card V since ostriches are animals typical of that country and are consistent with the inkblot's contours. By contrast, this answer is so unlikely among the Italian population that it does not even appear in the form quality reference table (i.e., the table that includes the answers matching the blot's contours). This has repercussions both on a quantitative level (i.e., on the indices measuring the answers' content) and on a qualitative level (i.e., on the answers' interpretation and on their projective content). As regards the impact on indices, this difference in content inevitably leads to a difference in the number of popular responses (i.e., the most common answers for a particular inkblot).

For instance, in Scandinavia "Christmas elves" is a popular answer to Card II (Mattlar & Fried, 1993), whereas in Italy a common response is "Bear's, Dog's or Lamb's Head or Entire Animal." Evidently, the latter will not be a common answer for people who have been exposed to the typically Northern European story of Father Christmas and his helpers. In a similar way, for the Japanese population the popular response to Card VI is not "animal skin" but "musical instrument" (Nakamura et al., 2007). The strength of the contents is that they are a metaphor for how people perceive themselves, their emotions and sensations, and the world and relationships. Moreover, precisely because content tells us something about clients, it often provides qualitative responses to the assessment questions and valuable material for the discussion of test results. More specifically, the use of material that is not perceived as foreign or "too Italian" can aid the discussion of results, which are not perceived as alien from the client.

After experiencing problems with her husband, a Nigerian woman called Tambara was referred to us by the support workers of her residential home because of her communication difficulties and issues in interacting with the staff and the other women residing there. In general, Tambara seems isolated from her social environment and not very well integrated into Italian society.

To Card VI, she replies: "Submarine."

Where do you see it?

It's the entire image.

A submarine?

Because there are people inside, here it can take direction and communication.

Do you see people inside?

No, I don't see them.... This is the part that stays above water and this is the one that goes under water.... And this looks like the door to enter ...

In this card which is typically associated with the topic of contact, through a metaphor Tambara tells us about her relation and communication issues. Her inability to communicate with other people is evident and is certainly amplified by migration (which often leads to isolation) and by her poor command of Italian. People are present, but they are not seen and hence become inaccessible, hidden behind a door, and Tambara describes herself as alone and excluded from a context she is struggling to access. At the same time, she also describes her defences and her effort to protect herself by placing herself in an environment (the submarine) from which she cannot be seen but from which she can look out and monitor what is happening around her. Without realising it, Tambara provides a description of herself that answers the referring providers' questions ("Why does she struggle to form a connection with us and the other women in the home? Why can we not have a collaborative dialogue?").

The clinician should spend some time explaining—especially if the assessment has not been chosen by the client but has been imposed—that the test does not have right or wrong answers and that every answer is useful in order to collect information that can be of help to the client too. The assessor should also bear in mind that the task presented in the test is unfamiliar to people who come from other cultures. For this reason, it is essential to adopt a position of collaboration and of cultural decentering, to explain what is being done and the sense the test has in Italy, and to ask if there is something similar in the client's culture. In order to consolidate the diagnostic alliance and better explain the purpose of the test, the clinician can provide examples, such as, "It is like when we look at clouds and try to guess what they look like." Clients can also be asked which tasks are used in their home country to assess a specific personality trait or competence, or which process and which people are involved in answering the assessment question that is being investigated. A cultural decentering attitude should be maintained even during the interpretation phase, since—as highlighted by Dana (2005)—different configurations of certain personality variables can have advantages or disadvantages when it comes to adapting to different environments, which here coincide with home cultures.

In brief, one should always bear in mind that an attitude, a personality trait, a relational modality, or a particular schema of interaction with the outside world that makes sense and is functional in a specific cultural context could make no sense and may be dysfunctional in a different context. When interpreting data, in order to avoid falling into the trap of cultural bias, the clinician must pay close attention to the client's background and take into careful consideration every possible relationship between cultural variables and the test results (Meyer et al., 2015).

For instance, it makes sense to take into account whether the client belongs to a collectivistic or individualistic culture. Recently, while assessing a Chinese female client, we decided to interpret the absence of

Texture responses in light of her culture of origin. According to Exner's (1986) Comprehensive System, Texture responses include clients' perceptions of something as soft, hairy, or with a tactile effect due to the inkblot's nuances. Providing no Texture responses indicates fear of physical or psychological intimacy and is interpreted as a maladaptive value. However, in this specific case, not providing any Texture responses could actually be considered to be functional and adaptive since greater relational distance and greater confidentiality are typical of Chinese culture compared to Western society. It is thus possible that data that appear to be indicative of a distancing attitude simply suggest the presence of a modality that, according to Chinese culture, is respectful of interpersonal distance.

Finally, the linguistic-cultural mediator's presence is always essential. In the aforementioned case, the Chinese client provided a high number of responses with anatomical content (mostly pelvises, sexual organs, and uteri), which—according to Exner's system—signal anxiety and concern about one's body. The mediator highlighted, however, that this type of content is highly unusual for a Chinese person because it involves unspeakable content and taboos. Before the assessment takes place, it is important to allow the mediator time to familiarise herself with the inkblots, especially if she has never seen them before, so as to eliminate any interference from her initial perception of the test.

As Dana (2005) highlights, we believe that, overall, the Rorschach is a valuable tool in its collaborative use with people who come from different countries. In fact, regardless of the place and culture of origin, Rorschach's inkblots are able to activate projective responses that can be useful if properly interpreted. This, together with the nonverbal nature of the stimuli, enables clients to provide answers that give us a lot of information about them and their internal world, and that can be used in a collaborative way during the feedback session and in the final assessment reports. When clients are faced with a problem-solving task, the way in which they solve it provides information that can be generalised to the way in which they tackle challenges and unfamiliar situations in their daily lives. The way subjects approach the Rorschach test mirrors the way they tackle a strange, unusual, and unknown task and reveals their intrinsic resources, the feelings that this type of situation arouses, and the attitude that the person has when dealing with novel situations. From a collaborative point of view, the most valid material is content, which—because of its cultural influences—is a metaphor for how people perceive themselves, the internal and external world, in their language and with reference to their home culture. If a decentering and collaborative attitude is maintained, this material becomes useful for answering the assessment questions and feeding back to clients a description of themselves and of their way of functioning while also highlighting the cultural representations that are part of their background.

The Drawing That Tells a Story: Transcultural Use of the Wartegg Test

The Wartegg Test (Wartegg, 1939, 1953, 1959), better known as Wartegg Zeichentest or WZT, is a possible transcultural diagnostic tool and can be used in the field of clinical assessment because it is capable of exploring the same personal dimensions as the Rorschach, despite the differences in development and popularity. The test aims to collect the projections of the client's internal world through their spontaneous drawings, prompted by eight ambiguous and incomplete stimuli.[6] Free of verbal language, it is characterised by unfamiliarity and lack of organisation, despite being semi-structured. This forces subjects to reorganise the material in a very personal way, on the basis of their intrinsic motivations. The fact that the WZT provides a careful description of the individual's autoregulatory system (between the self, others, and the culture in which the individual is immersed) enables it to be used as a transcultural tool. The test is very easy to administer, and it is even possible to use mime, thus totally bypassing the language barrier.

The richness of information that can be obtained from the test has been corroborated by research carried out over a period of 20 years by the Italian Institute of Wartegg, which has developed the interpretative model of the Crisi Wartegg System (CWS; Crisi, 1998, 2013; Crisi et al., 2018). Its adequacy in transcultural settings was explored for the first time in a pilot study carried out by Oltolini and La Mela (2019) aimed at verifying its suitability to migrant populations.[7] The test was administered to an experimental sample of 41 migrant men whose performance was subsequently compared to that of an Italian control group. In the foreign group, the task was understood and completed by 93% of participants in around 10 minutes (which is the average time for this test). Seeing that the language barrier represents a significant limit to the validity of tasks administered to cultural minorities, the fact that only 7% of the sample did not understand the standardised instructions can be considered a success. Having excluded from the experimental group the three participants who did not seem to understand the indications provided by the assessor, the researchers were left with a number of participants who were capable of tackling the task without particular issues.

As far as qualitative observations are concerned, the participants experienced the test as a low-impact task, capable of revealing the areas in which migrants invest their psychological resources: Relationships, the need to act and produce (i.e., the importance of work and professional profile), attachment bonds, and their roots. A qualitative analysis showed that, compared to Italians, some migrants displayed slightly altered indices, which we hypothesised were the evident result of migration-related distress, such as a greater reactivity to the environment, the activation of alarm systems, and a reality testing impoverished by hyper-arousal, with original if not always elaborate thoughts. The test also identified a generalised state of inner tension, since the migrants' protocols exhibited an above-average anxiety index and a higher number of special scores, which informed us of the presence of sometimes confused or tangential thought processes and verbalisations. Acculturation stress was detected through an alarming increase in the suicidal tendency index that almost reached cut-off levels and called for ongoing mental health care. The intergroup comparison highlighted the role of culture and the weight it exerts on cognitive functions and thought processes; verbalised answers abounded with less vital and more pragmatic—sometimes pathological—content. However, this did not affect global cognitive resources since both groups obtained a good score in box 6, which is usually linked to the cognitive sphere. These data were reassuring and explained why 60% of the experimental group placed themselves in an adaptive area with sufficient coping strategies to face difficulties.

To sum up, the WZT enables us to paint a clearer picture of the people who enter our country, and it can be used as input to promote a more profitable therapeutic alliance. When used together with the Rorschach test, in addition to making the diagnostic hypotheses more robust, it helps the clinician to formulate relevant and comprehensive answers to the client's questions.

The Use of Cognitive Tests in Transcultural Assessment

In order for a cognitive test to be effective and useful in the context of transcultural assessment, firstly it has to be able to overcome the language barrier. In fact, if the client is not fluent in the language the assessment is carried out in, there is a risk of obtaining a performance and results that are not representative of the client's actual abilities. This is why we administer tests and subtests that, thanks to their structure, enable us to investigate clients' cognitive resources, the way they approach the task and their strategies, without the use of the verbal channel. For instance, this is the case with the Cognitive Assessment System (CAS; Naglieri & Das, 2005); the performance subtests of the Wechsler Intelligence Scale for Children (WISC-III; Orsini & Picone, 2006) and the Wechsler Adult Intelligence Scale (WAIS-IV; Orsini & Pezzuti, 2013); the Test di Intelligenza Non Verbale, which is the Italian version of the Comprehensive Test of Nonverbal Intelligence (CTONI; Hammill et al., 1998); and the Rey-Osterrieth Complex Figure Test (ROCF; Stern et al., 1994).

A second essential element in our use of cognitive tests relates to the purely qualitative way in which we analyse results; in fact, the tests we use do not have normative data that are adapted to migrant clients' cultural characteristics and it would thus be impossible to compare quantitative results to the normative data. However, the administration of performance subtests is carried out in a way similar to cross-battery assessment[8] (Flanagan et al., 2013), which allows the clinician to observe *how* the client approaches the task, which strategies they implement, and, above all, whether such elements prove to be functional and adaptive to the task's purpose. The underlying idea here is the parallelism between the solution of the task in the here and now and day-to-day life. Tests allow us to witness which behaviours are carried out in a situation that is stressful, ambiguous, and apparently simple but difficult to carry out until the end; they also allow us to understand our clients' real potential.

The CAS is a cognitive protocol based on the PASS theory of intelligence (Das et al., 1975), which means it evaluates the processes of planning, attention, simultaneity, and succession with the aim of highlighting the client's strengths and weaknesses. As previously mentioned, because of the particular context of transcultural assessment, only those tasks that can be carried out without a predominant use of language are administered (the only area that cannot be investigated is succession as it requires the client to repeat unrelated words or meaningless sentences). The CAS has many strengths, such as the fact that simple requests gradually become more complex, which enables the clinician to see if the client reacts with greater commitment and tenacity or with anxiety, worry, and surrender. Moreover, some tasks require time to be measured, thus adding another source of discomfort and apprehension. Finally, both an observational and an explicit analysis of strategies[9] are carried out; this enables the assessor to explore the client's schemas and understand whether the client is aware of them and is able to verbalise them as well as to determine whether the clinician's observations are consistent with what is reported by the client. The analysis of strategies is a valuable opportunity for the assessor to introduce a collaborative element to the assessment; in fact, it might be difficult for the client to independently find solution strategies while facing a test, thus risking a stalemate or stunted progress. This is what happened to Yana, a Russian woman referred to us for assessment following an extremely conflictual relationship with her partner.

Yana approaches testing with great commitment and seriousness; she deals with the initial clear and simple items in a confident and agile way. However, when the task becomes more complex, Yana's confidence wavers, giving way to anxiety, perhaps in line with a strong success-oriented approach linked to her home culture. A growing dissatisfaction with her performance begins to take shape, together with growing stress caused by her awareness of the passing of time, which cannot be controlled and hence makes Yana aware of the likelihood of making mistakes. To protect herself from these uncomfortable sensations, she tries to discredit the task, which she defines as childish. This enables her to continue the assessment, but only to a certain point because, in the middle of a more complex matrix reasoning task, Yana stalls: Time is pressuring her and she does not know how to proceed. The only thing she manages to verbalise is her own shame over not knowing what to do.

When something like this happens, the assessor needs to understand how to overcome the block; it is clear that, in the moment, Yana is incapable of organising her thoughts and planning her actions. What if we provided her with a suggestion about how to proceed? Would she be able to accept the advice? Would she be able to use it? Would she be able to interiorise it and reuse it in similar situations? It is at moments like this that the assessor needs to guide the client in overcoming the impasse by carrying out what is referred to as *scaffolding* (Wood et al., 1976). In this way, it is possible to verify whether the client's inner resources are sufficient and can be supported in order to reach more satisfying results. This is what happened with Yana; once provided with a possible strategy, not only does she appear capable of accepting it and correctly implementing it, but she also appears capable of using it again autonomously in similar tasks. Interrupting the test at the first signs of struggle and interpreting them as Yana's inability to overcome a problem would not have allowed us to witness her ability to accept help and, subsequently, to plan a tailored intervention enabling her to fully exert her parenting role. While being able to follow external suggestions can indicate a functional tendency towards collaboration, it can sometimes hide a dependence on external reassurance and fuel a demeaning self-concept.

As previously mentioned, parts of the WISC-III and WAIS-IV can also be administered; more specifically, performance subtests enabling the calculation of the Processing Speed Index measure the extent to which the client is able to follow external instructions and reason in a strategic way without being influenced by the worry caused by the stopwatch. Furthermore, these types of tasks are definitely less demanding compared to other tests—especially projective tests—and can thus be used in an attempt to lower the client's defences, which can understandably be raised in an assessment setting.

Sasindu is a middle-aged Sri Lankan man referred to our service because of his abusive conduct towards his wife and daughter; defensive and prejudiced, he completely devalues the CAS protocol and avoids all the emotional stimuli proposed by the Wartegg and Rorschach tests. Because of his lack of openness, we decide to administer the WISC-III Picture

Arrangement subtest (which requires the sequential arrangement of pictures to tell a story) with the aim of breaching Sasindu's defences and understanding the way in which he arranges time and causality in relationships. Once he has arranged the pictures, we ask him to tell us what happens in the sequence, in order to verify that he has actually understood the represented interaction. However, Sasindu does not seize this opportunity; he arranges the cards in a confused manner, and the stories he tells have no real rationale.

In addition to the impossibility of establishing a relationship with Mr. Sasindu because of his defensiveness, it is interesting to notice the consistency in his performance on all tests, which mirrors the way in which he faces everyday life: Sasindu is not capable of being in tune with himself or using his resources because he is too busy hiding, an attitude conveying a partial and coarse perception of the world and producing inadequate behavioural responses. We are thus aware that we will have to work hard with him and reassure him in order to reach the minimal alliance needed to conduct a realistic and useful evaluation of his resources.

Feedback Techniques: A Few Ideas

In feedback and discussion sessions with migrant clients, it is necessary to bear in mind a few important elements to successfully complete an assessment. In addition to the essential presence of the linguistic-cultural mediator, it is important to tailor the use of language, tone of voice, and examples to each individual client. In other words, the clinician's language should adapt to the client's way of expressing themselves and interacting, with the aim of establishing a dialogue, of rendering understandable what has been collected throughout the assessment, and of answering the initial assessment questions.

The Use of Metaphorical Images

An example of the use of symbols and metaphors—especially well-suited to work with children and teenagers—is the drafting of a story, a fable, individualised according to the client's age, emotional and cognitive development, and sex as well as the context and family dynamics (Dana, 2005). The story is drafted not only on the basis of the information provided by the child but also based on the assessment results, and it contains a message conveying how the protagonist makes some positive changes, usually thanks to their family's support. Most children ask for the story to be put in writing; not many migrant children are accustomed to having "gifts" that are as personalised and tuned into their emotional world. Parents are encouraged to place the story in a place that is easily accessible to the child.

The use of metaphorical images is useful with adults, too, when writing the final report because it renders information more accessible and understandable. For instance, in the aforementioned case of Yana, we thought of a lunar landscape with cold tones, capable of representing her tendency to avoid emotional situations that she feels are destabilising. This metaphor of her inner world was chosen after discussing with her how, during the Rorschach, seeing colours had generated in her such anguish that she had started crying. Thanks to the metaphor, it was possible to widen the conversation and discuss the important role of colours in life.

In feedback and discussion sessions, starting from what the clients themselves produced throughout the assessment process facilitates discussion as it makes clients feel comfortable, valued, and respected and does not require them to navigate uncharted waters.

Collaborative Feedback

The discussion of results contributes to building a dialogic dimension that could not be more different from a mere communication of data. According to Finn's (2007) model, collaboration means sharing and negotiating with the client every piece of information and all diagnostic hypotheses. As a means and tool to explore new possibilities, communication between the clinician and the client takes on new meanings. If we implement this way of working with migrant people, it is not difficult to imagine the positive impact on self-esteem, self-efficacy, and sense of self, triggered by providing a mirroring that differs entirely from the one they receive in a life often full of struggles and humble tasks and devoid of acknowledgement.

We arrange discussion sessions with the utmost care and sensitivity. Throughout our work—and especially during the feedback session—we bear in mind Swann's self-verification theory (Swann et al., 1992) and, more specifically, the articulation of information on three levels. In Yana's case, at the first level, we confirmed her need to reach a high performance on cognitive tests since that is what is taught in schools in her home country. At the second level, we chose to introduce her constant attempt to satisfy her personal needs, and at the third level, we included her emotion-avoiding attitude, which enabled her to justify her involvement with abusive men and her defensive attempt to demean herself and others. It is easy to understand that Yana would not have been able to accept this information straightaway and immediately imagine the changes she could make; hence, we decided to begin a therapeutic process and help her, in due time, to face her defensive system with greater awareness.

The Bilingual Letter

The bilingual letter is another useful tool (Dana, 2005). It is necessarily brief in order to allow an easier and more immediate understanding of the contents. In the letter, we thank the people who enabled us to get to know the client and to establish a good relationship with them, and we subsequently sum up what we have learnt from the tests and their history. With their personal history, cultural background, and resources, migrant people are an example of tenacity and courage in facing difficulties, as well as of faith and hope for the future. In other words, we clinicians explain what we have learnt thanks to our encounter with the client, therefore reversing the idea that they are the one learning from us. It is important to bear in mind that the letter, written in both the client's native language and Italian, is in itself a message to convey openness to the client's diversity and to welcome them to our society.

A Couple of Examples

Mary and the Lost Diamond

Mary, a mature-aged woman from the Philippines, is referred to us by social services for an assessment of her parenting skills. After reporting her husband for abuse, she is temporarily placed in a residential home with her two children, a pre-adolescent and a 7-year-old girl. Support workers and social services have doubts regarding her capability to handle problems encountered in raising her children; it seems as if Mary is always in need of support, is not autonomous, and cannot handle school, work, or relationships on her own. The social services' assessment question has to do with Mary's global psychological functioning; like many other migrant women struggling with marital abuse, she is alone and has no support network. She appears particularly scared during the first assessment session, but she is also collaborative and curious to better understand her struggles; in fact, she asks the following questions: Why do I feel sad when my husband offends me? Why am I incapable of defending myself? Why am I struggling to learn Italian?

Thus, Mary herself seems to recognise that she has a certain degree of fragility, a tardiness in taking action, and a tendency to look for external support and protection. With these questions, she admits to experiencing dysphoric feelings and to looking for a "crutch" (on an emotional and behavioural level) that can help her deal with everyday life.

From a cognitive point of view, her fragility emerges on performance tasks; she proceeds quite slowly, struggles with tasks that require planning, displays a limited range of strategies (probably due to the few opportunities to experiment that she has had), and appears more oriented towards practical things. She asks for reassurance, encouragement, and confirmation; she has to be encouraged to take risks and change her view when there is nothing on the horizon. When she feels she has received good instructions, she follows them almost literally, which leaves little space for flexibility and personal initiative. This behaviour, on the one hand, reassures her and enables her to overcome difficult situations, while on the other hand, it fuels a demeaning vision of herself as a weak person in constant need of reinforcement.

In less structured and more emotionally demanding tasks, such as the Rorschach and the WZT, a range of negative emotions appears, a depressive core based on the observation that so far nobody has been able to consider her a valuable person. B6, the box of the Wartegg Test that best describes these processes, requires the client to use the mind's natural predisposition to close open figures by joining two separate marks into a single drawing (generally a geometric figure or a construction). Mary draws "a diamond," thus possibly expressing her desire to have more transparent and sharper mental faculties that would help her be functional in her daily life. On a symbolic level, she seems to be telling us that she wants to "shine" in terms of cognitive efficacy and also reasoning. Formal quality, however, cannot support this ambition, and she is aware of this to the point that she attempts a new drawing that is even less precise than the first one. Mary actually considers herself to be more similar to a "worm," a figure she draws in box B2, which seems to contradict her grandiose ambition.

In parallel, in the Rorschach test topics emerge linked to self-esteem and self-efficacy, Mary's weak personality traits, probably linked to depressive aspects. The sadness Mary states she experiences when she does not feel valued re-emerges when she is confronted by "impacting" inkblots, which arouse anxiety precisely because they suggest situations of discomfort, which she feels she has to defend herself from. In these situations, in which she senses a demeaning of herself, she resorts to imagining and simplifying reality in an attempt to escape from a feeling of impotence and of not knowing what to do, which would be a confirmation of her poor competences. Because of her anxiety, generated by complicated and complex experiences, and because of culturally determined aspects (such as the gender role attributed to Asian women), her comfort zone is represented by all those moments when somebody else takes charge of the situation. In self-report tasks, Mary reports an absence of aspects of suffering. However, this is her answer to Card I (traditionally considered to be a self-introduction): "Something old and crumpled. Around it are broken pieces. As if they broke the pieces and spread them around." Dealing with these experiences cannot be pain-free; Mary dreams of someone who values her, of an expert capable of recognising "the diamond's purity" and of highlighting its beauty.

Going back to Mary's questions, it would be possible to answer her by providing the image of a paper boat which is sometimes at the mercy of negative emotions.

Why do I feel sad when my husband offends me? For Mary, it is very important to feel appreciated and valued. At the moment, she is incapable of finding anything good inside herself; she feels like a "worm," and she looks for sources of external support capable of protecting her vulnerable self-esteem. When people whom she has tried to build a strong relationship with disappoint her (such as her husband, whom she married at the age of 36 and from whom she hoped to receive rather than give), a vicious cycle of negative thoughts begins, providing confirmation for her sad self-narration. Shame, guilt, and inadequacy are feelings that characterise her experiences as an incapable and undeserving person. Anyone would feel deeply hurt and sad if they constantly thought of themselves as inferior to everybody else.

Why am I incapable of defending myself? While at the mercy of both "freezing" and painful emotions, Mary tries to turn her gaze elsewhere. She does not react, perhaps because she does not have faith in her own possibilities. A basic level of trust seems to be missing and to have been replaced by a kind of resignation, of fatalistic waiting, of redemption fantasies. Her gaze matches the inactivity of someone waiting for something or someone to change the situation.

Why am I struggling to learn Italian? Mary is tired and exhausted from the mental operation of simplification aimed at avoiding painful emotions, so she sometimes acts in a delegating manner that does not stimulate her cognitive dimension. She accumulates no new experiences; she acts according to scripts she has already experienced and fails to encounter new opportunities to learn. Acquiring a language has a wider meaning that goes beyond simply possessing command of a language; she would like to partially give up her certainties (her home culture) and launch herself into new explorations. From a certain perspective, the discovery of new ways of being is more the beginning rather than the end of her story, but she first needs to recover her energy level and faith in a world that is not always so threatening.

The final session with Mary is an emotionally charged moment for all those involved. Assessor, mediator, and client discuss openly the difficulties she has encountered in recent years and also the many things she has done to overcome her problems. She has never previously found herself in the position of being able to openly express all her thoughts; nobody has ever asked her what is important to her, and thus she finds it surprising to be asked such questions. We agree that the test results suggest that she is like a paper boat facing a storm at sea. She herself previously recognised her vulnerabilities, but she has never thought of herself as brave; facing the waves takes a lot of strength and courage, and sometimes this strength can waver in the face of great difficulties—migration, problems with a language she seems incapable of learning, a job and a marriage that are not working, children who are growing up. Through the analysis of the tasks and of the test results, Mary is able to recognise the many things that she has managed to do and the energy she has used to control the boat and try to overcome the storm. She recognises that, when focussing on the need to achieve a goal, she can make impulsive decisions, but her mistakes decrease when she is given clear and comprehensible instructions. She has never thought that facing the waves—especially high and dangerous ones—can be exhausting, which is why one might let oneself be carried away by the currents, just like Mary, who on many occasions has let herself be guided by others with no energy left to control the tiller. Exhausted, she seems to have given up on her goals, which makes her feel very sad. Allowing herself to feel these feelings starts to make her shame disappear as well as helps her realise that no paper boat can survive alone in the middle of the sea. Mary feels appreciated, understood, and valued; more confident in herself and her abilities, she accepts getting help, and says she will not give up expressing her thoughts and wishes. She is—and will always be—the only real tillerman of her boat.

Some Kids' Intelligence Lies in their Hands

Boiken, an Albanese pre-adolescent, is referred to social services by his school because of his behavioural difficulties, which have led him to encounter numerous—sometimes even legal—problems as well as to prematurely drop out of school. It is suspected that he might have an anti-social disorder, and a psycho-diagnostic assessment is arranged to respond to this particular question. During the first session with Boiken and his father, we learn that he has been in Italy for 2 years and that, before that, he lived for 11 years in Albania, where he attended school before moving to Italy and being placed in a lower grade because of his poor Italian. Boiken says he does not like going to school and has no intention of going back; he would prefer to start working. His father tells us that the boy began speaking very late, around the age of 6, and that he has always struggled to learn. He asks: "What is wrong inside his head? Why does he not remember things? Why is his school performance in Italy poor? Why was his performance poor in Albania too?"

We initially hypothesised the presence of an attention and concentration disorder, which is why we selected neuropsychological tasks to evaluate inhibitory control, memory, and visuo-spatial reasoning. Boiken exhibits a poor performance, poor planning abilities, and no functional strategies in solving tasks. Furthermore, despite the presence of the linguistic-cultural mediator, he seems incapable of understanding the instructions, and the mediator raises doubts regarding his command of his native language. Despite the numerous difficulties, Boiken is collaborative, involved in the tasks, and determined to better understand his struggles. Moreover, his attention holds for the tasks' entire duration, and we manage to administer a good number of tasks in just one sitting. The information collected thus far suggests the need for the hypothesis to be reformulated, for the idea of an attention deficit to be abandoned, and for the potential presence of a linguistic and cognitive deficit to be explored. We hence administer neuropsychological language tests in both Italian and his native language, as well as some WISC-III performance subtests. On these tasks, too, Boiken obtains poor results: Fluency is poor in both Albanese and Italian (with scores inferior to those of an average 8-year-old), but we are surprised by his ability to gradually manage the increasing complexity on the cognitive tasks. In fact, he somehow manages to interrupt the accumulation of negative and frustrating results. He himself is satisfied and fulfilled: During the administration of the Mazes Subtest, he states he is happy because those are the things he likes and knows he can do well. The assessment detects a consistent deficit involving many cognitive domains, and it seems clear that Boiken struggles to understand the external world. His problematic behaviours could be regarded as a dysfunctional response to not feeling sufficiently valued and understood.

Boiken's intelligence lies in his hands; he likes making, building, and creating. He needs to attend a school that welcomes his abilities in an inclusive way and to be supported in a personalised way in order to experience life, especially in a work environment, by developing personal values and feeling an active part of society. Boiken's case is testimony that sometimes there can be a discrepancy between the question raised by social services and that raised by the family, sometimes due to culturally different—but not irreconcilable—representations. This case also demonstrates that carrying out an assessment is a continuous process of adjustments and changes, even during the administration itself. We clinicians should not be afraid of being overwhelmed by the load that this flexibility requires, nor of opening up to what is new and surprising.

Creating a Process

In conclusion, so far, our group has experimented with the tools and modalities that we described throughout the chapter, but we are aware that this work will never end and that we will have to redesign our interventions from time to time in light of the encounters that will take place in the future and of the stories that we will be able to create together with our clients.

Notes

1 For more information on Crinali, see our website: www.crinali.org.
2 Cultural decentering consists in being aware that migrants can have different cultural representations from the clinician, which the clinician needs to get closer to and try to understand (Moro, 2000).
3 Berry (1997) identifies four acculturation strategies: *Marginalisation* takes place when one neither maintains one's own culture nor tries to become part of the host society; *separation* is the strategy through which migrants maintain their culture of origin while avoiding interaction with the society they entered; *assimilation* happens when the desire to maintain the home culture is weak and that of interacting with the host society is strong; and finally, *integration* is the strategy through which one tries to maintain one's own culture while also becoming part of the host society.
4 The ASIC can be administered to children between the ages of 8 and 12. It comprises two main factors: *Perceived Discrimination* and *Immigration-Related Stress*. The former includes injustices the child feels they have been a victim of and feelings of exclusion and marginalisation, while the latter relates to feelings linked to the experience of living in a new country, far away from one's country of origin, and to potential difficulties caused by having to communicate in a new language.
5 The Rorschach test is a well-known projective psychological test in which subjects are asked to interpret ten inkblots presented on ten separate cards.
6 The eight stimuli (dots, lines, and shapes) are presented in eight separate boxes on a single sheet of paper; each of them differs from the others and aims to be suggestive of a specific design. The client is instructed to complete the drawings using the stimuli.
7 This pilot study was conducted with the collaboration of the Italian Institute of Wartegg, which supervised the scoring and marking procedures and processed the statistical data by comparing them with the data contained in the Italian archive.
8 Cross-battery assessment is a methodology that was introduced in the 1990s and involves the use of information collected from a variety of tests in order to gain more specific and detailed information.
9 The idea underlying the analysis of strategies is partially based on Kaplan's (1988) Boston process approach, which "warrants close observation of behaviour en route to a solution" (p. 309) and involves an analysis of the mistakes and processes through which the client tries to solve a problem (Libon et al., 2013). Our assessment group investigates strategies once the task is completed and not while it is being carried out (as suggested by the Boston Process Approach), but the purpose remains the same: Understanding how the client solved the task and identifying potential blocks or inaccuracies that hinder the achievement of a satisfying performance.

References

Aballouche, S. (2002). La mediación intercultural [Intercultural mediation]. *Anuario de Psicologia*, *33*(4), 593–596. https://revistes.ub.edu/index.php/Anuario-psicologia/article/view/8765/10972
Berry, J. W. (1997). Immigration, acculturation, and adaptation. *Applied Psychology: An International Review*, *46*(1), 5–34. https://doi.org/10.1111/j.1464-0597.1997.tb01087.x

Bevilacqua, P., Caccialupi, M. G., Cattaneo, M. L., dal Verme, S., Finzi, I., Parolari, L., Ruspa, M., Russomando, P., & Sacchetti, G. (2001). *Professione mediatrice culturale: Un'esperienza di formazione nel settore materno infantile* [*The profession of the cultural mediator: A training experience in the maternal and infant sector*]. Franco Angeli.

Caritas & Fondazione Migrantes. (2019). *XXVIII Rapporto Immigrazione 2018–2019: Non si tratta solo di migranti* [*28th report on immigration in 2018–2019: It is not just about migrants*]. Tau Editrice.

Caritas Italiana Fondazione Migrantes, & Caritas Diocesana di Roma. (2004). *Dossier Statistico Immigrazione Caritas-Migrantes 2004: XIV Rapporto* [*The Caritas-Migrantes 2004 statistical dossier on immigration: 14th report*]. Edizioni Idos.

Cattaneo, M. L. (2015). Elementi di base della clinica transculturale [Basic elements of transcultural consultation]. In S. dal Verme, *Quaderno di formazione alla clinica transculturale* [*Transcultural consultation training notebook*] (pp. 9–23). Crinali Cooperativa Sociale Onlus. http://www.crinali.org/wp-content/uploads/2015/02/Elementi-base-della-clinica-transculturale.pdf

Cattaneo, M. L., & dal Verme, S. (2005). *Donne e madri nella migrazione: Prospettive transculturali e di genere* [*Women and mothers in migration: Transcultural and gender perspectives*]. Unicopli.

Cattaneo, M. L., & dal Verme, S. (2009). *Terapia transculturale per le famiglie migranti* [*Transcultural therapy for migrant families*]. Franco Angeli.

Cattaneo, M. L., & dal Verme, S. (2020). *Sviluppi della clinica transculturale nelle relazioni di cura* [*Developments of transcultural consultation in care relationships*]. Franco Angeli.

Crisi, A. (1998). *Manuale del test di Wartegg: Norme per la raccolta, la siglatura e l'interpretazione* [Wartegg test manual: Rules for collection, scoring and interpretation]. Magi Edizioni.

Crisi, A. (2013). The Wartegg drawing completion test. In L. Handler & A. D. Thomas (Ed.), *Drawing in assessment and psychotherapy: Research and application*. Routledge.

Crisi, A., Carlesimo, S., & Maio, S. (2018). *Manuale di siglatura del test di Wartegg secondo il CWS* [*Wartegg test scoring manual according to the CWS*]. Magi Edizioni.

Dana, R. H. (2005). *Multicultural assessment: Principles, applications, and examples*. Lawrence Erlbaum Associates.

Das, J. P., Kirby, J., & Jarman, R. F. (1975). Simultaneous and successive synthesis: An alternative model for cognitive abilities. *Psychological Bulletin*, *82*(1), 87–103. https://doi.org/10.1037/h0076163

ECRI. (2020). *Annual report on ECRI's activities covering the period from 1 January to 31 December 2019*. https://rm.coe.int/ecri-annual-report-2019/16809ca3e1

European Commission. (2019). *Rapporto Nazionale Italia: Opinione pubblica nell'Unione Europea* [*Italian national report: Public opinion in the European Union*]. Standard Eurobarometer 92. https://europa.eu/eurobarometer/surveys/detail/2255

Exner, J. E. (1986). *The Rorschach: A comprehensive system* (Vol. 1, 2nd ed.). Wiley.

Finn, S. E. (2007). *In our clients' shoes: Theory and techniques of therapeutic assessment.* Erlbaum.

Flanagan, D. P., Ortiz, S. O., & Alfonso, V. C. (2013). *Essentials of cross-battery assessment* (3rd ed.). John Wiley & Sons.

Fondazione ISMU. (2021). *Ventiseiesimo Rapporto sulle migrazioni 2020* [*26th report on migration in 2020*]. Franco Angeli.

Hammill, D. D., Pearson, N. A., & Wiederholt, J. L. (1998). *Test TINV: Test di Intelligenza Non Verbale* [*CTONI: Comprehensive Test of Nonverbal Intelligence*]. Erikson.

Kaplan, E. (1988). A process approach to neuropsychological assessment. *Aphasiology, 2*(3/4), 309–312. https://doi.org/10.1080/02687038808248930

Libon, D. J., Swenson, R., Ashendorf, L., Bauer, R. M., & Bowers, D. (2013). Edith Kaplan and the Boston process approach. *Clinical Neuropsychologist, 27*(8), 1223–1233. https://doi.org/10.1080/13854046.2013.833295

Mattlar, C., & Fried, R. (1993). The Rorschach in Finland. *Rorschachiana, 18*, 105–125. https://doi.org/10.1027/1192-5604.18.1.105

Médecins Sans Frontières. (2016). *Traumi Ignorati – Richiedenti Asilo in Italia: Un'indagine sul disagio mentale e l'accesso ai servizi sanitari territoriali* [*Ignored traumas – Asylum seekers in Italy: An investigation into mental distress and access to territorial healthcare services*]. https://archivio.medicisenzafrontiere.it/pdf/Rapp_Traumi_Ignorati_140716B.pdf

Meyer, G. J., Giromini, L., Viglione, D. J., Reese, J. B., & Mihura, J. L. (2015). The association of gender, ethnicity, age, and education with Rorschach scores. *Assessment, 22*(1), 46–64. https://doi.org/10.1177/1073191114544358

Moro, M. R. (1994). *Parents en exil: Psychopathologie et migrations* [*Parents in exile: Psychopathology and migrations*]. Presses Universitaires de France.

Moro, M. R. (1998). *Psychothèrapie transculturelle des enfants des migrants* [*Transcultural psychotherapy for children of migrants*]. Dunod.

Moro, M. R. (2000). *Seminario introduttivo alla clinica transculturale* [*Introductory seminar to transcultural consultation*]. Crinali Cooperativa Sociale Onlus. http://www.crinali.org/wp-content/uploads/2015/02/Introduzione-alla-clinica-transculturale.pdf

Naglieri, J. A., & Das, J. P. (2005). *Cognitive assessment system.* Giunti.

Nakamura, N., Fuchigami, Y., & Tsugawa, R. (2007). Rorschach comprehensive system data for a sample of 240 adult nonpatients from Japan. *Journal of Personality Assessment, 89*(Suppl. 1), 97–102. https://doi.org/10.1080/00223 890701583291

Noseda, C., & Bevilacqua, P. (2002). *Le difficoltà della valutazione multiculturale della personalità: Una ricerca sul livello di acculturazione in differenti gruppi etnici* [Issues in the multicultural assessment of personality: A research study on the acculturation levels in different ethnic groups]. (Publication No. 441127) [Master's thesis, Università Cattolica del Sacro Cuore]. Thesis/Dissertation Catalogue of the Università Cattolica del Sacro Cuore.

Oltolini, I., & La Mela, C. G. (2019). *Il disegno che racconta: L'assessment collaborativo con il WZT in situazione transculturale* [*The drawing that tells a story: Collaborative assessment with WZT in transcultural situations*] [Unpublished master's thesis]. Università degli Studi Guglielmo Marconi.

Orsini, A., & Picone, L. (2006). *Wechsler Intelligence Scale for Children – III*. Giunti.

Orsini, A., & Pezzuti, L. (2013). *Wechsler Adult Intelligence Scale – Fourth Edition*. Giunti.

Paniagua, F. A. (1998). *Assessing and treating culturally diverse clients: A practical guide* (2nd ed.). Sage.

Phinney, J. S. (1992). The Multigroup Ethnic Identity Measure: A new scale for use with diverse groups. *Journal of Adolescent Research, 7*(2), 156–176. https://doi.org/10.1177%2F074355489272003

Rorschach, H. (1942). *Psychodiagnostics: A diagnostic test based on perception* (3rd ed.). Hans Huber. (Original work published in 1921).

Stern, R. A., Singer, E. A., Duke, L. M., Singer, N. G., Morey, C. E., Daughtrey, E. W., & Kaplan, E. (1994). The Boston qualitative scoring system for the Rey-Osterrieth complex figure: Description and interrater reliability. *Clinical Neuropsychologist, 8*(3), 309–322. https://doi.org/10.1080/13854049408404137

Suarez-Morales, L., Dillon, F. R., & Szapocznik, J. (2007). Validation of the acculturative stress inventory for children. *Cultural Diversity and Ethnic Minority Psychology, 13*(3), 216–224. https://doi.org/10.1037/1099-9809.13.3.216

Swann, W. B., Stein-Seroussi, A., & Giesler, B. (1992). Why people self-verify. *Journal of Personality and Social Psychology, 62*(3), 392–401. https://doi.org/1 0.1037/0022-3514.62.3.392

Tribunale per i Minorenni di Milano e Procura della Repubblica presso il Tribunale per i Minorenni di Milano. (2018). *Bilancio di Responsabilità Sociale 2018* [*2018 Social Responsibility Report*]. http://www.ca.milano.giustizia.it/documentazione/D_17754.pdf

Wartegg, E. (1939). *Gestaltung und Charakter: Ausdrucksdeutung zeichnerischer Gestaltung und Entwurf einer charakterologischen Typologie* [*Form and character: Interpretation of expression from drawings and outline of a characterological typology*]. Verlag von Johann Ambrosius Barth.

Wartegg, E. (1953). *Schichtdiagnostik: Der Zeichentest (WZT): Einführung in die experimentelle Graphoskopie* [*Layered diagnosis: The Drawing Test (WZT): An introduction to experimental graphoscopy*]. Verlag Für Psychologie.

Wartegg, E. (1959). *Reattivo di disegno per la diagnostica degli strati della personalità: Manuale: Adattamento italiano* [*The use of drawings in the diagnosis of personality layers: Manual – Italian adaptation*]. Organizzazioni Speciali.

Wood, D., Bruner, J. S., & Ross, G. (1976). The role of tutoring in problem solving. *The Journal of Child Psychology, 17*, 89–100. https://doi.org/10.1111/j.1469-7610.1976.tb00381.x

Chapter 8

"Different Cultures Wear Different Shoes!" Therapeutic Assessment with a 17-Year-Old Immigrant Boy in the Netherlands

Hilde De Saeger and Inge Van Laer

In practicing Therapeutic Assessment (TA) over the past 10 years, we have worked with many different clients and their families. As has been said several times, you keep your TA clients with you. This is especially true for this Dutch Moroccan boy and his mom. TA helped them to find each other again as well as enlarged their hope and trust in the flexibility of human beings. At De Viersprong, a center for adults and adolescents with severe personality and conduct disorders in the Netherlands, we have several evidenced-based treatments. Although we operate in the larger cities of the Netherlands, only a minority of our client population has a non-Dutch, non-White ethnic background. The exception is the families who are referred by the court to get multi-system therapy and functional family therapy because of their behaviors which cause problems. The fact that we get few referrals is not unusual as only 5% of Moroccan adolescents find their way to mental health care vs. 9.3% of native Dutch adolescents (Tierolf et al., 2017). Research shows that there are several reasons for this phenomenon. First, the Moroccan culture is less action prone than the Dutch culture. In addition, there is fear about mental health care in general; the recognition of the problem is different and limited; and, last but not least, the expectations differ greatly towards mental health care. Distrust and negative experiences keep the Moroccan community at home (Tierolf et al., 2017). Mental health problems generally are not accepted in the Moroccan community—thus, they are more frequently expressed as physical complaints.

Since 2011, we have been using the TA model at De Viersprong to conduct our assessments. TA is a semi-structured model developed by Stephen Finn based on the early work by Constance Fischer (Fischer, 1985). The core value is a close collaboration between the assessor and the assessed in combination with respect, compassion, and openness (Finn, 2009). In Therapeutic Assessment with adolescents (TA-A), we try to encourage the parents to commit to the assessment because of the importance that both the adolescent and their system make a shift in their

DOI: 10.4324/9781003124061-12

existing story. TA-A starts with an initial session with the adolescent and the parents to strengthen the alliance with the multiple participants, who often have a hard time understanding each other. All the members are invited to formulate their own questions for the assessment. This initial session is followed by several test sessions, depending on the questions. In our centre, we use a variety of instruments, such as basic intelligence testing and screening and testing for developmental disorders, along with self-report and performance-based tests. After each test, we offer the extended inquiry in which both the adolescent and the parents are asked about their experience of the test and are invited to explain further questions the psychologist may have.

The next step is the assessment intervention session with the adolescent. This is often a more creative session in which hypotheses are checked by bringing the problem into the room and exploring some new, alternative behavior. It is followed by a session with the parents in which we check the same hypotheses to get some idea about their understanding of the problem. We focus on the interaction between the parents and the adolescent. Finally, we hold a summary/discussion session with the adolescent individually and then with the parents in which we discuss the answers to the assessment question. We then write letters to each participant (Finn 2007; Tharinger et al., 2013). Importantly, in the Netherlands we were in the past limited in the number of hours we could spend on an assessment, and this was the case in the assessment described below. For the same reason, we always work with only one assessor on a case, and that assessor works in close collaboration with their colleagues.

We are charmed by this model because it helps us and our clients to understand their dilemma of change[1] and the power of their maladaptive coping strategies. TA also gives words to the strengths and the flexibility of the family systems. This approach helps our clients discover their focus and need for therapy, it provides hope, and it helps to restore the epistemic trust that is so powerful in therapy (De Saeger et al., 2016; Kamphuis & Finn, 2019). Epistemic trust (ET) is "trust in the authenticity and personal relevance of interpersonally transmitted knowledge" (Fonagy & Allison, 2014). Needless to say, this degree of trust is extremely different when you have to rely on a community that differs greatly from your own and that has not always treated you respectfully. Some healthy mistrust is to be expected. This becomes even more complex when clients start to develop epistemic hypervigilance (EH) in reaction to their attachment trauma. We believe that TA can be of great use in the restoration of ET (see Kamphuis & Finn, 2019).

In working with clients with different ethnic backgrounds, Therapeutic Assessment has proved to be more useful than the traditional assessment model. Assessments with these clients are complex because the cultural factors must be checked continuously. The case conceptualization needs to be well-founded due to the different problem analyses and different understandings of behavior in different communities. These clients need an understandable explanation about the procedures and the tests. It is important to pay attention to the different health visions to deepen the understanding of the problem (Finn, 2007 Hoogsteder & Dias, 2017; Mercer, 2011; Tharinger et al., 2013).

Therapeutic Case Study

Referral and Phone Contact

A few years ago, Rayan,[2] a 17-year-old Moroccan boy, was referred to De Viersprong by his social worker. Rayan's social worker told the assessor she could not understand why Rayan was behaving badly, knowing that his mother was working hard to create a good life for her and her kids and trying to become integrated into and accepted in Dutch society. This meant Rayan's mother was in a constant fight against pre-conceptions about being Moroccan. Recently, Rayan had rejected every offer of help despite his suffering and the worries of his mother. To get a better understanding about what was going on and why previous help had not succeeded, his social worker referred him for an adolescent-focused TA.

Rayan was born in the Netherlands in a Moroccan family; both his parents were first-generation immigrants. It is important to note that although Rayan was born in the Netherlands, he is considered an immigrant and does not automatically acquire Dutch citizenship, but retains his Moroccan nationality. In Holland, there are strict government policies regarding foreigners attaining citizenship. Rayan had been in different kinds of therapy for 8 years because of behavioral problems and more recently more internalizing problems as well. He had received individual therapy, creative therapy, training to improve his social skills, and resilience training. In the past, he had had several psychological assessments, which included IQ testing and attention deficit assessment (ADHD testing). He was diagnosed with ADHD, which didn't feel right to him. For some reason, however, the problems kept on increasing; he became "locked in," became more and more disobliging, and became verbally aggressive. During the social worker's phone conversation with the assessor, Rayan was described as quickly irritated, impulsive, arrogant, and verbally aggressive, which could end up with him being vindictive. The way Rayan was described matched the stereotyped ideas that exist in West Europe—that Moroccan boys are aggressive, vindictive, and externalizing. Besides this aggressive attitude and behavior, Rayan's social worker also mentioned that Rayan felt rejected as soon as anyone gave him feedback. She mentioned low self-esteem, suicidal ideations, threats to commit suicide, and troubled relationships. At the time of the referral, everyone, including Rayan's family, was giving up on him, and he in return was giving up on himself and the world.

During the phone contact with Rayan's mother, the assessor could feel the mom's fear and despair. She told the assessor that Rayan was completely demoralized, that he was convinced he was a lost cause. He had lost all confidence in people wanting to help him, therapists in particular. In her description of Rayan, his mother mentioned a lot of what we would describe as epistemic hypervigilance in Rayan's attitude towards the world. Mother was exhausted, desperately looking for some kind of solution. She felt that she couldn't recognize her son anymore—he was slipping through her fingers. She felt ashamed about the behavior of her son and what it said about her "failure" as a mother. Although she agreed to the assessment, and expected Rayan would do the same, she did so not out of hope but out of guilt. The assessor felt that the mother felt she had to be the superior version of herself. At the same time, the assessor felt her own demoralization; what could she possibly offer that no one had already offered?

During the phone contact with Rayan, the assessor noticed that Rayan was kind and friendly but didn't talk much. Because the assessor knew about his demoralization, she didn't push Rayan too much and instead explained to him what TA was like and what he could expect. He agreed to make the appointments and assured her that he would show up.

Initial Session: Alliance and Assessment Questions

When the assessor met Rayan for the first time, she was surprised. Rayan was charming, open, made contact very easily, and had a big smile on his face. This was a huge difference from the assessor's expectations. Rayan did not meet the expectations of a 17-year-old troubled boy, and he did not at all present as the rejecting, suicidal, desperate boy described by his mother and the social worker. The assessor had expected him to be withdrawn, irritated, hypervigilant, not wanting to be there, and maybe aggressive and arrogant towards a female assessor. Apparently, the description of Rayan's problems activated stereotyped ideas in the assessor and made her feel a little hypervigilant herself. Although the assessor liked Rayan, she also struggled with the discrepancy and grew curious. She wondered: What was Rayan's reason for presenting himself in an open way with a big smile, knowing that he really didn't want to be there? Was Rayan's charming attitude a smokescreen, a way to hide and mislead the assessor, to "get away"? After all, he was quite experienced with therapy. She decided to write down the discrepancies and keep them in mind—to go slow and stay close to the "not-knowing stance." She planned to include Rayan and his mom in every interpretation and to check in with colleagues about her own "racial enactments." She fell back on her main values of staying emotionally attuned, being aware of any disruption, and being as transparent as needed.

To understand the health care history of Rayan, the assessor told Rayan what she knew and how she understood the information about his past therapies. She invited Rayan and his mother to tell their understanding of the past 8 years in mental health care. The assessor focused on Rayan's experience and tried to figure out his narrative about his sense of martyrdom. His mother helped him to remember all the different therapists. At the end, Rayan told the assessor he was done with all these people, saying they knew him and wanted the best for him. But, in reality, they all failed to make things better, just like his family, who had tried to start all over again a few times in their lives to achieve a better life. At this point, Rayan was describing his deep disappointment not only in mental health care but also in the entire society, thus confirming the hypothesis of elevated epistemic hypervigilance the assessor had formed.

The demoralization entered the room in the purest form it could be. Because of the family's deep disappointment in previous helpers, the assessor decided to be transparent in what she thought she had to offer. She told Rayan that it was not her intention to make him better, to repair him. Her only intention was to try to understand him and his mother and how things had ended up the way they were. The assessor gave them the opportunity to stop at any time they wished. Both of them were very clear they did not want to have a variety of therapies any more. The assessor was clear she wanted to give it a try but that she could only do this in collaboration.

Rayan was invited to formulate assessment questions, and he came up with one question:

1   How can I deal better with emotionally difficult situations?
     Rayan's mother had three questions:
2   How can I understand how we end up so frequently fighting or in conflict?
3   What can I do to help Rayan not get so angry?
4   What kind of therapy will help Rayan the most?
     Rayan agreed on only two questions different from everyone elses:
5   How can we understand my problems concentrating and being restless?
6   What kind of therapy would help me the most?

Next, the assessor discussed the question posed by Rayan's social worker. She wanted to know, how should we understand why Rayan is taking care of everyone but himself? Rayan was upset by this question as well as question #3 about his anger. He seemed to lose hope again and wanted to stop. The assessor took the time to explore Rayan's feelings about this question. Rayan told her that a lot of people around him seemed to think he couldn't take care of himself, but they didn't get it and that made him feel angry. This feeling of not being understood and "seen" seemed to be of great importance to him. Without completely understanding, the assessor decided to stay close to Rayan's feelings and checked to see if he was willing to modify this question in a way to make it useful to him. Rayan ended up with the following question:

Why do others think I'm neglecting myself?

By modifying this question and making it his own, Rayan was able to rejoin the assessor. For the second time, she was surprised as she had expected Rayan to reject the questions related to ADHD since he did not agree with this diagnosis. To her, the question about self-neglect felt positive, but Rayan seemed unaware of this aspect of it. This was also the first time she had heard that people found Rayan to be caring towards others. At the same time, she did feel the big disconnection between Rayan and the world.

The initial session ended with Rayan, mother, and the assessor looking back on the session. Rayan said he somehow had become curious about what kind of questionnaires and tests could possibly help to find answers to the questions. Rayan also wanted to know what the assessor was thinking about everything they had discussed before. The assessor decided to tell him she was surprised by his willingness to participate as well his curiosity and thanked him for wanting to work with her. For the assessor, it felt Rayan was moving towards an ambivalent state regarding the assessment. He wasn't yet rejecting her, and he even had gotten a little curious, but he was still cautious because of his previous experiences.

Test Sessions, Timeline, and Family Tree

In the next meeting, Rayan, his mother, and the assessor first discussed complementary reactions to the initial session to address any concerns and to check if they still felt all right with the questions. Rayan and his mother both felt understood during the previous session and were still feeling comfortable with the assessment questions, the way they were formulated and put on paper. Reassured by the words of Rayan and his mother, the assessor asked Rayan to complete the Minnesota Multiphasic Personality Inventory-Adolescent (MMPI-A; Butcher, 1992) after explaining to him that this questionnaire could give information about how he usually deals with emotions. It could offer some ideas towards answering Rayan's question as well as the question his mother formulated about the anger and the conflict between them. We carefully thought about his taking the MMPI-A and the Dutch norms. Rayan was verbally intelligent, he was born in the Netherlands, raised speaking both Moroccan and Dutch, and had always been in school. We did think about the different culture he lived in and how this could influence the results as there are not a lot of Moroccan boys in the norms. The MMPI-A manual (Archer, 2015) states that 20% of the normative group had a different ethnic background than the original standardization sample, which is comparable to the percentage in Dutch society.

After finishing the MMPI-A, the assessor invited Rayan to share with her how he had experienced completing the questionnaire. As many adolescents do, he told her that there were a lot of questions. Rayan responded that some of the test questions made sense and others were, as he put it, very strange. The assessor explored with him whether there were questions he felt ambivalent about. Rayan told her he found it difficult to make a choice between true or false for items that were about feeling comfortable among a group of people. He felt the need for more nuance in his answers.

Looking at the MMPI-A profile, the validity scales showed that he had taken the test honestly and seriously, with F-scale 51, TRIN 67 F, and VRIN 54. This not only gave the assessor some news about the test attitude but also about how Rayan was feeling about the proce-dure so far. The MMPI-A clinical scales showed an elevated scale 2 (Depression) with 85 as well as an elevated scale 1 (Dealing with physical complaints) with 81 and scale 3 (Suppression of pain) with 84. Without going into too much detail, Rayan revealed throughout the MMPI-A that he was feeling down most of the time as well as ex-periencing many physical complaints. He indicated physical complaints and health concerns that might be related to some psychological components, such as tension and discomfort, which was a little beyond what the assessor expected because of the rather low results on the F scale. It seemed that Rayan did not really make the connection with the burden inside of him. This code type often refers to clients who have learned to hide their negative emotions and avoid conflict in relationships. This way of coping with emotions must have been useful during earlier periods in his life. The backside of dealing with emotions this way is that depression is overlooked, that negative emotions keep being labeled as weak, and that physical complaints show that things are not okay. This MMPI-A profile gave the assessor a sense of what was going on. It gave her some empathy for the long history of ne-gative emotions that must be locked inside of Rayan, and it made her curious about why he had to keep up appearances. It also gave an understanding of the social worker's assessment question "How can we understand why Rayan is taking care of everyone except himself?" and why Rayan got so angry about this assessment question. It was still "level 25"[3] at this moment in the assessment.

While Rayan was completing the MMPI-A, his mother was asked to draw a family tree. When the assessor met the mother, she was wearing a headscarf, which was traditional in her culture, yet she also had a strong drive for equality between men and women. She spoke perfect Dutch and could handle both cultures in a collaborative way. The mother explained that she came to the Netherlands at the age of 3 together with her parents. Some years later, her parents brought her back to Morocco, where they left her. She was raised by her grandparents without having any contact with her parents, brothers, or sisters. When she turned 18, her parents brought her back to the Netherlands to take care of the younger children because a younger brother was behaving badly. Back in the Netherlands, she discovered her father's addiction to alcohol and drugs. Due to the addiction, there was a lot of aggression at home as well as financial problems. Mother said she felt ashamed as her father and brother met the stereotypes about Moroccan males. This conflicted with the traditional values she brought with her from her grandparents and her life in Morocco. She expected everything to be better in the Netherlands and found out that she had been misled by her parents.

Secretly, with help from a neighbor, she managed to learn Dutch, and after a lot of difficulties due to a lack of support from her family, she managed to go to school and get her first job as a translator. At the age of 21, her family arranged a marriage for her. She didn't want to give up the freedom she had been fighting for and contacted a Moroccan man she had met sometime before whom she thought her family would agree to. She asked whether he wanted to marry her, so at least she was in charge. This man became her first husband and Rayan's father. They had three children, of whom Rayan is the youngest (brother +3 and sister +7). History repeated itself; her husband became physically and verbally violent towards her and the children as the result of alcohol abuse. In addition, there were a lot financial problems as her husband refused to work. Despite her ethnic background and her role as a mother, she kept working as a medical secretary. When Rayan was 4, mother decided to divorce, although she was afraid of her family's reaction and the possibility that the family of Rayan's father could become vindictive. The divorce took about 6 years before it was finalized. During these 6 years, there were many conflicts that Rayan witnessed. Right after the official divorce, when Rayan was about 10 years old, his father abducted him to get back at the mother. After a few weeks trying to get her child back, mother informed the police, and they found Rayan severely neglected. This is about the time Rayan came into mental health care.

While the mother was describing these traumatic life events, the assessor noticed she expressed no emotion at all. When asked whether she recognized this observation, the mother told the assessor that this was the only way she could deal with all the bad things that had happened in her life. This seemed to be the same coping strategy the MMPI-A revealed about Rayan when he had to deal with emotional situations. Despite mother's detachment, the assessor felt deep respect for her and some connection.

After this period, at the age of 11, mother decided to marry a new man. Mother herself described her second marriage as another escape. She knew about the poverty single mothers had to deal with and wanted a better future for her children. (In the Netherlands, 15% of Moroccans live in one-parent families. Research shows that 16% of Moroccans living in the Netherlands have severe financial problems, and in the slipstream children of single mothers develop more conduct and emotional problems [Colpin et al., 2000].) Mother met her husband in Morocco. They had known each other from their youth. He told her he had always been in love with her, and she felt the opportunity to start all over again. She felt protected from her ex-husband, who was threatening her and the children. From the start, Rayan and his stepfather had a troubled relationship. Rayan did not accept the new father figure in his life. He was afraid that the new man in the family would be aggressive as well, so he felt the need to protect his family against this danger.

When Rayan was 14, his biological father suddenly left for Morocco without saying goodbye. Since then he has had no contact at all with his father or extended family in the Netherlands. Rayan is very upset and angry with his father's disappearance and abandonment. Mother thinks Rayan is projecting all his anger about his father onto his stepfather. Because of the troubled relationship between Rayan and his stepfather, mother decided that Rayan did not have to help in the family business despite the expectations in their community, where it is very common that children start working in the family business once they are old enough. Instead, she wanted Rayan to study hard to get a university degree so he could have a better and easier life than she had. The traumatic events mother talked about, like the abandonment by her parents, the prohibition against learning Dutch and going to school, the expectation of an arranged marriage, and Rayan's abduction were related to culture and did raise a lot of questions. Although the assessor was trained in using her curiosity by asking questions and trying to get in mother's shoes, she also noticed afterwards she had been more hesitant than she would have been with a Dutch family. After completing the family tree, mother was asked to complete some questionnaires to screen Rayan for ADHD criteria. The results showed few signs specifically suggesting ADHD. No criteria were met for hyperactivity, nor for attention problems. The only thing mother did endorse was Rayan's restlessness.

The assessor reviewed this information and thought carefully about various hypotheses. She started thinking about trauma and anxiety, which had not been mentioned anywhere, as well as the same coping strategy that mother and Rayan used in which they hid their negative emotions by always looking on the bright side of life, working hard, and taking care of others. She decided to introduce a performance-based test, expecting this would help to gather information about Rayan's coping strategies as well as his strengths. Because of time limitations, she decided to do only the Rorschach.

In the next session, the Rorschach was introduced and administered according to the R-PAS system (Meyer et al., 2011). When he was being introduced to the Rorschach, Rayan told the assessor that it seemed like a really strange test to him. The assessor agreed with him and told him she could definitely understand his feeling since she had had the same kind of feeling several years ago when she had been introduced to the Rorschach. So, the assessor decided to share with Rayan the doubts she had herself about the Rorschach when she was asked to get trained in it. She told him that, ever since then, she had respected this test more and more because every time she noticed that the information the Rorschach revealed was very useful. In fact, this test had become one of her favorites. The assessor noticed her self-disclosure was appreciated by Rayan. After finishing the Rorschach, Rayan was asked (among other questions) if there might be some answers that had crossed his mind but he had not verbalized. The following exchange ensued, with the assessor being careful to take half steps:

Rayan: There was one indeed on this card. [He pointed to card X.]
Assessor: Do you want to share your response with me about that card?
Rayan: That card makes me think I am standing alone in the middle with all the others standing around me. I don't like that much.
Assessor: You don't like that much?
Rayan: All those people are looking at me. It makes me feel uncomfortable because they might see what's going on inside of me.
Assessor: Oh, that sounds uncomfortable indeed. What I often hear from teenagers I'm working with is that most of the time they're quite inventive and have their own tricks to deal with this kind of uncomfortable situation. Is that something you recognize in yourself?
Rayan: Maybe some kind of wall?
Assessor: Maybe some kind of wall, and what does this wall look like for you?
Rayan: I don't know. I do know I push other people away.
Assessor: You push other people away?!?

Rayan: By being angry, maybe aggressive sometimes ...
Assessor: So being angry, aggressive, sometimes helps you to build a wall that keeps others away so they can't see what's going on inside of you?
Rayan: Yeah, may be ...

Next, the assessor asked Rayan to draw a timeline and write down all the important moments in his life to get a better understanding of why this wall needed to be there and to get a glimpse of what was behind the wall. The things Rayan pointed out were a good childhood, his parents' fighting, the new marriage of his mother, and the abandonment by his father. He just touched on the abduction, and he did not mention the addiction. In discussing his timeline, Rayan told the assessor he had a good childhood, although he was often frightened by the yelling downstairs between his parents. His mother used the words "playing rough" instead of "fighting" to describe what was going on downstairs. Although Rayan was the youngest sibling, most of the time he was the one who went downstairs in an effort to intervene and make his parents stop fighting. He spoke very briefly about the abduction by his father and then switched to the time his mother married his stepfather. He said he had never liked his stepfather because he only paid attention to Rayan when he needed him to help in the family business. This made him feel not accepted and understood by his stepfather. Rayan said he felt abandoned by his father. When he was telling this, he realized that this must have been about the time he started getting angry and verbally aggressive and developed an arrogant attitude. He wrote down the word "wall" on his timeline. At that moment, Rayan told the assessor he was tired. Although the assessor still had a lot of questions, she decided to listen to Rayan and not push too much because he had worked tremendously hard, and she remembered from his responses on the MMPI-A self-report measure that his being tired was probably a reflection of his being emotionally overwhelmed and possibly feeling ashamed as well.

Results of the Rorschach indicated that Rayan was a sensitive boy who was able to notice nuances and subtle details (elevated perception of small, unusual details, Dd%), which could help explain why Rayan was always the first one who noticed there was something going on between his parents. Rayan was interested in connections with others and saw relationships as potentially supportive and collaborative (elevated Cooperative Movement, COP, and Mutuality of Autonomy Health, MAH). There appeared to be a somewhat egocentric presentation (elevated Card Turnings and Reflection responses), which matched the arrogant attitude described by Rayan's social worker and his mother. Rayan seemed to cope by spontaneously, maybe even impulsively, reacting to and interacting with the world (low Human Movement

Proportion, M/MC), which often resulted in the conflicts and fights mother had described in her assessment question. The R-Pas gave us more "personality in action." It revealed a part of Rayan that had not been seen in the assessment before. It helped make the assessor understand that his gentle and kind presentation was not just socially desirable behavior. This was a strength as well as a characteristic that was important to Rayan because he liked to help and take care of other people and was good at it as well. This, combined with Rayan's sensitivity and his spontaneity and, at times, his impulsive reactions to what is going on around him can result in anger, which is expressed in an aggressive and arrogant attitude. Rayan's behavior seems to distract other people; he seems to serve as the ideal lightning rod.

Assessment Intervention Session

In preparing for the assessment intervention session, the team discussed an intervention that could help Rayan better understand the function of his "wall" because the hypotheses at that moment were that his wall could protect him from experiencing negative emotions (Rayan's question) and could avoid or decrease family conflict and fights (question form the social worker about Rayan taking care of everyone). Besides having a better understanding of his behavior, the team hoped that Rayan could also become more compassionate towards himself. They came up with the idea of asking Rayan to show how each individual in his family was related to him. In his arrogant stance, he might put some people far away, the ones who annoyed him. We hoped to help him understand how important they were to him, how he was devoted to them, and how much this perspective might cost him.

When the assessor met with Rayan for the assessment intervention session, she asked if he had anything to add to the previous session since that had seemed a pretty heavy session. Once again, he gave her a big smile and he told her that he felt really tired after that session and got curious about the wall they had discussed together in the previous session. She asked him if he was willing to continue the search for what was behind his wall, which he agreed to. She asked him to write down the names of his family members on cups and place them on the table in a way that felt good to him. As the assessor expected, Rayan took a cup for himself, mother, stepfather, sister, sister's daughter (his niece), and brother. He chose not to mention the ex-husband of his sister because they had got divorced recently and Rayan felt her ex-husband had failed in his role as a father and husband. As he had told us during the extended inquiry of the Rorschach, he put himself in the center with everyone around him with more or less distance between them. Rayan said he was very sensitive to what others felt, which was consistent with the results of the Rorschach and what he wrote down on his timeline. He disclosed he didn't like the feeling of two people being in conflict, so quite often he tried to fix it, but as he was the youngest he had no idea how to achieve this. Most of the time this ended up with him being angry and/or arrogant and, in doing so, taking away the focus on the distress between the others and becoming the problem himself. He discovered that in order to help others he became a problem not only for himself but also for others.

As Rayan discovered all these insights by himself, something started to shift. Rayan looked at the assessor and asked if he could take a cup for his biological father as well. The assessor told him it was his choice. He did so, and he put his father on the edge of the little table in between them. He said that it didn't feel right. He took the cup and placed it somewhere else in the room because that was the place his father "deserved." The assessor asked Rayan what this was like for him. Rayan said he didn't care, again with his lovely big smile. The assessor decided to tell Rayan she didn't believe him. Rayan looked surprised and maybe a little shocked. She explained why she didn't believe him. During the assessment, she had gotten to know him as someone who had had a rough time. But despite this, he was also looking for someone he could trust, someone who paid attention to him and found him worthwhile. She truly could not believe that Rayan just didn't care about his father, who had left him and was living his life without looking back. She told him she did not believe the arrogant "I don't give a shit" attitude. When she explained this to him, she saw he was touched. The big smile on his face disappeared, and tears were visible in his eyes. Rayan could hear the information and was able to open up to it. The assessor gave him some time to process this. After a while, he asked whether they could show the representation of his family on the table to his mother. He felt it was important to share it with her. Rayan himself proposed taking the next step planned in a therapeutic assessment with adolescents!

Because mother and the assessor had worked intensively together in the previous sessions, the assessor hoped mother would be able to take in all this new information. Rayan himself started to explain that he had discovered that he is sensitive to conflicts between family members. When this happens he feels terrible, which makes him start acting out because he doesn't know what to do else, but he desperately needs it to stop. Last but not the least, he told his mom how complicated things were with his father, how he felt angry and abandoned. They both took the time to sit with this new information, a little sad but also excited. Then, Rayan's mother told him she recognized herself in his story. She was also very sensitive, with the difference that she did not act out like Rayan when she felt nothing was helping to solve the conflict or tension between family members. Her strategy was to keep trying to talk to each one of them and look for some openings so they would talk to each other again, but she got completely detached from herself so that others could not feel her emotions anymore and thought she didn't care.

This recognition by his mother was incredibly helpful to Rayan. It not only confirmed the new narrative Rayan had just created in that session, but it also changed mother's narrative about Rayan's behavior as well. She finally started to understand Rayan's anger and aggressive/arrogant attitude as his way to decrease family conflict. She could look at him with more compassion than before. She could see he was taking another way of dealing with the same painful situation, and Rayan could understand his mom in her rational way of dealing with all the difficulties. Because of all the work the two of them had done during this session, their new narrative about how Rayan dealt with emotional situations, and the link with the regular fights, anger, and conflicts at home, the assessor decided not to plan a family intervention session but to organize the summary/discussion session.

Summary/Discussion Session

During the summary/discussion session, the assessor asked Rayan and his mother if they had any idea about possible answers to their assessment questions. The two of them could answer all the questions by themselves. The only question they needed help with was the question about what type of therapy would be helpful. They said it felt really important to them that the other family members got to know this new narrative, so they asked whether they could get support during therapy to help the others understand this new narrative. The assessor agreed to this with a big smile, feeling proud of both of them.

Reflection

Looking back on this assessment, the cultural differences made this TA even more challenging than usual. Although the assessor was an experienced TA assessor who respected the TA values greatly (curiosity, transparency, respect, etc.), she discovered that she also got stuck in her Western European values and prejudices. She expected her views to be greatly different from Rayan and his mom, and instead of asking questions and being curious, she kept silent. When the assessor and mother completed the family tree, the assessor realized that she hadn't invited Rayan's father nor his stepfather to the assessment, although she normally puts a lot of effort into trying to commit all parents and stepparents to the assessment. Apparently, she intuitively followed her idea that in Moroccan families the mothers take care of their children, and she was afraid of not being able to start the assessment if she insisted on seeing Rayan's father by videoconference and/or Rayan's stepfather in person.

She found out later that Moroccan society aims much more at a "we" culture than Western culture. In Western culture, children are taught psychological values in which well-being is the highest good. Individuality is above the community. In a "we" culture, togetherness is the most important thing, responsibilities are shared, and the individuals derive their strength from the contributions they make to the community. The task of children in Western culture is to be happy; in a "we" culture the task of children is to make others happy and the focus is material and not psychological because they have to work with the others to ensure that the group survives.

In the Netherlands, there are few concentrated Moroccan communities. This means that families are apt to be integrated into the broader Dutch community. However, a person's challenge of integration exists in a context where one's immigration status is still one of an outsider. Rayan's mother imported some of the Moroccan but also some of the Dutch values and norms, and they changed over time. Rayan shared some of these values but changed some of them and even rejected some of them. It was important for the assessor to be aware of her own values and norms and her own preconceptions about Moroccan people and immigrant families and to be open to the personalized values and norms of Rayan and his mother. She learned that true transparency and true curiosity is asking, sharing, and being in the not-knowing stance.

The main goal during TA is to try to make a shift in the existing story of the adolescent and his parents. Looking back at this TA, Rayan and his mother succeeded in making this shift, but that wasn't without consequences. Rayan and his mother made this shift together, which brought them closer to each other. After the assessment intervention session, they both told the assessor they thought the rest of the family should learn the information as well in order to have an understanding of what was going on. They decided they would like some family sessions to talk together. The consequence was they all had to be willing to talk with each other about mental health, acknowledging that Rayan was feeling sad instead of just behaving badly.

This was very different from what they were used to in their family as well as in their community. By proposing talking about mental health problems with their family, they took the risk of being rejected by their family and/or community. Not only did this mean they could lose their connection with them, but being part of a minority and not being accepted by other members of this minority could make them very alone and vulnerable. So, the shift in their existing story was one step. Trying to make this shift together with their family was another step, with risks that needed a lot of attention. Rayan and his mother tried to invite their family to talk about Rayan's behavior. Despite their efforts, his stepfather and brother tried it once but decided it wasn't helping at all and never showed up again. Rayan, his mother, and his sister continued with some therapy that helped Rayan not to feel alone anymore and gave him the opportunity to open up a little bit more about what he was feeling.

Notes

1 The dilemma of change is the way clients keep on doing the same things over and over again because they perceive all alternative ways as more painful (Finn 2007).
2 The client name and all potentially identifying information have been altered to protect the client's identity.
3 By level 25, we mean that this information is seriously conflicting with the way the client thinks about themselves, a lot more than the level 3 Finn writes about. The questions are often anxiety provoking for clients and mobilizes their defense mechanisms (Finn, 2007).

References

Archer, R. P. (2015). *Using the MMPI with adolescents.* Routledge.

Butcher, J. N. (1992). *Minnesota multiphasic personality inventory-adolescent.* University of Minnesota Press.

Colpin, H., Vandemeulebroecke, G., & De Munter, A. (2000). Opvoeding in ee-noudergezinnen. Een overzicht van de onderzoeksliteratuur [Education in single-parent families. An overview of the research literature]. *TOKK: Tijdschrift voor Orthopedagogiek, Kinderpsychiatrie en Klinische Kinderpsychologie, 25*(1), 31–44.

De Saeger, H., Bartak, A., Eder, E. E., & Kamphuis, J. H. (2016). Memorable experiences in therapeutic assessment: Inviting the patient's perspective following a pretreatment randomized controlled trial. *Journal of Personality Assessment, 98*(5), 472–479.

Finn, S. E. (2009). The many faces of empathy in experiential, person-centered, collaborative assessment. *Journal of Personality Assessment, 91*(1), 20–23.

Finn, S. E. (2007). *In our clients' shoes: Theory and techniques of therapeutic assessment.* Routledge.

Fischer, C. T. (1985). *Individualizing psychological assessment.* Laurence Erlbaum Associates.

Fonagy, P., & Allison, E. (2014). The role of mentalizing and epistemic trust in the therapeutic relationship. *Psychotherapy, 51*(3), 372.

Hoogsteder, M., & Dias, E. B. (2017). Diagnostiek bij patiënten met een migratieachtergrond [Diagnostics in patients with a migration background]. *GZ-Psychologie, 9*(6), 16–21.

Kamphuis, J. H., & Finn, S. E. (2019). Therapeutic assessment in personality disorders: Toward the restoration of epistemic trust. *Journal of Personality Assessment, 101*(6), 662–674.

Mercer, B. L. (2011). Psychological assessment of children in a community mental health clinic. *Journal of Personality Assessment, 93*(1), 1–6

Meyer, G. J., Erard, R. E., Erdberg, P., Mihura, J. L., & Viglione, D. J. (2011). *Rorschach performance assessment system: Administration, coding, interpretation, and technical manual.* Rorschach Performance Assessment Systems.

Tharinger, D. J., Gentry, L. B., & Finn, S. E. (2013). Therapeutic assessment with adolescents and their parents: A comprehensive model. In D. H. Saklofske, V. L. Schwean, & C. R. Reynolds (Eds.), *The Oxford handbook of child psychological assessment* (pp. 385–420). Oxford University Press.

Tierolf, B., Steketee, M., Gilsing, R., & Bellaart, H. (2017). Leefomstandigheden van kinderen met een migratieachtergrond [Living conditions of children with migration background]. Kennisplatform Integratie & Rayanenleving.

Chapter 9

Psychological Assessment of South Sudanese Persons in Mental Health Treatment in the United States

John Chuol Kuek

The South Sudanese Context

South Sudanese persons, children and adults, are now some of the most displaced persons in the world because of continuing political and social upheaval in the Republic of South Sudan. The United Nations Refugee Agency 2020) estimated that there are 4.3 million South Sudanese citizens now living in other parts of the world, including the United States and Australia. Most of these persons are political refugees who cannot return to their homeland because of political persecution. Many of the families who have fled South Sudan are incomplete or broken families that have lost a parent, the mother or father, and children. A look into the internal politics of the Republic of South Sudan since the country's establishment in 2011 indicates that many persons who fought for a democratic form of government have disappeared or been murdered. The primary purpose of this chapter is to introduce mental health professionals to the mental health needs of South Sudanese persons who are now residing in countries such as the United States and to traditional healing mechanisms or transpersonal elements in the culture that have been helping those with psychological illnesses recover. As with many previous immigrant and refugee groups that have come to this country in the past, there is an absence of research on the mental health needs of the South Sudanese. In this chapter, I focus on key assessment issues and therapy approaches when working with South Sudanese in clinical mental health settings.

Persons of South Sudanese background, both immigrants and US-born, are one of the newest groups seeking mental health services in the United States and other developed countries (Kuek, 2012). Throughout this country, for example, an increasing number of South Sudanese are entering the mental health system for assistance related to past trauma experienced in their homeland and in their journey to the United States. They are seeking services for many unresolved issues related to being displaced refugees in other African countries, emotional hardships experienced while immigrating, loss of family members along the way,

DOI: 10.4324/9781003124061-13

separation from kinships and community, problems in adjusting to life in the United States (or other countries), and issues related to family life, including intergenerational distress (Kuek, 2015).

In the United States, there are growing South Sudanese communities in Des Moines, Iowa, Detroit, Michigan, and San Diego, California, and other cities, and in each of these communities these persons are in desperate need of culturally and linguistically competent mental health services. South Sudanese persons, like persons from other cultural, racial, and ethnic minority backgrounds, especially immigrants and refugees, present with many *Diagnostic and Statistical Manual of Mental Disorders* (5th ed.; DSM-5; American Psychiatric Association, 2013) disorders. Unfortunately, although this has not yet been empirically documented, it is anecdotally reported that a majority present with disorders related to severe traumatic experiences. Being one of the most recent groups to immigrate to this country, and because South Sudan only came into existence as a sovereign country in 2011, there is limited research on the impact of ongoing civil war, interethnic violence, political and religious persecution, and terrorism on the population. Yet, the small body of research on the prevalence of mental disorders in South Sudan post-2011 does suggest that a significant proportion of the population, both children and adults, has experienced many incidents of trauma during their lifetime (Kuek, 2012). For the majority of those who have fled their homeland to seek a better life, including those coming to the United States, these refugees and migrants come with "active" cases of trauma that present in the form of post-traumatic stress disorder (PTSD), mood disorders, anxiety, substance abuse, and other more severe disorders (Lien et al., 2016).

Trauma-Informed Treatment

> One of the ongoing problems in the South Sudanese community is post-traumatic stress disorder (PTSD), which is often not discussed openly, but it is a significant issue when it comes to wellbeing of family and community.
>
> —Abur & Mphande (2020, p. 10)

It is my contention that trauma must be considered at the beginning of treatment and during the "assessment phase" for all South Sudanese persons. In the following pages, I discuss some of the literature that examines the extent of trauma in the South Sudanese population and how it presents itself through formal diagnostic categories. By logical extension and clinical observation in the United States, it is evident that persons who have been affected by the ongoing civil strife in South Sudan did not leave their trauma "behind" in their homeland or in a third country on the way to the United States. That is, for many South Sudanese, the trauma of experiencing war and atrocities remains just as real today as the day they actually experienced a traumatic event. For others, they come to this country having experienced multiple traumatic incidents that have piled on top of each other only to overwhelm them psychologically.

Researchers such as Ayazi and colleagues (see Ayazi et al., 2013; Ayazi et al., 2015), who are the most notable researchers on the impact of civil war post-2011 in South Sudan, have primarily documented the presence of PTSD in their studies on the prevalence of mental disorders. Based on their findings over a series of studies, one can conclude that PTSD appears to be the "signature disorder" for this population in South Sudan and by extension for the many persons who have fled their country. Moreover, in therapy, South Sudanese persons are more likely to focus on the traumatic event or incident that occurred in their homeland that has drastically changed their life. For many, the trauma experienced in South Sudan was continuous from day to day, with no moments of respite in order to heal. For others, the trauma has been inescapable and is related to witnessing death and mutilation, rape and sexual assault, death threats and coercion, destruction of property, and kidnapping, as in the case of the "lost boys" and "lost girls" of South Sudan (see Bowles, 2010).

Oftentimes, there is a "disconnect" between South Sudanese persons who have experienced trauma in their homeland and their children who were born in countries such as the United States. That is, US-born children may not understand, or want to understand, the trauma and lingering pain experienced by their parents. They may want to ignore or minimize their parent's experience for many reasons, including not having to "relive" the trauma or have it affect their lives. For other children, they may be experiencing historical or "intergenerational" trauma that passes from one generation to another. That is, they may be highly affected by their parents' experience in their homeland to the point that their empathy also affects them. This can include having feelings of despair, hopelessness, and worthlessness. Of course, it is important to note that this trauma may not be reflective only of the post-2011 years but may also go back to the European colonization of South Sudan and most of Africa and how colonization breaks people (see Memmi, 1991).

In addition, these authors have witnessed an additional condition that has yet to be included in the DSM-5 classification system but that is very real for many South Sudanese who are displaced within, or outside of, their homeland. This condition, discussed by Keller et al. (2017) in relation to Central American refugees, is "prolonged grief disorder."

It is important to note that leaving one's homeland, whether as a child or an adult, does not automatically cure one of mental health problems that began back home. For example, Keller et al. (2017) examined the pre-migration trauma experience of 234 persons from Guatemala, El

Salvador, and Honduras seeking refuge/asylum at the United States border and found that 83% cited violence as the primary reason for leaving their homeland. More importantly, the researchers found that 32% of these persons met the diagnostic criteria for PTSD, 24% for depression, and 17% for both disorders simultaneously. Although the historical and political experiences differ significantly between these countries and South Sudan, it is clear that persons living in countries with extreme violence and war are likely to develop significant negative psychological outcomes such as PTSD.

In addition, prolonged grief disorder (PGD), while not included in the DSM-5, is likely to be present in South Sudanese persons who seek out mental health services. Heeke et al. (2017) studied persons in Columbia who experienced either direct trauma or a loss from armed conflict in that country. They defined this condition as "a maladaptive reaction to loss ... marked by separation distress, feelings of emptiness, and difficulties moving on over a period of at least 6 months" (p. 2). They observed that "while PTSD is characterized by intrusions of the even, avoidance of reminders of the event, and persistent symptoms of increased arousal, the dominant element in PGD is separation distress in relation to the lost person" (p. 2). Muller et al. (2017) studied interethnic violence and its impact on children in South Sudan and found that high numbers of children throughout the country had experienced the loss of at least one parent and were in one-parent households, with extended family, or under the care of a non-governmental organization. We contend that, in addition to PTSD, many South Sudanese persons who are seeking mental health treatment in the United States and other countries may be presenting with PGD singularly or in combination with PTSD.

Arrival of the South Sudanese in the United States: Origins

Estimates suggest that over 100,000 South Sudanese persons have settled in the United States, especially over the past 20 years. Their main reason for coming to the United States, as well as to other Western countries such as Australia and Canada and neighboring countries in Africa, has to do with the continuing civil war in South Sudan. In December 2011, South Sudan gained its independence from the greater Republic of Sudan. Unfortunately, the transition into nationhood was bloody and full of false promises about democracy, unity, and freedom. Almost one decade later, the country remains torn by a war that is largely tribal and interethnic and manipulated by the country's leadership (see Breidlid, 2014; Christopher, 2011; Johnson, 2016; Jok, 2011; Leonardi, 2013; LeRiche & Arnold, 2013; Thomas, 2015).

It is sad to say that actions, both internal and international, taken toward peace and reconciliation have ended with no resolution and instead have resulted in heightened political, social, and economic oppression (see Kuek et al., 2014). Moreover, persons who do not support the current government are psychologically tortured through displacement from their ancestors' lands, including the confiscation of land, cattle, and other possessions (Kuek, 2015). Others are jailed, exiled, tortured, or simply disappear from their community or village (see Johnson, 2016; Leonardi, 2013).

Today, the United Nations Refugee Agency website, from the United Nations High Commissioner for Refugees, reports that while South Sudan has a population of over 11 million persons, there are 4.3 million South Sudanese persons, including refugees and asylum-seekers, outside of South Sudan. Over 1.5 million South Sudanese reside in the neighboring countries in Africa, with the majority in Uganda and Sudan. More startling is that 63% of these persons are children or minors who face many hardships due to broken families, poor education, limited medical care, housing instability, and famine. According to 2020 statistics from the United Nations Refugee Agency, almost 300,000 persons, or 67,000 households, are considered "refugees" within the country, with 82% of this group being women and children. Sadly, many of these persons are likely to migrate in search of a stable and healthy life within South Sudan or across many countries. Ameresekere and Henderson (2012a) observed that "mental health is significantly important for South Sudan as the majority of the population has been exposed to high rates of violence, displacement, and political and social insecurity" (p. 4). The fortunate few may end up in a country like the United States, where access to mental health services is more likely to be available.

There is no doubt that the immigrants from South Sudan, like those from other recent war-torn countries such as Iraq, Somalia, and Afghanistan, come to this country with significant "psychological baggage" that remains unresolved and interferes with all aspects of daily living, from relationships to work. This "baggage" impacts their ability to manage the stress associated with adjusting to life in this country as well their coping skills and psychological well-being. It also affects their ability to be resilient and manage the many challenges of daily living in their new country (Kuek, 2012). Moreover, unresolved problems related to trauma that evolve from acute to chronic states become more difficult for the mental health professional to treat.

As will be discussed shortly, research has been conducted in South Sudan regarding the prevalence of mental disorders, especially trauma and PTSD. This research, while limited, does suggest that a large proportion of the South Sudanese population has developed trauma, from mild to severe and acute to chronic, because of the continuing violence and aggression in their country. A systematic review of the research literature in the United States indicates no studies on the presence of trauma or PTSD in persons of South Sudanese background. The few studies that exist are in the form of doctoral dissertations and have limited visibility (Bowles, 2010; Jal, 2016; Jaysane-Darr, 2014; Tutlam, 2017; Yoon, 2019). A review of these studies indicates that while all focused on particular aspects of South Sudanese subgroups' adjustment to living in the United States, none focused on direct mental health assessment or treatment. Thus, one has to look at the research conducted in South Sudan and extend those findings to persons who immigrate to the United States.

Mental Health Problems of South Sudanese Persons: Empirical Research in South Sudan

A review of the literature indicates that the majority of the studies that have been conducted on the mental health status of South Sudanese citizens focus on the presence of mental disorders or symptoms in the population. That is, the studies are epidemiological in nature and use tools that are specifically designed to assess and identify certain mental disorders or conditions (e.g., the Harvard Trauma Questionnaire). For example, Ayazi et al. (2012) found that out of 1,200 persons living in South Sudan in their sample, 28% met the diagnostic criteria for PTSD and 6.4% for depression. They also found that 9.5% met the criteria for co-morbid PTSD and depression. In a different study, Ayazi et al. (2016) found that up to 23% of their sample reported "psychotic-like experiences" as reactions to traumatic events. In 2014, Ayazi, Lien, Eide, Swartz, et al. found in a large sample that 5.5% met the criteria for generalized anxiety disorder and 3.1% for panic disorder, again reactions to experiencing traumatic life events. Roberts et al. (2009), prior to South Sudanese independence in 2011, found in their sample that up to 36% of South Sudanese persons met the criteria for PTSD and 50% for depression.

In a study prior to South Sudan's independence, Baron (2002) examined the mental health status of persons from South Sudan in long-term exile in Uganda and found family breakdown, suicide, "excessive family responsibility," and "no future possibilities" as mental health problems for this group. That is, South Sudanese identified these problems as significant stressors that caused not only worry but also trauma and psychological maladjustment. Adaku et al. (2016) also studied South Sudanese refugees in Northern Uganda and found that "overthinking," ethnic conflict, and child abuse were identified as mental health problems by their sample. Ng et al. (2017) found that up to 40.7% of a total sample of 1,525 persons in South Sudan, with 20% from Juba, qualified for PTSD. They also found that 40% of the sample had been forced to leave their home or had witnessed seeing their property destroyed by other tribes or government soldiers, which caused much trauma. Moreover, they observed, "Mental health patients [in South Sudan] are often neglected or imprisoned" (p. 56).

Ayazi, Lien, Eide, Shador, et al. (2014), in a study on the "stigma" of being labeled mentally ill, reported that up to 80% of a sample of 1,200 South Sudanese adults believed that persons with mental illness were dangerous and should be generally isolated from the rest of society. These findings suggested an interesting contradiction: persons who may be traumatized by continued civil arrest and are labeled as mentally ill are likely to be scorned and avoided by fellow South Sudanese. Persons from rural settings, with lower levels of education, believed that these persons were more likely to suffer from spirit possession than traumatic events.

Courtney et al. (2017) studied a sample of 1,058 members of the South Sudanese People's Liberation Army for HIV prevalence and behavioral risk factors, primarily in Bilfam, Mogiri, and JIU, which are communities in Juba. The researchers found that the sample, primarily made up of men, had a 5% infection rate for HIV. Regarding mental health status, 23% met the diagnostic criteria for PTSD, 15.3% for depression, and 37.4% for alcohol dependence.

Janowski, Wessels, Boj, Monday, Maloney, Achut, and Ward (2020) found that evidence-based parenting programs, especially for children who had lost one or both parents in the civil conflict, served to strengthen the resilience of these children since many had symptoms of depression, helplessness, and trauma. They found that engaging children in storytelling promoted the healing process in children, especially those with PTSD. Jordans et al. (2013) found that while mental health services were rare in South Sudan, those children who did participate in counseling were not only engaged in treatment but also motivated to increase their well-being and manage trauma, including parental loss.

In a 2018 editorial, Majok labeled the mental health situation in South Sudan as a "ticking time bomb" and noted that the South Sudanese populace was in dire need not only of mental health services but also of systems that would immediately address this need. Majok noted that the populace likely suffered from high rates of depression, anxiety, schizophrenia, and PTSD because of ongoing chronic stress due to war, violence, and aggression. Majok warned that the constant stress experienced by South Sudanese, with no period of healing or mental health assistance, made for potentially higher rates of mental illness and maladjustment in the population, including chronic trauma, substance abuse, suicide, and even psychosis. Sadly, Singh and Singh (2014) found only two practicing psychiatrists in the country of South Sudan.

Strohmeier et al. (2018), in a study on the mental health status of humanitarian workers in South Sudan, concluded that between 2015 and 2016 the country was the most dangerous country for such workers because of the high emotional toll of their work. The researchers assessed 277 workers, mostly in Juba, and found that 24% met the diagnostic criteria for PTSD, 39% for depression, and 38% for anxiety. Moreover, 24% met the criteria for high burn-out. Of note, South Sudanese humanitarian workers were more likely to report greater levels of maladjustment than those from foreign countries, suggesting that "empathy" possessed by those from the homeland is likely to take a larger toll. There is no doubt that many of these workers, while not mental health professionals, attempted to cope in the best manner possible yet developed significant emotional and behavioral problems, including alcohol abuse.

Mental Health Problems Unique to the South Sudanese: Culture-Defined Syndromes

Ventevogel et al. (2013) conducted a landmark study in four communities impacted by civil strife in Africa, including South Sudan. Using various methods of data collection, including focus groups and interviews, the re-searchers outlined a set of mental health problems or syndromes that are unique to the South Sudanese in Kwajena Payam and Yei. In their study, Ventevogel et al. (2013) identified the "cultural syndromes" that have existed in these communities over time and are not associated with Western DSM-type conditions. While not going into detail about each of the syndromes, the authors did identify and describe basic aspects or behaviors related to these conditions. These conditions are present not only in communities in South Sudan but are likely to be present in South Sudanese living in the United States. That is, mental health professionals should expect South Sudanese persons presenting for mental health services to describe their "existential crises" related to trauma, including leaving home due to force or violence, through culture-defined concepts such as the following.

Moul is a syndrome related to aggressive behavior and is frequently accompanied by bizarre ideas and thoughts. In addition, Ng et al. (2017) described persons with *Moul* as aggressive, wandering naked, and de-stroying objects.

Wehie arenjo is a syndrome that reflects a "destroyed mind" and suggests that the person has lost a sense of purpose and meaning in life, with sadness, apathy, and isolation being key accompanying behaviors.

Nger yec is a somatic or physical-based condition in which the person experiences stomach problems, especially cramping, and may reflect the impact of chronic stress on the body, especially the stomach.

Mamali, like *wehi arenjo*, is a concept used to describe persons with a "disturbed mind" Persons with this problem or condition are likely to have lost touch with many aspects of reality.

Ngengere, similar to *moul*, is a problem that relates to the person being violent and aggressive, often with no purpose or direction.

Yeyersi reflects a condition or problem in which the person has many intrusive thoughts and is likely to be overwhelmed by obsessive thinking and rumination, especially thoughts considered bad or negative.

Ng et al. (2017) identified two additional culturally defined syndromes: *Raanjok* refers to people who are possessed by demons and evil spirits.

Jue or *nok* refers to persons who may experience medically unexplained seizures because of stress and sadness.

This author advises that mental health professionals employ the DSM-5 "cultural formulation" interview as well as other tools when assessing South Sudanese persons since many symptoms reported during the assessment phase may reflect indigenous, religious/spiritual, and folk beliefs. Moreover, mental health professionals should be careful in understanding symptoms since they may overlap with different DSM-5 disorders, including depression and anxiety.

Cultural Treatment Modality: Transpersonal Psychology

I have used transpersonal psychology as the foundation for the treatment of persons of South Sudanese origin who seek mental health services in the United States. This approach, which I have discussed extensively in a separate publication (Kuek, 2015), considers what Lajoie and Shapiro (1992) described as "the study of humanity's highest potential, and with the recognition, understanding, and realization of unitive, spiritual, and transcendent states of consciousness." Moreover, according to Walsh and Vaughan (1993), "Transpersonal psychology's orientation is inclusive, valuing and integrating psychological and spiritual development." In South Sudanese culture, like many other African cultures, spirituality, community, extended family, kinship, religion, oral history and narrative, and centeredness on the earth are consistent with the foundations of transpersonal psychology. This approach is appropriate for working with diverse indigenous-based persons from various parts of the world, including persons with South Sudanese roots.

The following South Sudanese- and African-based concepts are grounded in this culture and must be understood in order to understand the mental health issues confronted by this population in and outside of South Sudan. These concepts are some of the basic "building blocks" of the South Sudanese existential experience in this world.

Nath. *Nath* refers to a traditional spiritually based coping mechanism based on the idea that each person is a pivotal part of life, which includes one's family, community, and the universe. Thus, when assessing and treating South Sudanese persons, the starting point is evaluating the person's "psychological standing" within their existence in the "here and now."

Nɑth kɛ mi bi bɛn nɔ̤ŋɛ dhiɛl. This concept refers to the belief that one's psychological evolution includes difficulties and challenges that must be confronted by the person. This spiritual perspective is an element used as a therapeutic intervention across South Sudanese ethnic traditions. Thus, instead of using Westernized medical concepts, including psychiatric concepts and ideas, the South Sudanese person is asked to reflect on the balance, or imbalance, of a universal collective identity that is valued over their individual identity. Therefore, the South Sudanese person cannot view themselves as simply an "individual" who is independent of their family, kinship, or community.

Dhiɛl. This term refers to resilience. For example, as in many parts of the world, some indigenous cultures come and go while others are re-silient enough to survive. South Sudanese persons look back at their history, both oral and written, and take both ownership and pride in knowing that since their culture has survived, they are also likely to survive or be resilient in the face of dramatic social change. Cultural resilience refers to a culture's capacity to maintain and develop cultural identity and critical cultural knowledge and practices over time in spite of profound efforts to change, modify, or destroy the culture, as has been the case through colonization. Despite challenges and difficulties, Sudanese culture is capable of modifying a painful situation to one that is more ordinary with the notion that "nothing is permanent in life" (*Thiɛlɛ mi bä kɛ pɛk*). This transformative philosophy and psychological strategy help South Sudanese persons engage various types of chal-lenges, such as natural disasters, warfare, poverty and famine, and the death of loved ones.

Working with South Sudanese Persons in San Diego, California: Culturally Related Assessment and the Transpersonal Approach

The following two brief case studies illustrate the challenges that many mental health professionals may encounter when working with South Sudanese persons in the United States.

As will be addressed later in this chapter, a major challenge for mental health professionals is finding the "right fit" in terms of psychological treatment for a South Sudanese client. In normal circumstances, when a client is in a room with a therapist, a therapist would expect to gather information in order to come up with a provisional diagnosis in order to consider the best psychotherapeutic intervention(s). During this assess-ment process, the therapist would ask symptom-related questions related to hearing voices, suicidal ideations, sleeplessness, loss of appetite, delusions, hallucinations, etc. The therapist would likely accomplish this assessment with the client answering questions honestly, openly, and with an absence of reticence. To most South Sudanese clients, these questions are quickly "personalized" and are considered intrusive and "personal" questions about one's personhood, identity, or place in this world. Thus, the person can quickly become annoyed, upset, defensive, guarded, and suspicious.

Assessing a South Sudanese client is different from assessing a Western client. For example, a South Sudanese person is likely to speak in third person and not use "I" statements, as is the case in English. The focus of responsibility may also be dramatically different in South Sudanese persons, with many expressing a belief that there are external factors, similar to an external locus of control, that are responsible for one's problems. Thus, the therapist must consider not asking the South Sudanese client to take responsibility for a problem that they may have caused without first listening and understanding their perspective. This should not be confused with the psychological process that many persons employ when they present themselves as victims to avoid responsibility.

Case Study on Trauma: Michael

Michael was born and raised in South Sudan. He is from the Jonglei region of South Sudan and is a member of the Dinka tribe. He studied veterinary medicine and practiced in the Republic of Sudan. He eventually left Sudan because of war and went to the Middle East. He has been living in the United States for 10 years. He described growing up in the town of Malakal in South Sudan, which at that time was still a part of the Republic of Sudan. He recalled a traumatic moment in his life while he was a student. The town was under the control of the Sudan People's Liberation Army (SPLA). He recalled losing a friend, who was murdered by the SPLA. He recalled:

> We were searching the next morning for what happened. So, apparently, after we left, like less than half an hour, he tried to come back to go to the dorm, but unfortunately, he was caught by the security patrol and was taken to the area where he was tortured and killed, so people began to search everywhere. Three days later, his body was uncovered there, thrown out there.

He then reflected on the impact of this horrible event and stated:

> You will have this intrusive thought coming back whether you like it or not, you could just be sitting, and all of a sudden, any incident will

remind you of this one, they will come and expose themselves, those things on your thoughts.

Michael's solution to this problem was to pray to God all the time to help him move on in his life. He then fell back on memories of growing up in South Sudan and talked about the healing of trauma within the culture:

> In rural areas of South Sudan, people go through their spiritual things that they know have been helping them treat mental illnesses, including trauma. They usually sacrifice cows, goats, wine, and alcohol to their gods. Dancing and drumming were the big part of their rituals. People would spend days in ceremonies trying to drive away trauma or other psychological illnesses as their common solution for anything that happens; whenever evil things happen, somebody's sick, someone will say, OK, we need to sacrifice. Yes, there are practices in my culture that deal with mental crisis or trauma, such as slaughtering a cow or goat, while people form a ring, the victim sits inside the ring. The traditional healer or medicine man would be the one leading the ceremony by calling on the ancestors' spirits to come and rescue their descendant. The medicine man would then give herbal medicine and encourage the individual to drink it all. People pray simultaneously until the condition has improved.

Michael concluded:

> When this illness progresses, indigenous people will not look at the cause, as it has to do about a tragic killing that occurred. It manifests in people. It could be in the form of somebody not focusing … they try to do something about it; maybe do sacrifice, but they don't actually look at the cause of the trauma. Maybe the ancestors are not happy. In my ethnic background, we do not have a word for trauma and relate it to a mental illness caused by demons or something else and deal with it accordingly.

In this case study, Michael presented what every South Sudanese has gone through. The information presented above demonstrates the psychosocial impact of the Sudanese civil war on the general public in terms of the widespread escalation of psychological traumatization everywhere in South Sudan. The South Sudanese worldview is based on spiritual and collective methods that are useful approaches to trauma healing and overall well-being. Doing nothing after a traumatic event occurs is indeed a human reaction, which the South Sudanese people have used as one of their healing mechanisms, in addition to traditional and Christian rituals.

Case Study in a Cultural Context: Peter

Peter is a 48-year-old South Sudanese male who is married and has eight children. He is a trusted leader in the community whom fellow South Sudanese persons seek out for support and guidance. Peter was court-ordered to seek therapy in order to reunite with his family after an arrest for domestic violence. On the day of his appointment with me, he walked to the office with downcast eyes and a shuffling gait. At this meeting, per the mental health clinic's policy, Peter was administered the Patient Health Questionnaire-9 (PHQ-9) (Kroenke & Spitzer, 2002, 2011) and GAD-7 Generalized Anxiety Disorder-7 (2006). The former self-rating scale identifies the presence of depression while the latter identifies anxiety. To date, there is not a standard linguistic adaptation of either instrument for use with South Sudanese persons in this country, and thus I had to translate both measures for Peter.

It is important to note that I have observed, in hundreds of interviews with South Sudanese persons, that they are likely to minimize or deny any type of psychiatric problems because of the stigma that comes with admitting to having a mental disorder. Moreover, they are likely to score very low on both measures, suggesting the absence of either depression or anxiety. Thus, the mental health professional is advised to re-administer these measures in future therapy meetings once rapport, trust, and openness has been established. Of great concern in the case of Peter is that while he appeared suicidal in his demeanor and mode of communication, including his speech, he denied having such a desire. He did endorse items on the PHQ-9 that deal with sleep disturbance and poor appetite, which was not expected given that many South Sudanese, especially men, view sleep disturbance and poor appetite as greed and laziness and not as mental health concerns.

In the sessions that followed, Peter appeared to feel comfortable with me because a "cultural connection" was clearly established. Peter opened up more and admitted to not understanding many of the questions asked at the first meeting. He stated that "the questions made no sense to me. I don't know what you were trying to ask of me." He noted that he felt good about being with a fellow South Sudanese and began to talk about the feelings of despair and desperation that he has felt since moving to this country. Peter focused on how his family life had changed dramatically since moving to the United States. He noted that his 28-year marriage had suffered and, in his opinion, "has fallen apart." He noted that he feels that his children are against him and resent his more traditional approach toward life. He feels betrayed, criticized, and humiliated by his family, especially since he is a man and the "supposed" leader of his family.

As a trusted leader in his community, Peter felt ashamed and isolated from family members and friends because he was no longer living with his family. In his isolation, he no longer took any interest in South Sudanese politics back home. Peter had lost much weight and did not know why this was the case. He observed, "I know I need to eat a little more to get some meat on these bones." He acknowledged the fact that he had lost weight, but he continued to justify it by saying, "But after dealing with so many family issues, I just can't seem to find the energy to eat like those folks with an appetite and who gorged in chunks of foods every few hours." Peter was referring to his overweight friends from the community.

In subsequent sessions, Peter narrated a scenario where he had a fight with his cousin who was younger and bigger than him. Another younger man, who was bigger than the man Peter was fighting with, came to the rescue after Peter was down on the ground. Once Peter picked himself up, he yelled, "You see now how a man who eats five chickens in one meal pulled you off my back like a baby!" This is a typical stereotype when it comes to weight gain in the Sudanese culture.

In taking apart this scenario in a subsequent therapy session, it was discovered that Peter's underlying mental health concern related to PTSD from being imprisoned and tortured during the civil war. He talked about almost dying. Eventually, he left prison and moved to South Sudan, where he joined the rebellion as a soldier for the SPLA. While he was fighting the regime in the Sudan, he witnessed his comrades killed on the frontlines, and he sustained multiple gunshot wounds and survived.

In the mental health assessment of Peter, the issue of weight gain or loss, which can be indicative of depression in South Sudanese culture, was not relevant in this case. Instead, I observed that Peter had lost hope and was projecting himself as being victimized by external factors, including family, community, and the US government. He talked about being on the verge of committing suicide because he had lost any hope that things would get better for him. Ironically, what contributed to saving his life was the heavy use of alcohol. His alcohol consumption had increased, in part to help numb his continual distress and in part to combat the chronic insomnia that was robbing him of restful sleep. In one session, Peter asked for the first time with tears in his eyes, "Why does the American government act out against South Sudanese men in this country? I don't care about anything anymore. I am just done." Peter's trauma has taken decades to reach this magnitude. Although he struggled to maintain his cultural resilience, the trauma has taken its toll on him.

From a clinical standpoint, Peter's unprocessed chronic trauma re-sulted in a substance use disorder that was a direct threat to his own health and the safety of others. Peter was impacted by the trauma so much that it ultimately undermined his health, marriage, and lifestyle. In applying a transpersonal approach such as attending religious services, joining a social circle of friends to talk politics and play dominos, Peter's faith and hope in life turned around. Over the course of a year and a half, the patient returned to his family and now feels that his leadership is back.

The Importance of a Psychoeducation Program in the South Sudanese Community

I have been very active in providing psychoeducation to the South Sudanese community as well as other African communities, including Somalis, in San Diego, California. I have focused on bridging indigenous-based concepts of mental health with those of traditional Western psychology and psychiatry. For example, Figures 9.1–9.4 depict common misunderstandings:

Text inside: "I hear voices all the time and often respond to them, but my community think I have a Jinn in me."

Jinn or genie: In Arab mythology, a supernatural spirit below the level of angels and devils. Another word for shape-shifting spirits that are known in Arab culture.

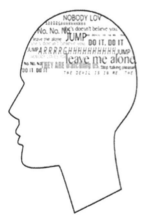

I hear voices all the time and often respond to them, but my community think I have a Jinn in me.

Figure 9.1 Indigenous translation of schizophrenia.

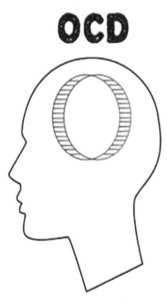

I have to repeat my Wudu 8 times everytime
I pray. My family and friends think that
I'm being "too religious".

Figure 9.2 Indigenous translation of OCD.

Text inside: I have to repeat my Wudu 8 times every time I pray. My family and friends think that I'm being "too religious."

Obsessive-compulsive disorder: This type of behavior is often misunderstood as just being religious because it's in line with the excessive hand- and foot-washing prayer rituals in the Muslim tradition.

Text inside: I suffer from anorexia, but my friends and family think I'm trying to lose weight so that I can find a husband who will find me attractive.

Anorexia: This is an eating disorder that mostly affects teenager girls and is often misunderstood as part of weight-loss activities.

Text inside: I suffer from anxiety and depression, but my community think I'm hopeless and ungrateful.

Anxiety and depression: These are mental disorders and symptoms of PTSD that affect many East African community members in the United States.

The East Africa region, which is referred to as the Horn of Africa, has been hard hit by the violent conflict that destroyed the social fabric and people's livelihoods during the past couple of years. The violent conflicts

EATING DISORDERS

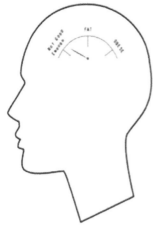

I suffer from Anorexia, but my friends and
family think I'm trying to lose weight
so that I can find a husband who will find
me attractive.

Figure 9.3 Indigenous translation of eating disorder.

have not only created social and political destruction but have also
contributed to massive displacements of people. Countries such as Sudan
and Somali have been destabilized and destroyed beyond imagination.
Thousands of people have lost their lives, others have been displaced, and
many have fled the country. San Diego is home to thousands of East
African groups.

In my work with East African community members in San Diego,
especially with South Sudanese, social kinships can be very healing and
curative. This includes the social circle of friends and family as well as
the community. In San Diego, there are few identified locations where
people congregate in a large number of all day to play cards and dominos. The City of San Diego has provided benches under trees where
Somali men congregate all day long. South Sudanese congregate at
Starbucks coffeehouses and community centers. Some individuals sit
there without playing any of the games but converse about issues facing
them on a daily basis in the United States and well as politics back in their
home countries. Activities such as social circles of friends and families,
playing cards and dominos, and religious gatherings are what I have

ANXIETY & DEPRESSION

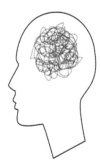

I suffer from anxiety and depression.
but my community think I'm hopeless
and ungrateful.

Figure 9.4 Indigenous translation of anxiety and depression.

labeled "transpersonal elements of the South Sudanese culture." Social gatherings like these help distract people from their cognitive distortions and desensitize those with social anxiety issues.

Assessing South Sudanese Persons in Mental Health Settings: Key Questions for Mental Health Professionals

The following is a list of key questions that mental health professionals should consider when assessing and treating South Sudanese persons in clinics in the United States. While not an exhaustive list, the question taps into the essence of South Sudanese people both in their home country and in their new or adoptive country.

1   Was the South Sudanese person born in the United States or South Sudan? This is important for many reasons related to language, values, beliefs, and the extent of acculturation stress that the person may be experiencing. In other words, it is important to assess the generation status of a South Sudanese person at the onset of treatment because those born in the United States are likely to prefer therapy in English while those born in South Sudan are more likely to communicate in their language or dialect. Goldsmith and Cockcroft-McKay (2019) noted that there are up to 400 dialects in South Sudan, even though English and Arabic are the most common

languages in that country. Thus, language or dialect is critical in the delivery of mental health services to South Sudanese persons.

2 Does the South Sudanese person identify with a particular tribe, community, or region of South Sudan? Goldsmith and Cockcroft-McKay (2019) stated that there are up to 600 ethnic groups in South Sudan, of which many are also active tribes. Tribal membership remains an integral part of a person's identity, as does their connection to a particular community or geographic region of South Sudan. More importantly, tribal rivalries continue outside of South Sudan, and it is important for the mental health professional to be very sensitive when asking any questions related to tribal membership so as to not offend the person.

3 How did the South Sudanese person leave their homeland? Did the person escape from their country because of political, social, and/or economic persecution or did they immigrate in a legal manner to other countries, including the United States? If the person fled their country, do they fall within the category of political refugee? Moreover, if they fled their country, what country did they temporarily settle in before coming to the United States? Did the person experience human trafficking, religious persecution, death threats, incarceration, and/or starvation? How long did the person stay in a third country prior to coming to the United States? Did the person experience the loss of a loved one through natural death, murder, or abduction?

4 Was the overall journey from South Sudan to the United States dangerous and perilous, with stops in refugee resettlement camps in other countries that may have included persecution, isolation, prejudice, violence, aggression, rape, human trafficking, and even torture? Is the person reporting chronic stress and trauma from living in and outside of South Sudan or is their history of trauma restricted to living in South Sudan? That is, has the person experienced stressful and traumatic events on a frequent or ongoing basis for most of their life? Ng et al. (2017) identified high numbers of lifetime traumatic events in both men and women in South Sudan that produce severe cases of PTSD when contrasted to persons who have experienced single incidents. Savic et al. (2013), in a study with Sudanese refugees in Australia, including those from South Sudan, observed that "the cumulative effects of pre-migration and post-migration experiences are thought to render refugees vulnerable to mental illness and psychosocial distress" (p. 383). Tutlam (2017) studied South Sudanese women who had experienced trauma in their homeland and who settled in the United States. The researcher studied both the mothers and their U.S.-born children. Tutlam found that 26% of the mothers met the criteria for PTSD, 32% for depression, and 39.5%

for anxiety. The percentage of children who met the criteria for PTSD was 10.5%, 6.6% for depression, and 7.9% for anxiety. These findings support the notion that trauma can have an intergenerational component and be observed in the children of mothers who experienced significant trauma in a war-torn homeland. At the same time, while the few studies that have examined mental health status have focused on PTSD as the "signature disorder" in South Sudanese persons, the mental health professional must not assume that each person with a South Sudanese background has this disorder. The individual might be expressing feelings and emotions related to prolonged grief disorder, discussed earlier.

5   In the United States, does the South Sudanese person live in a community that includes other persons from their country or are they completely isolated to the point that they feel no cultural connection to that community? What social support systems does the person have in their community, and do the systems help manage or alleviate both stress and trauma? Has the South Sudanese person been assisted by community-based organizations, including churches or mosques? Is the person homeless, unemployed, and/or without their family? Abur and Mphande (2020) observed in the Dinka, which is one of the largest of all tribes in South Sudan, that "togetherness" is a powerful concept that extends beyond the nuclear family. They stated that "Dinka people live in large groups or extended families that reach beyond 12 families in a kinship chain of close blood relations" (p. 7). Jal (2016) investigated the role of South Sudanese leaders in assisting and preventing suicide amongst South Sudanese community members in the state of Nebraska. The researcher found that South Sudanese community organizations had devised programs to aid those immigrants who were considering suicide.

6   What is the degree of acculturation stress experienced by the South Sudanese person at any given time in the United States? To what extent is the person struggling to be a part of their community and the country? Are they struggling with language, urban or rural life, laws and regulations, American customs and values, religious association, and/or finding a fit in the community? Yoon (2019) studied a group of unaccompanied refugee minors from South Sudan who settled in the United States in 2001 and found that this group experienced significant challenges in acculturating to the new society and that it was a multidimensional process similar to that experienced by many other immigrants. Khawaja and Milner (2012) studied South Sudanese couples in Australia and found that acculturation stress, or the stress associated with adjusting to life in a new and foreign country, caused significant hardship, including the dissolution of marriages and psychological distress.

7 Related to tribal membership, especially in men, has the person lost a special role or place that he held back home? That is, does the person feel displaced because they are no longer in a position of responsibility or leadership within their tribe? In turn, has this caused the person to feel empty and with no purpose in life?

8 If one is working with a South Sudanese family, is there significant intergenerational distress between parents born in South Sudan and children born or raised in this country? Have the children abandoned culturally and religiously based values, mores, customs, and rituals in favor of "American ways"? Like other immigrants to this country, it is very common to witness intergenerational conflict between children and their parents that causes pain and division and causes parents to wish they were back home. Abur and Mphande (2020), in studying the mental health of South Sudanese Australians and their children, observed that "clashes… arise around such issues as mode of dress and behavior, differences in child-rearing practices, and in particular, a greater sense of independence amongst young people" (p. 8).

9 To what extent do religion and/or spirituality play a role in the South Sudanese person's view of everyday life? For example, like in many other African countries, the populace of South Sudan practices many religions, from Islamic to Christian. In addition, many South Sudanese persons have blended pre-Christian or pre-Islamic beliefs into their own personal practices. This may include spirit possession and other more indigenous beliefs. Ng et al. (2017) examined mental health-seeking behaviors in persons in South Sudan and found that 28% of their sample sought traditional healers, 20.5% sought witch doctors, and only 8.7% sought religious leaders from organized religions such as pastors and priests. This is very important not only when assessing a South Sudanese person but also when working with the person in therapy.

10 To what extent do South Sudanese feel accepted by other ethnic and cultural minority groups in the United States, especially African Americans? Many immigrants from African countries feel a psychological distance between themselves and Black Americans and do not see their experience as similar to that of the latter group.

11 Are South Sudanese expressing their psychological struggles using Western concepts such as "depression" and "anxiety" or are they describing their problems from within their culture, such as *moul* and *ngengere*? If they are using the latter terms, then the mental health professional has to avoid immediately linking the description offered by the person to a DSM-5 disorder. As with culture-bound syndromes included in the DSM-5, the mental health professional is cautioned from "translating" an indigenous-defined mental health problem into a Western disorder as this can lead to misdiagnosis.

12   What are the coping skills possessed by South Sudanese in therapy? Tankink and Richters (2007) discussed "silence" as a coping mechanism for many South Sudanese women who had experienced violence. The authors cited the case of "Ajak," a 36-year-old Dinka woman who was living as a refugee in the Netherlands. Ajak had witnessed constant violence and aggression due to war, including the murder of most of her siblings as well as sexual violence, and when she was allowed to talk about her experiences she lamented that "talking means remembering and pain. Forgetting is the best I can do, but it is difficult" (p. 196). For many South Sudanese persons, silence may be the initial step in addressing past emotional wounds ranging from rape to torture, human trafficking, and kidnapping. Silence, in traditional Western modes of psychotherapy, is considered resistance, but it should not always be viewed this way when working with South Sudanese persons, especially women who have been traumatized through physical, emotional, and sexual abuse.

13   What type of assistance are South Sudanese persons seeking in mental health programs? Like many other immigrants and refugees, as well as newer generations of persons born in this country, South Sudanese persons often come to treatment to resolve immediate problems or issues that may relate to daily living and do not appear to be mental health-related. For example, it is common for South Sudanese persons to ask for assistance in completing certain types of documents or paperwork related to healthcare, immigration, education, or other social services. The identified "stress" may relate to meeting a deadline and may be recognized as a stressor by the person. Once the stressor is resolved, it is not unusual for the South Sudanese person to not return to therapy until the next stressor appears in that person's life.

14   Should mental health professionals use standard measures such as the PHQ-9 to evaluate South Sudanese persons? I have found that using such measures can frequently produce limited, useless, or obsolete information, for many reasons. For example, South Sudanese persons struggle with yes/no or discrete questions as well as rating scales. At this time, the best method to assess a South Sudanese person, especially a recent immigrant, is to engage them in a conversation that allows for trust and openness over time. The conversation should not focus on the reason why the person is seeking mental health services but on the challenges in adjusting to life in this country. In addition, South Sudanese persons are highly verbal or oral in how they share their personal narrative or story and should be allowed sufficient time to express themselves. Allowing this narrative to be shared increases trust not only in the work of the mental health professional but in the mental health system itself. The

majority of the research studies cited in this chapter that address trauma and PTSD in South Sudan have employed the Harvard Trauma Questionnaire (Ayazi et al., 2013).

Conclusions

The primary purpose of this chapter was to introduce mental health professionals to some of the mental health issues that persons of South Sudanese backgrounds are presenting in treatment, especially in the United States and other Western countries. South Sudanese persons come from a country that came into existence in 2011. Unfortunately, the transition to a sovereign and democratic country remains tainted by the ongoing war, political, social, and economic turmoil, rebellion, terrorism, inter-ethnic hostilities, and civil unrest. As a result, South Sudanese persons have experienced multiple traumatic events that continue to affect their mental health status, even outside of their homeland. This chapter has focused on identifying some of the challenges that this population continues to have as new arrivals to the United States. The focus of this chapter has been on assessing and getting to know this population in a manner that can promote both linguistic and cultural competence, as well as political understanding. I have successfully applied transpersonal psychological principles in helping fellow South Sudanese persons heal from trauma (see Kuek, 2015). My work is currently the only work that considers a therapeutic approach.

Postscript: Reflections on Visiting South Sudan in 2016

In 2016, I traveled to my homeland after a 25-year absence. I had immigrated to the United States and established roots in San Diego, California. Yet, I had dreamt of someday going back home to aid in the building of democracy in the new country of South Sudan. As part of this trip, I visited a military camp in the eastern part of South Sudan, near the border with Ethiopia. In the 2 months that I spent in this camp, I visited a refugee camp, where I witnessed the "collateral damage" of war. I met many children who were orphans and had no family, widows, and widowers, and parents who had lost their children because they were kidnapped and forced to be child soldiers. I also witnessed significant poverty, hunger, and medical illnesses amongst the populace of the camp. Persons presented diverse mental disorders, including severe depression, anxiety, substance use, psychosis, and PTSD. They displayed fear, trauma, anger, suspicion, crying spells, hopelessness, isolation, despair, and alienation. Many shared with me their disbelief in God or a greater power and felt abandoned by their ancestors and proud history. I too felt powerless and helpless as I listened to the many narratives that reflected the cruelty that humans can inflict on fellow humans. I cried with the many victims and prayed with them with the goal of instilling hope in life. At times, as I walked through the refugee camp, I felt that many of the persons living in the camp were walking around with no soul in an almost robotic fashion, traumatized by war, anarchy, and oppression.

I chose to stay at the camp and devoted the rest of my time there to help these refugees in many different ways. For example, I held classes under trees and in tents on first aid, self-care, trauma and its sequelae, stress management, suicide prevention, parenting, nutrition, anger management, psychiatric treatment, and improving help-seeking behaviors, especially for medical and mental health assistance. In the short period of time that I was there, I sensed a "re-awakening" amongst many of the refugees and began to see them smile and talk about their future instead of their past. They were grateful and optimistic about their lives and even about returning to their ancestors' lands.

In the short time that I was there, I also learned much about the many challenges of this young country that is struggling to become a democracy where every person counts equally. As I noted at the beginning of this chapter, there is much to do in South Sudan. Involvement, but not interference, has to come from all parts of the world, including the United States. In my observations of "my country," there is much work that is needed to create a solid yet fluid infrastructure that will support not only the education but also the medical and mental health needs of South Sudanese citizens. At this time, there is no such infrastructure, and without it, there is a strong likelihood that South Sudanese persons in their homeland and in other countries will remain at high risk for severe mental illness.

References

Abur, W., & Mphande, C. (2020). Mental health and wellbeing of South Sudanese-Australians. *Journal of Asian and African Studies*, *55*(3), 412–428.

Adaku, A., Okello, J., Lowry, B., Kane, J. C., Alderman, S., Musisi, S., & Tol, W. A. (2016). Mental health and psychosocial support for South Sudanese refugees in northern Uganda: A needs and resource assessment. *Conflict and Health*, *10*, 18. https://doi.org/10.1186/s1303-016-0085-6

Ameresekere, M., & Henderson, D. C. (2012a). Post-conflict mental health in South Sudan: Overview of common psychiatric disorders—Part 1: Depression and PTSD. *South Sudan Medical Journal*, *5*(1), 4–8. www.southsudanmedical journal.com

American Psychiatric Association. (2013). Diagnostic and statistical manual of mental disorders (DSM-5). https://doi.org/10.1176/appi.books.9780890425596

Ayazi, T., Lien, L., Eide, A. H., Jenkins, R., Albino, R. A., & Hauff, E. (2013). Disability associated with exposure to traumatic events: Results from a cross-sectional community survey in South Sudan. *BMC Public Health*, *13*, 469. https://doi.org/10.1186/1471-2458-13-469

Ayazi, T., Lien, L., Eide, A. H., Ruom, M. M., & Hauff, E. (2012). What are the risk factors for the comorbidity of posttraumatic stress disorder and depression in a war-affected population? A cross-sectional community study in South Sudan. *BMC Psychiatry*, *12*, 175. https://doi.org/10.1186/1471-244 x-12-175

Ayazi, T., Lien, L., Eide, A., Shadar, E. J. S., & Hauff, E. (2014). Community attitudes and social distance towards the mentally ill in South Sudan: A survey from a post-conflict setting with no mental health services. *Social Psychiatry and Psychiatric Epidemiology*, *45*, 771–780. https://doi.org/10.1007/s00127-013-0775-y

Ayazi, T., Lien, L., Eide, A., Swartz, L., & Hauff, E. (2014). Association between exposure to traumatic events and anxiety disorders in a post-conflict setting: A cross-sectional community study in South Sudan. *BMC Psychiatry*, *14*, 6.

Ayazi, T., Swartz, L., Eide, A. H., Lien, L., & Hauff, E. (2015). Perceived current needs, psychological distress and functional impairment in a war-affected setting: cross-sectional study in South Sudan. *BMJ Open*, *5*, 1–10. https://doi.org/10.1136/bmjopen.2014-007534

Ayazi, T., Swartz, L., Eide, A. H., Lien, L., & Hauff, E. (2016). Psychotic-like experiences in a conflict-affected population: A cross-sectional study in South Sudan. *Social Psychiatry and Psychiatric Epidemiology*, *5*, 971–979. https://doi.org/10.1007/s00127-016-1243-2

Baron N. (2002). Community based psychosocial and mental health services for Southern Sudanese refugees in long term exile in Uganda. In J. De Jong (Ed.), *Trauma, war, and violence: Public mental health in socio-cultural context* (pp. 1577–203). Springer. https://doi.org/10.1007/0-306-47675-4_3

Bowles, M. E. (2010). Culture care beliefs, meanings and practices related to health and well-being of South Sudanese 'lost boy and lost girl' refugees. *Dissertation Abstracts International: Section B: The Sciences and Engineering, 70*, 9-B.

Breidlid, A. (Ed.). (2014). *A concise history of South Sudan* (Rev. ed.). Fountain Publishers.

Christopher, A. J. (2011). Secession and South Sudan: An African precedent for the future? *South African Geographical Journal*, *93*, 125–132. https://doi.org/10.1080/037362245.2011.619322

Courtney, L. P., Goco N., Woja J., Farris T., Cummiskey C., Smith E., Makuach, L., & Chun, H. M. (2017). HIV prevalence and behavioral risk factors in the Sudan People's Liberation Army: Data from South Sudan. *PLoS ONE, 12*. https://doi.org/10.1371/journal.pone.0187689

GAD-7 Generalized Anxiety Disorder-7 (2006). Arch Intern Med. 22;166(10):1092-7. https://doi.org/10.1001/archinte

Goldsmith, A., & Cockcroft-McKay, C. (2019). Mental health in South Sudan: A case for community-based support. *Disasters*, *43*, 534–554. https://doi.org/10.1111/disa.12373

Heeke, C., Stammel, N., Heinrich, M., & Knaevelsrud, C. (2017). Conflict-related trauma and bereavement: Exploring differential symptom profiles of prolonged grief and posttraumatic stress disorder. *BMC Psychiatry, 17*, 118. https://doi.org/10.1186/s12888-017-1286-2

Jal, D. (2016). *Exploring South Sudanese leaders' lived experiences managing organizational suicide crises in the state of Nebraska* (Unpublished Doctoral dissertation). Colorado Technical University.

Janowski, R. K., Wessels, I., Bojo, S., Monday, F., Maloney, K., Achut, V., Oliver, D., Lachman, J. M., Cluver, L., & Ward, C. L. (2020). Transferability of evidence-based parenting programs to routine implementation in postconflict South Sudan. *Research on Social Work Practice, 30*(8), 858–869

Jaysane-Darr, A. (2014). National bodies: Raising South Sudanese in America. *Dissertation Abstracts International: Humanities and Social Sciences, 74*, 9-A.

Johnson, H. F. (2016). *South Sudan: The untold story from independence to civil war*. Bloomsbury.

Jok, J. M. (2011). *Diversity, unity, and nation building in South Sudan: Special Report*. Institute of Peace. www.usip.org

Jordans, M. J. D., Komproe, I. H., Tol, W. A., Nsereko, J., & De Jong, J. T. V. M. (2013). Treatment processes of counseling for children in South Sudan: A multiple n = 1 design. *Community Mental Health Journal, 49*, 354–367. https://doi.org/10.1007/s10597-01309591-9

Keller, A., Joscelyne, A., Granski, M., & Rosenfeld, B. (2017). Pre-Migration trauma exposure and mental health functioning among Central American migrants arriving at the U.S. border. *PLoS ONE, 12*. https://doi.org/10.1371/journal.pone.0168692

Khawaja, N. G., & Milner, K. (2012). Acculturation stress in South Sudanese refugees: Impact on marital relationships. *International Journal of Intercultural Relations, 36*, 624–636.

Kroenke, K., Spitzer, R. L. (2002). PHQ-9 Personal Health Questionnaire-9 (2011). *Journal of General Internal Medicine*, 16(9), 606–613.

Kuek, J. C. (2012). *South Sudanese community insights: A cross-generational cross-cultural rescue model for families and family counselors*. CreateSpace.

Kuek, J. C. (2015). *Culture, trauma and transpersonal psychology: A contemporary study of South Sudanese*. CreateSpace.

Kuek, J. C., Velasquez, R. J., Castellanos, J., Velasquez, D. R., & Nogales, E. (2014). Hunger for an education: A research essay on the case of South Sudan and the voices of its people. *FIRE: Forum for International Research in Education, 1*(2). https://doi.org/10.18275/fire201401021004

Lajoie, D. H., & Shapiro, S. I. (1992). Definitions of transpersonal psychology: The first twenty-three years. *Journal of Transpersonal Psychology, 24*, 79–98.

Leonardi, C. (2013). *Dealing with government in South Sudan: Histories of chiefship, community and state*. Boydell & Brewer.

LeRiche, M., & Arnold, M. (2013). *South Sudan: From revolution to independence*. Oxford University Press.

Lien, L., Hauff, E., Martinez, P., Eide, A. H., Swartz, L., & Ayazi, T. (2016). Alcohol use in South Sudan in relation to social factors, mental distress and traumatic events. *BMC Public Health, 16*, 937. https://doi.org/10.1186/s12889-016-3605-9

Majok, S. A. (2018). Mental health in South Sudan: A ticking time bomb. *South Sudan Medical Journal, 11*(3), 55.

Memmi, A. (1991). *The colonizer and colonized*. Beacon Press.

Muller, B., Munslow, B., & O'Dempsey, T. (2017). When community reintegration is not the best option: Interethnic violence and the trauma of parental loss in South Sudan. *International Journal of Health Planning and Management*, *32*(1), 91–109.

Ng, L. C., López, B., Pritchard, M., & Deng, D. (2017). Posttraumatic stress disorder, trauma, and reconciliation in South Sudan. *Social Psychiatry and Psychiatric Epidemiology*, *52*, 705–714. https://doi.org/10.1007/s00127-017-1376-y

Roberts, B., Damundu, E. Y., Lomoro, O., & Sondorp, E. (2009). Post-conflict mental health needs: A cross-sectional survey of trauma, depression and associated factors in Juba, Southern Sudan. *BMC Psychiatry*, *9*, 7. https://doi.org/10.1186/1471-244X-9-7

Savic, M., Chur-Hansen, A., Mahmood, M.A., & Moore, V. (2013). Separation from family and its impact on the mental health of Sudanese refugees in Australia: A qualitative study. *Australian and New Zealand Journal of Public Health*, *37*, 383–388. https://doi.org/10-1111/1753-6405.12088.

Singh, A. N., & Singh, S. (2014). Mental health services in South Sudan. *The Lancet*, *383*, 1291. https://doi.org/10.1016/S0140-6736(14)60636-X

Strohmeier, H., Scholte, W. F., & Agard, A. (2018). Factors associated with common mental health problems of humanitarian workers in South Sudan. *PLoS ONE*, *13*(10). https://doi.org/10.1371/journal.pone.0205333

Tankink, M., & Richters, A. (2007). Silence as a coping strategy: The case of refugee women in the Netherlands from South-Sudan who experienced sexual violence in the context of war. In B. Drozdek & J. P. Wilson (Eds.), *Voices of Trauma: Treating survivors across cultures* (pp. 191–210). Springer.

Thomas, E. (2015). *South Sudan: A slow liberation*. Zed Books.

Tutlam, N. T. (2017). *The impact of maternal war trauma on children: A study of South Sudanese* families resettled in the U.S (Unpublished Doctoral dissertation). Saint Louis University.

United Nations Refugee Agency. (2020). South Sudan refugee crisis. https://www.unrefugees.org/emergencies/south-sudan/

Ventevogel, P., Jordans, M., Reis, R., & de Jong, J. (2013). Madness or sadness? Local concepts of mental illness in four conflict-affected African communities. *Conflict and Health*, *7*, 3. https://doi.org/10.1186/1752-1505-7-3

Walsh, R., & Vaughan, F. (1993). *Paths beyond ego: The transpersonal vision*. Penguin Putnam.

Yoon, J. (2019). Purpose development, acculturation, and identity among South Sudanese unaccompanied refugee minors: A multimethod analysis of longitudinal adjustment outcomes. *Dissertation Abstracts International, 80*.

New Measures, Alternative Interventions, and Indigenous Inclusion

Chapter 10

Singing to the Lions: Culturally Relevant Intervention in Zimbabwe and Beyond

Jonathan Brakarsh, Lucy Y. Steinitz,
Jane Chidzungu, Eugenia Mpande, and
Lightwell Mpofu

This chapter is an exploration of our efforts, challenges, and reflections in creating a program to address the needs of children affected by fear and violence in their lives, specifically in Africa, but also, how it has spread to other countries as diverse as India, Jordan, and El Salvador. The hope is that this chapter will introduce readers to the Singing to the Lions program (see Brakarsh with Steinitz, 2017a) and—based on our experience and the lessons learned—that it can serve as a guide to creating a dynamic intervention from conception to implementation and, finally, to evaluation.

Violence occurs around the world—in our countries, neighborhoods, homes, and schools. There is considerable research on the impact of violence on children's psychological and physical health. If not addressed, violence upon children can affect their adult lives as well as future generations. This is illustrated by the Adverse Child Events Study (Centers for Disease Control and Prevention, 2021) and many others. Programs are needed to mitigate the effects of violence on children, especially those which can be used cross-culturally.

Singing to the Lions is an 18-hour psychosocial workshop that was developed for children and youth by Jonathan Brakarsh and Lucy Steinitz, in collaboration with community members, parents, and professionals, based on findings from a research study (Brakarsh & Fisher, 2013) with Zimbabwean children on the impact of fear and violence in their lives. The workshop uses interdisciplinary methods to build understanding, skills, and adaptive behaviors that respond constructively to anxiety, trauma, and loss. Accordingly, the activities of the workshop were carefully designed, using the principles of cognitive behavioral psychology and narrative therapy, and are expressed through music, movement, drawing, storytelling, and visualization. Following a period of pre-testing in three countries, a facilitators' manual titled *Singing to the Lions* (Brakarsh with Steinitz, 2017a) was published in early 2017 with

DOI: 10.4324/9781003124061-15

funding from the Africa Justice and Peacebuilding Working Group of Catholic Relief Services (CRS), a widely respected international humanitarian organization. Since that time, Singing to the Lions has been implemented in 26 countries. An assessment of Singing to the Lions was conducted in 2019 utilizing 2 years of monitoring and evaluation data plus interviews with implementers and participants in 10 countries (Wachira & Steinitz, 2019). The assessment also included preliminary data on the 1-day adult community adaptation, which is called Rising from Resilient Roots. (Catholic Relief Services, 2019).

Origins: Dreaming the Idea

The concept for Singing to the Lions began with my (Jonathan's) work, over a period of two decades, with sexually abused children in Zimbabwe. As co-founder of Family Support Trust, a hospital-based NGO, I observed the impact of abuse on children's development. In addition, I saw how other significant events—political conflict, war, famine, domestic violence—caused long-lasting effects on children's lives that influenced their health in adulthood. There was a need to give children the skills to protect themselves psychologically, build resilience, and find effective ways to change their situation. Singing to the Lions evolved from the development of techniques with children and adults to reduce their fear in the presence of violence and to create greater resilience. This led to small group work with diverse African populations and later evolved to larger community interventions. In moving from individual work to larger community interventions, the emphasis was on three areas: Experiential, psycho-educational, and community activism. In contrast, individual work with children and adults emphasized the experiential aspect of the therapeutic process.

Three previous books and programs, *The Journey of Life* (Brakarsh & Community Inspiration Team, 2004), *The Journey of Life Series* (Brakarsh, 2005), and *Say and Play* (Brakarsh, 2010) contained the seeds of this community intervention model and its three principles: Giving children a voice, children as experts on their lives, and community action where children and adults work together to respond to issues that children have identified. In Singing to the Lions, these ideas came to fruition.

The title Singing to the Lions appeared in a dream that I had during the politically tense time leading up to the 2008 election in Zimbabwe when all citizens were under threat:

> My fears coming in the form of lions surrounded me, I was trapped. And I knew this was the end. Suddenly children came singing down the street and a calm settled over everything, and the lions

actually began purring. The children came singing to the lions and started petting them and I knew I was free. (Catholic Relief Services, 2018)

The dream showed me the way to respond to fear, that we can "sing to the lions"—that is, that we can sing to our fears and that children could learn these skills, perhaps better than adults could. Fear does not have to dominate our lives.

My collaboration with Lucy Steinitz from CRS—a long-time friend and colleague who lived in Africa for 17 years—turned the dream into reality. By working together, in collaboration with three Zimbabwean senior trainers and with community input, the program and the manual *Singing to the Lions: A Facilitator's Guide to Overcoming Fear and Violence in Our Lives* (Brakarsh with Steinitz, 2017a) was finally born (Figure 10.1).

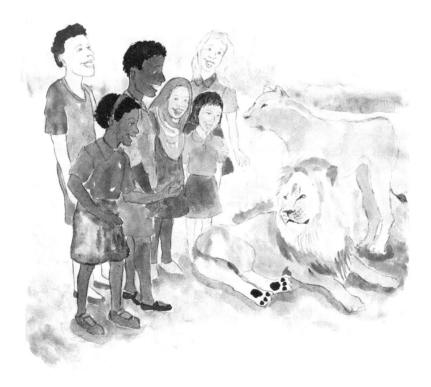

Figure 10.1 Singing to the lions.

Collaborative Development and Implementation

Even before we got started, the need for this kind of intervention was identified by the UNICEF-Zimbabwe Child Protection Group, a consortium of social welfare NGOs, in addition to personal communications with a wide variety of Zimbabwean NGOs dealing with child welfare issues, and Jonathan's own experience in providing therapy to Zimbabweans and training seminars to mental health and social service professionals over two decades. Lucy came to the same conclusion, having worked closely with grass-roots organizations in Namibia since 1997 that provided care and support to orphans and other vulnerable children affected by HIV and AIDS.

Practitioners from a wide variety of disciplines offered consultation on techniques as diverse as yoga, meditation, mindfulness, eye movement desensitization and reprocessing (EMDR), hypnotherapy, medical visualization, dance and art therapy, somatic therapies, and education. Throughout the various stages of development, a reference committee composed of academics, researchers, and practitioners from several countries also reviewed the Singing to the Lions manual and provided input.

The program's objective is for children's voices to be heard on the issues that impact their lives and for children and adults working together to implement change in their community on these issues. For the community, it is important to explain the goals of the program, obtain their consent, hear what concerns or issues should be addressed, and at the conclusion of the workshop have an opportunity to discuss what has been learned. After the workshop, it is also important to hold follow-up sessions to reinforce the skills and lessons learned—whether as a new Singing to the Lions group or as part of an existing group from which the Singing to the Lions participants were drawn. Hence, there are both "before" and "after" sessions with parents, guardians, community leaders, and the children (i.e., the workshop participants). Specifically, we designed a brief pre-workshop meeting where facilitators meet with children together with parents and members of the community to obtain their input regarding the key issues that involve their children and to discuss the planned workshop activities. Then there is a post-workshop meeting where the workshop participants present what they have learned to the wider community for further discussion and plans for action.

What emerged from the Singing to the Lions workshops and the post-workshop discussion groups, both in Zimbabwe and later in workshops across Africa, India, the Philippines, and Central America, was the wide range of challenges facing children in growing up and the pervasive presence of fear in their lives (Wachira & Steinitz, 2019). Over time, we learned that the Singing to the Lions workshop program could be easily adapted to a variety of groups and settings.

Target groups include orphaned and vulnerable children, children affected by political or family conflict, refugee children, children at risk of or targeted by sexual and physical abuse, juvenile offenders, and children affected by natural disasters. The common denominator is that almost all have experienced multiple adverse childhood experiences that, if not addressed, could have a negative impact on their future.

School staff, field officers from child welfare NGOs, and community members are often asked "Who are the children you are concerned about?" to help identify children who could benefit from this intervention. After trying out different methods, facilitators in this program prefer to have a mixture of children in terms of their psychological functioning so that the workshop participants can witness a range of responses to life's challenges. When possible, as part of the selection process, children are also asked "Who are the children you are worried about? Who is the most liked?" Their responses do not always concur with that of the adults, demonstrating that children's perceptions can be very different from those of adults and need to be included in selecting children for the program. What continued to surprise us was the pervasiveness of fear and trauma in children's lives because even some of the "well-adjusted" children had fears and traumas that they had not revealed until the workshop.

Singing to the Lions takes place in schools, community settings, prisons, staff offices, training centers, churches, mosques, and, at least in part, under trees. Most participants have been 10 to 18 years old, but youth group members are often older (up to age 25). Ideally, the age range of each workshop should encompass children within a 3-year age span, and the children should be from the same school or community so that friendships and bonds formed during the program can be sustained.

Initially, we heard concerns from some teachers, parents, and community members that recently traumatized youngsters may fall victim to re-traumatization through Singing to the Lions, even though there were safeguards in the program. Although two facilitators and a local resource person should always be present, Singing to the Lions is generally not recommended for participants who have very recently undergone a severe trauma. As this cannot always be screened for in advance, however, we have undertaken an extra precaution in the manual to recommend that local health/mental health resources should be identified before a workshop begins for a possible referral. In addition, all participants are told that all activities are voluntary and that a one-on-one meeting with a facilitator can be requested at any time. Finally, activities use analogies and metaphors rather than directly confronting a person's past experience, and workshop sessions are interspersed with mindfulness, dance, music, and breathing techniques to relieve tension. These precautions seem to work. Of the more than 6,000 children who have participated in a Singing to the Lions workshop as of December 2020, there have been no reports of a renewed mental health crisis related to their Singing to the Lions experience.

Working with Trauma

Trauma work requires a holistic approach. It has a bio-psycho-social impact that affects all aspects of the Self (Wyatt, 2020). If trauma is not resolved, it may be passed on to the next generation. A trauma that is resolved is passed on to the next generation as a story. A trauma-kept secret is passed on to the next generation as a trauma to be experienced again (Dr. Michael Silvestre, EMDR trainer and therapist, personal communication, 2016).

In refining the ideas in this program, we pondered the question, "What do children need to respond effectively to fear and violence?" Based on a review of the work of Peter Levine (Levine & Kline, 2008), we agreed that several types of support are necessary between children, parents, and their environment. Levine posits that adults can provide consistency, the capacity to soothe and regulate, the ability to help the child in the moment, and the support to help children create a story of resilience focusing on the strengths in their lives.

The Singing to the Lions program incorporates six areas of skills and knowledge (Brakarsh with Steinitz, 2017a, p. 3) to help children to

a   learn self-calming skills, which include breathing, movement, and meditation—the objective is for children to make rapid and effective decisions based on reasoning rather than fear;
b   alter their negative view of themselves as the one deserving abuse and instead discover their strengths and positive attributes;
c   learn to decrease their social isolation and stigma by realizing that they are not alone but are part of a larger social network;
d   understand the impact of fear and violence on their lives and identify resources both internal and external (knowing who to go to in time of crisis);
e   identify ways to overcome violence and fear in their lives by analyzing problems and implementing plans of action; and
f   have hopes and develop goals for the future.

These six areas are interwoven into the six themes or teaching modules of the workshop: Welcome, Discovering Who We Are, Understanding Fear and Violence, Strengthening Who We Are, Making Connections, and Moving Forward. Each of the modules interlink to form a more powerful whole, taking the child on a journey from understanding of self to recognizing their strength, learning the importance of social connections that make them stronger, and applying what they have learned. The illustrations in the manual provide a visual guide to the facilitator of how the activity might look when implemented. There is also a monitoring and evaluation form.

The workshop format is flexible. For example, it can be conducted as a 3-day workshop, divided into half-day workshops, or adapted for schools in a program of 3-hour periods.

Bringing the Workshop to Life

Trauma work requires a physical component. The body needs to be activated, for trauma creates a disconnection, a dissociation, between one's feelings and sensations. It creates a disengagement, so the objective is to help the person slowly and safely to begin to re-engage with their bodies, feelings, and sensations (van der Kolk, 2015).

Several of the exercises in the program illustrated below go beyond words and concepts to work with the body and the breath, for example, by "sweeping away fears" in Letting Go of Problems, drawing The Four Squares to diminish the threats, and visualizing strengths in Treasure Tree and Mountain, Water, Wind, Fire (Figure 10.2).

In the Singing to the Lions program, we observed that working with trauma means working with the body, the story the person has about the trauma, and how the trauma influences their life. Based on our observations, three components are interwoven into the therapeutic process of Singing to the Lions—breathwork and movement, narrative therapy, and the power of the imagination.

Breathwork and movement are important components in this program to help reduce anxiety and the fight, flight, or freeze response. Children with feelings of being overwhelmed by an event can learn the sensations that their body sends them, acknowledge them, and then through breathing and movement learn to release these sensations to relieve the body and mind (Brakarsh with Steinitz, 2017a). Breathwork and movement are used from the very beginning of the workshop as part of the Welcome activity. When the participants enter the room, local music is playing and the facilitators are dancing and invite everyone to join them. In the next activity, Learn about Lions, the children use the Lion's Breath pose, adapted from yoga, to *roar* like lions, feeling their strength and ferocity (Figure 10.3).

When trauma occurs, it is not only the event itself but also how the event lands in our nervous system that creates the trauma. The techniques of cognitive behavioral therapy (CBT), which focus on gradually shifting negative thoughts toward more adaptive, functional

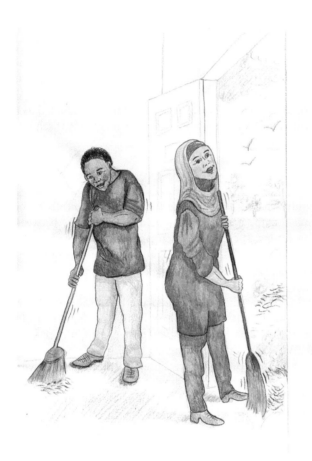

Figure 10.2 Letting go of problems.

perspectives, are interwoven into many activities in the program. Based on our interpretation of the event, we create a story around it. Narrative therapy focuses on exploring our current story and creating an alternative story that allows new possibilities and new ways of understanding to take root. Narrative therapy's Australian and New Zealand origins (White & Epston, 1990) are a natural complement to our workshop due to the model's community premise in its focus on the ability to create one's own story, identity, and its awareness of the social constructs impacting human problems. Children's stories are highlighted in one of the longest activities, Tree of Life, where participants draw a tree representing their life, starting from the roots and reaching upwards. In this way, they can identify and clearly see their heritage—the roots that they connect with their parents, relatives, and

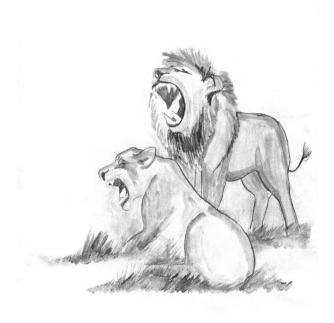

Figure 10.3 Roaring lions.

ancestors as well as their place of birth or home village; the trunk re-presenting both difficult and positive times in their life as they have grown up; the branches representing their hopes and dreams and ulti-mately their talents, skills, and the good things in their life now, which they write or draw on the leaves and fruits of the tree.[1] (Catholic Relief Services, REPSSI, 2018) (Figure 10.4).

We hold on to core beliefs about ourselves. From our core beliefs, we create a story that influences how we live our lives and understand the various events that happen to us. Both logic and imagination can create these new possibilities and realities. While Cognitive Behavioral Therapy (CBT) and narrative therapy primarily utilize logic, imagination, the third modality, can also be a powerful force for change.

During the Singing to the Lions workshop, imagination manifests through drawing and visualization, guided conversations with each other, and drama activities. In the next phase of the workshop, the children use their imagination to create a safe place inside them (The Safe Place Inside Us) and then use a sheet with four squares showing big lions getting

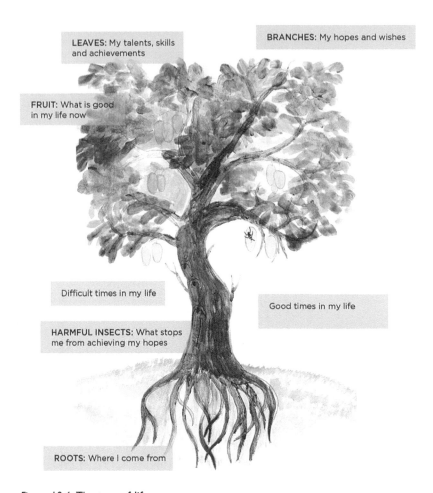

LEAVES: My talents, skills and achievements

BRANCHES: My hopes and wishes

FRUIT: What is good in my life now

Difficult times in my life

Good times in my life

HARMFUL INSECTS: What stops me from achieving my hopes

ROOTS: Where I come from

Figure 10.4 The tree of life.

smaller in each square. They go through the process of shrinking their fears and then returning to their safe place (The Four Squares). Finally, they work in groups and with a drama exercise "take on" the qualities of different powerful elements of nature—fire, wind, mountain, water—to access their strengths and imagine new abilities and possibilities in their lives. (Figure 10.5)

A study from the University of Colorado-Boulder's Cognitive and Affective Neuroscience Laboratory (Reddan et al., 2018) shows that if you imagine a threat, the relevant parts of the brain light up as if you are actually experiencing it. The study describes how this effect can be used therapeutically. It concludes by confirming that "an internal

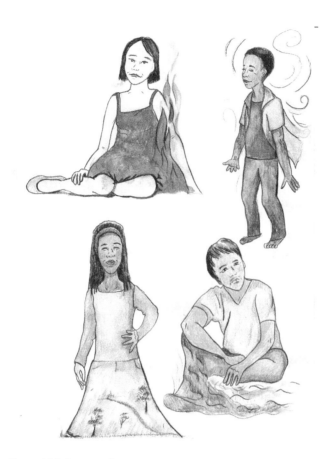

Figure 10.5 Fire, wind, mountain, water.

simulation of a real-world experience can alter the way one responds to that situation in the future." The authors continue, "Imagined exposures to threatening stimuli are effective in the reduction of learned threat responses" (p. 1003). The skill of imagination and visualization can be a protective barrier around the child that serves to reduce their fear when they interact with their environment and, consequently, can be a useful method in ameliorating post-traumatic stress.

People assume that the way to reduce fear or negative emotion is to imagine something good. In fact, what might be more effective is exactly the opposite: Imagining the threat, but without the negative consequences. ("Your Brain on Imagination," *Science Daily*, 2018)

Imagining the threat without the negative consequences is an important concept in this program. In Singing to the Lions, the workshop proceeds by having the participants collect all their problems in the form of sticks and stones, acknowledge them, put them in a sack, and participate in a ritual in which the contents of the sack are buried in the ground to allow Mother Earth to hear the problems and cleanse them (Letting Go of Problems).

In an earlier example, Learn about Lions, children face their fears metaphorically in the form of lions. Rather than be fearful and intimidated, the children sing louder and louder to create a wall of sound that overwhelms the ferocity of the lions.

After the sections Discovering Who We Are, Understanding Fear and Violence, and Strengthening Who We Are, the final phases of the workshop are Making Connections and Moving Forward. These include activities such as the Helpers Game, which explores who can help the children in various situations, such as when their mother is ill and can't work or a friend is being sexually abused. In Small Steps Up the Mountain, participants learn how to break big problems or challenges into smaller, more manageable sections. As one of the concluding activities, Honoring Each Other, the workshop participants write on a piece of paper taped to the person in front of them what they admire or like about them, exchanging places in line until all the participants have written their thoughts. For participants who have experienced abuse or violence in their lives, this provides a powerful document for each person of the positive ways in which they are seen (Figure 10.6).

Program Development

When we first offered the Singing with Lions program, the three senior trainers were Eugenia Mpande, Jane Chidzungu, and Lightwell Mpofu, all native to Zimbabwe. They all had been working in organizations Jonathan had collaborated with previously. All three trainers were chosen for their depth of experience in working on psychosocial issues, their demonstrated skills as facilitators, and their ability to speak Ndebele, Shona, and English, the primary languages spoken in Zimbabwe. The senior trainers were also instrumental in providing feedback during the development of Singing to the Lions.

Pre-testing was initially conducted in Zimbabwe by the senior trainers (two sites) and a couple of months later by Lucy with local collaborators in Uganda (one site) and Sierra Leone (one site). The program worked equally well across ages 11 through to adulthood. The process brought up both present fears and those from the past in the participants, and it helped highlight their achievements and strengthen their self-esteem. The participants found The Tree of Life activity especially meaningful in that

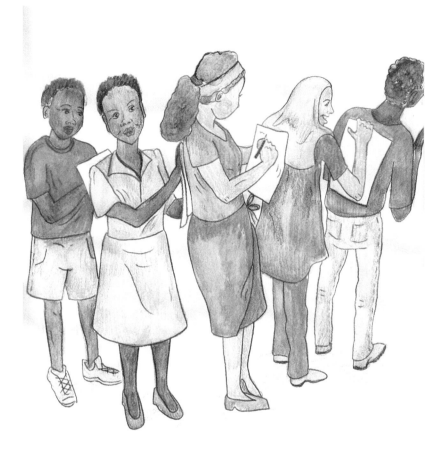

Figure 10.6 Honoring each other.

it allowed them to see a map of their lives and hopes in the form of a tree and its branches. We identified the need for a supplement to the workshop manual (which we later added) to explain the concepts further. We also incorporated more energizing activities to maintain the flow of the workshop and to help the children process difficult emotions. Overall, the participants found the process therapeutic and the content and skills relevant.

Lightwell Mpofu, senior trainer, writes:

The piloting process was an interesting experience; it was probably the best part of co-creation. Being the first to see the community reaction to ideas and concepts that you have only discussed is an unparalleled experience. Seeing the different ways in which different participants grasp and respond to concepts presents a chance to explore the universe that is a human being.

Through the process of co-creation with the workshop participants, Lucy Steinitz and the Zimbabwe-based senior trainers—Jane Chidzungu, Eugenia Mpande, and Lightwell Mpofu—Singing to the Lions could truly begin to sing.

The Training Experience

Given its focus on trauma and resilience, we agreed from the beginning that Singing to the Lions is not the kind of workshop where you can just pick up the manual and run with it. Facilitators don't need advanced degrees, but they should be carefully trained and should—ideally—co-facilitate several workshops with a more advanced trainer before venturing out on their own. We planned it so that persons who wanted to facilitate Singing to the Lions should first participate in a Singing to the Lions workshop, followed by two and a half days of learning facilitation skills, and then followed again by three to four workshops as an apprentice (co-facilitator). We sought to give equal weight to both the experiential and didactic components of the training. In some settings, however, this training process had to be shortened due to a shortage of time and funding as well as logistical constraints. Even after apprentices became qualified facilitators, we strongly recommended that two facilitators conduct the workshop together with a local resource person; we did not compromise around this structure.

Lightwell comments: "We encountered some unforeseen circumstances arising in the facilitator training program. Some of the facilitators wanted to inject their own interpretation into the material. This presented a challenge as new interpretations were added to the material which potentially confused or diluted the impact of the exercise." Our collective experience is that, especially in Africa, a new facilitator tends to believe that they should be able to master new material quickly and then transmit it to others without looking at notes, much less by reading or referring to a manual during the course of the exercises. But that is not how Singing to the Lions was structured; every written word or sentence was considered for its psychosocial impact. This resulted in a bit of an impasse. Without checking the manual during the course of the facilitation, the facilitators tended to communicate their own understanding of an exercise using their own words. Although this was well-intentioned, the problem is that sometimes those words skipped certain nuances or even important steps.

In March 2019, Cyclone Idai devastated Mozambique and large parts of Manicaland Province, Zimbabwe. The rain and winds were of such magnitude that villages were buried under rock avalanches and farming areas were destroyed, leaving people without food. As part of the disaster relief efforts in the Chimanimani area (Zimbabwe), a number of the new Singing to the Lions facilitators revealed that they had also been directly affected by the devastation, thus adding new traumas to those they had experienced from childhood. We were concerned whether working with material on violence and fear could reactivate their pre-existing traumas. But we discovered that the opposite was true; working on Singing to the Lions began a healing journey for those training to become facilitators. As Lightwell commented:

> When planning these workshops in Chimanimani, we could see that the facilitators/community volunteers we trained in Chimanimani, a district in Manicaland, were essentially traumatized themselves. At some point, I thought it was a bad idea to try and use the injured in a process of healing. "What if they relapsed during the workshops?" I asked myself. Looking back, I think that was the best thing about the Chimanimani projects. No one could have known the extent of damage as much as the ones who had experienced the damage, and as such it was good to have such people leading the healing efforts. I was also amazed at the healing journey that the facilitators took throughout the project inception. Some even testified that being involved in the project had been therapeutic to them and augmented their healing.

Eugenia and Jane describe their experience facilitating workshops as follows: "When children enter the Singing to the Lions space, they are greeted by local music and the facilitators already up and dancing. The greeting and welcoming process engaged the children by making them feel valuable, loved, and warm. They knew this was going to be something of a different experience." Lightwell adds,

> The introductory exercise Learn about Lions has some children in the group becoming the lions, and then the lions move steadily, roaring toward the rest of the children, who start singing to the lions. The wall of sound surrounds the lions and takes their power away. The children's singing becomes stronger and stronger. It is one of the most powerful moments of the workshop. The process reduced fear, showing the children that they could be brave, courageous, and together could overcome fear in their lives.

According to Eugenia and Jane:

> During the Tree of Life activity (activity #2), the metaphor of tree and forest always brought about immediate positive transformation and insights. With the children merely looking first at individual images of trees and then the forest—when trees were visualized together—they could identify themselves as members of the group, realize they are not alone, and make new connections in this new forest. They started opening up, smiling, and having supportive conversations among themselves. The power of this metaphor is that it works very well with people with different literacy levels.

The trainers continue:

> We have noted an amazing transformation of the children, even on the first day, and wondered if they are same children that we saw as they were coming into the room. When the children arrive at the workshop venue for the first time, in the morning they are tense, sad, withdrawn, and shy. Some of them will just sit on the chair and not behave like children despite the fact that they know each other. By lunch time of the first day, they will be so relaxed and fully present, enjoying all the activities. The children on the second day are on time, eagerly waiting for the workshop to start. They acknowledge that they will never be the same after the workshop and often talk about the need to share with other children the knowledge and skills they acquired during the workshop.

The training team of Eugenia Mpande, Lightwell Mpofu, and Jane Chidzungu has described their experiences facilitating workshops. For brief clips of a workshop and an overview of the workshop experience, please watch the 20-minute *Singing to the Lions* video (Catholic Relief Services, 2019).

How the Children Responded

According to Eugenia and Jane, the practical activities, which included grounding and calming exercises, helped children take ownership of the process, learning to calm themselves no matter what the situation. The trainers said: "We observed children seeing the need to help others and being more compassionate and supportive. The children become each other's keepers with empathy during the workshop and even after in situations where their peers are facing challenges of abuse or neglect. Involving an adult (teacher/guardian) as a resource person ensures that the children continue to meet and access support."

Lightwell reflects: "In my memory, there will always be the picture of peace that you can see in participants faces during the treasure tree exercise ... the picture of belonging in a place that can never be taken away from them is priceless. I think that is one of my favorite parts of the workshop." Eugenia and Jane describe the workshop impact: "Children have described *Singing to the Lions* as liberating, enlightening and fun. Many have even gone to the extent that on the last day or session of the workshop they explicitly express their sadness and wish to do more exercises." Lightwell summarizes, "The impact Singing to the Lions has in the community can never be overemphasized. Through the incorporation of community structures which include community leaders and resource persons, the process does not end when the workshop finishes but continues beyond the reach of the initial facilitator."

According to the children and youth, Singing to the Lions helps remove emotional obstacles so they can go forward with their lives. By sharing their experience within a group, there is a collective process where people can unburden themselves and be viewed with the respect and the commonality that we all are humans, and we all carry trauma and pain.

A young teenage commercial sex worker who was sexually abused as a young child said, "If I had gone through this process 2 years ago, I would not be where I am today, I would have been a better person. This process was very helpful; I will never be the same." A teenage girl with albinism mentioned to us after this exercise, "I used to spend all my life worrying about what people think about me given my condition. The Treasure Tree helped me realize that I am a very beautiful person. Now I don't have to worry about what people say anymore; no one can take away the goodness in me."

After a workshop in Bulawayo, a 10-year-old boy told his experience of when the army came to his house looking for his parents. He climbed out the window, went to the front of the house where a member of the army was knocking on the door, and said to the man, "I knocked on their door a while ago. I don't think they are home yet." The army left. The boy credited his actions to the breathing exercises and the strength he drew from being with others in the workshop. A woman whose grandchild attended the Singing to the Lions Disaster Relief Program in Chimanimani reported:

> Having attended the trauma healing workshop, Tawanda is a changed person. He now associates and mingles with other kids. Tawanda has developed the tendency of openness and accountability. The issue of bedwetting has just vanished away miraculously. His level of concentration and obedience has excessively improved to such an extent that I can send him to the shopping center without any hesitation and he can come back well in time.

We have included several of the activities in Singing to the Lions in the adult, one-day adaptation Rising from Resilient Roots. Of these, the Tree of Life exercise has had the biggest impact. One woman from the Democratic Republic of the Congo made the following comment during the workshop, after completing the Tree of Life exercise:

> At first, I was reluctant to participate in this exercise. I didn't want to share. But we started with our roots and worked our way up the tree, and gradually I found myself joining in. When we paired, the other person spoke first and then it was my turn. The first time I spoke about myself, it was really hard. I shared some things I had never spoken about to anybody. But the second time we told our stories, the good and the bad, it got easier. And by the third time, I felt I could speak freely, and I shared my whole story.... Then, last night [after the exercise], I slept very well, and today I feel so good. This experience has changed my life.

Cultural Adaptations and Spin-Offs

How do we create a therapeutic experience that can transcend cultures? In developing Singing to the Lions, our focus was on the human experience—fear, victory, humor, wisdom, and other aspects. This focus on human experience is what unites cultures and allows this program to transcend most cultural differences. Also, the use of universal forms of expression—art, dance, music, song—allows for the crossing of cultural barriers.

There were certain adaptations made when the image of the lion did not evoke fear. Since lions are not considered a dangerous animal in all countries of the world, Singing to the Lions became Charming the Snakes in India and Singing to the Wolves in Middle Eastern countries, each with culturally appropriate illustrations (Figure 10.7). With the recognition that cultural sensitivity and adaptation is critical for the program's success, CRS produced these variations in order to fit local contexts. To date, the program has been translated into French, Spanish, Arabic, and Odiya. Trained facilitators are also encouraged to make other adaptations in relation to specific activities, for example, in the songs and poems that are offered and in how boys and girls interact with each other. In some of the activities requiring a level of literacy, rather than writing their responses, especially with younger children and those with limited education, the facilitators encourage participants to draw symbols or small pictures instead.

As Singing to the Lions grew in popularity, older youth and adults began asking for a similar curriculum for themselves. Catholic Relief Services saw this as an opportunity to adapt the program to these

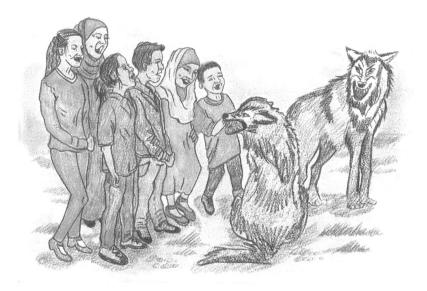

Figure 10.7 Singing to the wolves.

groups, with the recognition that they would probably not be able to devote three full days to the workshop as the children do. While working collaboratively with staff and migrant youth in West Africa, CRS launched Rising from Resilient Roots (RRR; Catholic Relief Services, 2020) as a 1-day resilience-strengthening workshop for youth and adult participants. Several of the activities in Rising from Resilient Roots—for example, Changing the Channel, Tree of Life, and some of the deep-breathing activities—are direct carryovers from Singing to the Lions.

Very quickly, Rising from Resilient Roots became integral to CRS's peacebuilding work in fragile and high-conflict areas. It is also used with youth and adults who experience a wide range of fears, losses, and anxiety by focusing on their inner goodness and capacities. We often say that to implement change, you have to change yourself first. Accordingly, Rising from Resilient Roots helps youth and adults with self-efficacy, stress reduction, and internal coping skills that foster hope, well-being, and social cohesion. Depending on the context, this workshop can also be adapted to help youth build their confidence while learning entrepreneurial skills or to provide emotional support to adults who have experienced significant loss, conflict, and violence. Although the workshop is not therapy, it can offer healing by helping participants to honor their identities, strengthen their relationships with others, and create a foundation for peace. In response to global demand, Rising from Resilient Roots has already been translated into French, Spanish, Arabic, and Portuguese.

How We Measured Our Successes

Between early 2017 and late 2019, Singing to the Lions was implemented in 24 countries (5,735 documented participants) by both CRS and non-CRS partner organizations. During the COVID-19 pandemic, the program slowed down, but it has now started picking up again in 2021—including adding two more countries—all with consistently positive feedback.

Prior to rolling out the program, CRS developed a theory of change for Singing to the Lions by way of a matrix (see Figure 10.8) that describes the changes we wished to see and which, we are happy to report, are corroborated by the feedback and other data that we have received to date. The matrix should be read from the bottom upwards, from outputs to the goal of the program. As written in the matrix, our ultimate goal is that children are more resilient when faced with situations of violence and fear in their lives. To support this goal, Singing to the Lions helps children gain knowledge and skills that lead to positive changes in their behavior and contribute to their improved well-being (Results 1-4).

The Singing to the Lions manual and facilitators' supplement (Brakarsh with Steinitz, 2017a, 2017b) contain detailed instructions on how the monitoring and evaluation can be implemented. We offer a 20-indicator assessment in three phases: (a) the pre-test, T-1, which takes place before the workshop, (b) T-2, the first post-test, which takes place immediately after the workshop, and (c) a second post-test T-3, 2 to 3 months later. The measures are intended to reflect changes in knowledge and behavior based on the insights and skills that are taught during the workshop. Unfortunately, the data has not always been collected or reported back to CRS. To date, our largest data set is from CRS's response to Cyclone Idai in Zimbabwe in 2019, where a statistical analysis was undertaken on 48 groups (1,103 participants), including T-3—which is the most important because it demonstrates lasting impact. Based on a chi-square test with a 95% confidence level, participating children demonstrated an average increase of 15% in their knowledge, skills, and behaviors 2 months after completing their Singing to the Lions workshop. The hope is that follow-up activities—in clubs, drop-in centers, and informal gatherings—can reinforce and even strengthen the gains. Although we don't know why this is, we observed that teachers, parents, and local community leaders often report a much greater impact than the children themselves.

In other countries, the data sets were often smaller, but results supported similar outcomes to Zimbabwe. In India, monitoring and evaluation data

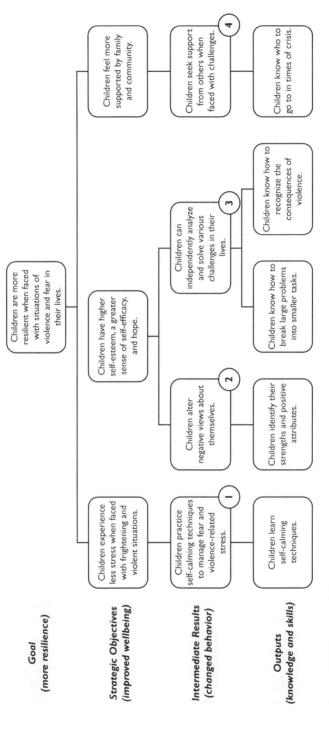

Figure 10.8 Theory of change.

for 254 children in India's Changing the Way We Care program showed a 20% increase in scores from T-1 to T-2, and T1-T3 evaluation data indicated a 26% increase for the same group 3 months after the workshop in September 2019. Although disaggregated data was not available, which precluded a more detailed statistical analysis, the results are both significant and encouraging. They reinforce the trend we have seen anecdotally and with much smaller sample sizes in other settings: the positive knowledge, skills, and behaviors learned during Singing to the Lions increase over time, even after the workshop has ended.

Beyond the numbers, there are the stories. How have the lives of children and adults changed since participating in the Singing to the Lions program? Almost immediately after Singing to the Lions was launched in 2017, the Archdiocese of Harare invited Lucy Steinitz, Eugenia Mpande, and Jane Chidzungu to train teachers from 12 of their schools. Two years later, they reported that "while other children were afraid during the January/February 2019 public violence, these children were able to "Change the Channel" and perceive the conflict in a different light" (Wachira & Steinitz, 2019).

Following the devastation caused by Cyclone Idai in March 2019, approximately 70 facilitators were trained to conduct Singing to the Lions with children from affected communities in Zimbabwe. Parents and children welcomed the program. One child said that the workshop gave her the skills she needed to deal with her fears and challenges. She also said that she learned how to draw strength from the community around her (Wachira & Steinitz, 2019). In a related "trauma healing program" in the Chimanimani and Chipinge districts of Eastern Zimbabwe, it was reported that children viewed the program as a safe haven where they could reveal and share their emotions and psychological challenges (Chikukwa, 2020). The facilitators also observed a large number of children came to the workshops uninvited, crowding around the periphery, having heard about the positive benefits from the children who were attending.

The original idea for Singing to the Lions was that there would be follow-up clubs and action-focused activities that could reinforce the workshop messages and that the children could apply directly to improve their lives and those of others around them. The follow-up program didn't happen very often, however, because of the additional cost or scheduling conflicts, but when it did the impact was powerful. Eugenia Mpande and Jane Chidzungu reported that in Hatcliffe, an informal settlement outside Harare, Zimbabwe, the Singing to the Lions Club in Success Academy initiated a one-dollar project following the Small Steps up a Mountain activity. Thirty children were each given a dollar investment as capital to start a business venture. Twenty-four of them invested and worked together to generate a revenue of $30 to $50 per month, demonstrating hope and resilience as the children learned together.

In Epworth, another nearby settlement, the workshop incorporated life skills training and was conducted for 40 women who were engaged in commercial sex work. Following these interventions, 15 of the women established a bakery as an alternative means of livelihood. In Gokwe, a rural town in Zimbabwe, the children in the Singing to the Lions group reported that girls were being attacked as they walked home from high school late in the day. The resource person, a teacher at the school, organized community volunteers to escort the girls to their homes.

For us, as the organizers, the best news about Singing to the Lions was how widely it spread and its impact in so many diverse settings. The facilitators in these varied settings told us that participants found the Singing to the Lions program to be "restorative," a place of safety, and an opportunity for the children to learn practical skills that they could immediately use in their families and communities. For example, in a program for orphans and other vulnerable children in Lesotho, the workshop was called "indeed a life changer, emotional healer and a life educator" (Wachira & Steinitz, 2019).

In Jordan, where a culturally adapted version of Singing to the Lions was implemented—called in Arabic Singing to the Wolves—child participants shared the experience of Singing to the Wolves with their siblings, extended family members, and neighbors. As a result, the parents of children who were not in the workshop requested that the experience be made available for their children as well.

As part of the Second Chances Program in El Salvador, CRS worked with women in prison, some of whom were able to care for their own children while still incarcerated (i.e., children under the age of 5). The participants explained that the Singing to the Lions program helped them put their own childhood experiences into perspective, which made them *more empathic and understanding toward the children in their care.* Upon seeing the impact of the Singing to the Lions activities on these adults, the University of Central America, Department of Psychology, took the workshop to younger people in juvenile detention (Wachira & Steinitz, 2019). When offered to 500 inmates in both an adult prison and a juvenile prison, the participants told the staff afterwards that they experienced a "notable behavior change in [the] management of their fears, and improved communication among inmates." Just as this chapter was being finalized, the Salvador government's Institute for the Comprehensive Development of Children and Adolescents asked CRS for assistance in training their entire program staff in Singing to the Lions so they could help incarcerated teenagers reintegrate successfully back into society. Funding has been obtained for CRS's Second Chances project, and three groups will be trained in late 2021.

In the Indian state of Odisha, Singing to the Lions was changed to Charming the Snakes, as there are no lions in India, and translated into

Odiya. The workshop was first rolled out as part of India's counter-trafficking work and was later used with children living in residential care institutions (i.e., orphanages) who were preparing for a return to community life. The children indicated *improved relations with peers and adults, knowing how to overcome fear and learning to be emotionally healthy by creating positive thoughts, and "letting go"of harmful thoughts.* An estimated 200 children have participated in the workshops.

Just prior to the writing of this chapter, training in Singing to the Wolves (the Arabic version) was offered in Iraq for the first time. In addition, Lucy periodically hears of "far-away" groups implementing Singing to the Lions without any initial contact with Catholic Relief Services or our senior trainers. Because the manuals and an explanatory video are on the Web, the program is accessible to all. This was a conscious choice by the staff at Catholic Relief Services, who felt that Singing to the Lions should not become a proprietary tool that would only be available to a select few. But as a result, we cannot properly evaluate how many people are implementing the workshop nor the quality and impact of their work.

Final Reflections

Through the past several years of implementation, from 2017 until the present, we have learned more about the program and its impact on children and adults. Because it integrates cognitive, emotional, somatic, and expressive arts methodology, it appeals to a wide range of ages and situations. It is gratifying that the knowledge and the skills of the children increase after the Singing to the Lions workshops.

One surprise is the power of analogy and metaphor. Children across most cultures were able to understand that the lions represent our fears. Local proverbs and idioms strengthened connections. The use of metaphors helped the children to tell their stories and provided a method to make meaning of their experiences.

Though very detailed, Singing to the Lions is not a rigid methodology. Through the use of songs, dance, and proverbs, it allows culture to play an important role in healing and psychosocial support. Moreover, its fluid nature allows for different cultures to relate to the manual in their own special ways while maintaining the underlying philosophy of the program. Using local culture, music, and dance rather than popular regional or international selections often evokes a stronger positive response from participants.

To create a bond between children and influential adults that would lead to greater action and attention to children's issues, we involve parents, guardians, community leaders, and relevant stakeholders from the onset and at the conclusion of the workshops. It is also hoped that the resource person will become the champion who will drive the process forward so that eventually community leaders will take over. This has occurred in a number of communities but not in as many as we had hoped, and the results are variable among different groups. From the feedback we have received, the reasons have to do with competing demands in the community, such as economic stressors, and the lack of funding (for example, for transport or snacks), as well as the lack of local leaders who could galvanize others and focus attention on the salient issues of children.

The workshops are nonthreatening and enable children to have fun through song, dance, and active participation. The amount of fun that the children have, despite the weight of the topics discussed, was a revelation to us. The ability of children to open up and voice their concerns while seeking support from adults to address these issues is a function of age. Most children are surprisingly unself-conscious, but requests for confidentiality increased among those over 17 years of age. It was also important that all children could identify external resources (helpers, supports) to realize that they were not alone and that support was available, sometimes from places they least expected it. It was clear to us from the beginning that Singing to the Lions was not a substitute when intensive treatment of trauma was needed. Individual support and referrals were made available; two trained facilitators and a community resource person were present at every workshop.

It is powerful to observe the strength of group process, watching children learn from one another and become empowered, being able to let go of what no longer serves them, and becoming more aware of their inner resources and acknowledging their skills and talents. They discover their commonality and so are able to connect, bond, and support each other. This gives them hope and boosts their confidence in the face of adversity.

Lightwell Mpofu summarizes:

> Participants have often described the workshop as a uniting force, and even those children known to be loners find themselves belonging in a peer group from which they can draw support in times of need. A great example of such unity is where some children who went through the workshop in Luveve, Bulawayo (Zimbabwe), decided to continue with their Singing to the Lions group after the workshop ended, and they took on seemingly insurmountable tasks like organizing school and community clean-up campaigns and organized a civvies day to fundraise for their friends without school stationery and uniforms.

Finally, once you have a program, how do you inspire others to be trained and to implement it? Basing a program within an NGO allows for considerably more resources to be dedicated to its development and dissemination than an individual might have at their disposal. What we have also learned is that every program needs a champion. Lucy Steinitz, CRS technical advisor on this project, fulfilled this role. She sourced the necessary start-up funding through CRS's Africa Justice and Peacebuilding Working Group and co-facilitated pilot testing. Over a 3-year period, she promoted the program through several international conferences and co-trained facilitators in various countries to which CRS and non-CRS staff were invited. Whenever opportunities arose to include the workshop in a grant proposal or project-design workshop, she advocated for it.

Lucy gives her insights on how to publicize and support a program:

> At Catholic Relief Services, we offered training to country program staff as an add-on to international gatherings within CRS (that included some of our partner organizations), held webinars, wrote news stories, and collaborated with our business-development colleagues to ensure that—as relevant—Singing to the Lions could be included in our proposals for project funding. You really have to eat, sleep, and dream a program like Singing to the Lions if you want it to take off. Within the first two years of publication, I also taught Singing to the Lions twice at Eastern Mennonite University, led multiple facilitator training workshops—in El Salvador, Tanzania (twice), the Philippines and India—and offered additional training, sometimes on my own time/money, whenever I traveled abroad for other CRS purposes.

Over time, several WhatsApp groups sprang up among youth participants and facilitators, and a Facebook page was established for facilitators to share experiences. Anyone who wants more information can download and print the manual and its supplement (Brakarsh with Steinitz, 2017a, 2017b) for free and watch the 20-minute *Singing to the Lions* training video on YouTube (Catholic Relief Services, 2018). Rising from Resilient Roots, our adult spin-off, is also available online for free (Catholic Relief Services, 2019). For questions or comments, write SingingtotheLions@crs.org.

Note

1 The concept for the Tree of Life came from a variety of sources, including the work of Anne Hope and Sally Timmel in their book: Training for Transformation. A Handbook for Community Workers (1999). Published by the Training for Transformation Institute, Kleinmond, South Africa. The Tree

of Life Trust (NGO) in Zimbabwe adapted this exercise as a healing and empowerment workshop model (www.treeoflifezimbabwe.org). The organization was developed in 2002 for unemployed youth and adapted in 2003 to address the psychosocial needs of Zimbabwean survivors of violence living in exile or still under threat (Reeler et al., 2009). Singing to the Lions also drew on an early version of Tree of Life that was subsequently co-developed with Catholic Relief Services (2018).

References

Brakarsh, J. (2005). *Journey of life series*. Regional Psychosocial Support Initiative.

Brakarsh, J. (2010). *Say and play: A tool for young children and those who care for them*. Project Concern International.

Brakarsh, J. & Community Inspiration Team (2004). *The journey of life*. Regional Psychosocial Support Initiative.

Brakarsh, J. & Fisher, J. (2013). *Singing to the Lions: Enhancing children's voices, participation and protection*. Africa Community Publishing Trust.

Brakarsh, J. with Steinitz, L. (2017a). *Singing to the Lions: A facilitator's guide to overcoming fear and violence in our lives*. Catholic Relief Services. https://www. crs.org/our-work-overseas/research-publications/singing-lions

Brakarsh, J., with Steinitz, L. (2017b). *Singing to the Lions supplement*. Catholic Relief Services.

Catholic Relief Services. (2018). *Singing to the Lions: Helping children and youth overcome fear and violence*. Singing to the Lions: Training Video. Bad Rabbit Studio. You Tube. https://youtu.be/QaIVH3aYD-c

Catholic Relief Services, REPSSI (2018). *Tree of Life: A workshop methodology for children, young people and adults*. Catholic Relief Services. https://www.crs. org/our-work-overseas/research-publications/tree-life

Catholic Relief Services. (2019). *Rising from resilient roots: Peacebuilding, migration, disaster relief, youth engagement and recovery from violence*. https:// www.crs.org/our-work-overseas/research-publications/rising-resilient-roots

Centers for Disease Control and Prevention. (2021). Adverse childhood experiences. www.cdc.gov/violenceprevention/acestudy

Chikukwa, M. (2020). Annual report for Rokpa Support Network: Chikukwa Trauma Healing Program done – January to December 2020. Unpublished paper.

Levine, P. & Kline, M. (2008). *Trauma-proofing your kids*. North Atlantic Books.

Reddan, M. C., Wager, T. D., & Schiller, D. (2018). Attenuating neural threat expression with imagination. *Neuron, 100* (4), 994–1005. https://doi.org/10.1016/ jneuron.2018.10.047

Reeler, T., Chitsike, K., Maizva, F. & Reeler, B. (2009). The Tree of Life: A community approach to empowerment and healing survivors of torture in Zimbabwe. *Torture, 19*(3), 108–193.

van der Kolk, B. (2015). *The body keeps the score: Brain, mind, and body in the healing of trauma*. Penguin Books.

Wachira, M. & Steinitz. L. (2019). Singing to the Lions: Who is singing and where – A global assessment. Catholic Relief Services. Unpublished paper.

White, M. & Epston, D. (1990). *Narrative means to a therapeutic end.* W. W. Norton and Co.

Wyatt, S. (2020, May 29). *Working with trauma.* Presentation at Boston Trauma Summit, Trauma Research Foundation, Boston, Massachusetts, USA.

Your brain on imagination: It's a lot like reality, study shows. (2018, December 10). *Science Daily.* https://www.sciencedaily.com/releases/2018/12/181210144943.htm

Chapter 11

Indigenous Inclusion and Intervention: The Flight of Eagles

Shaun Hains

This chapter is written from a North American Indigenous perspective and is based on work done in the Treaty Six area of Canada. The approach of this project is unique and has not been widely shared. I present our Indigenous psychological interventions at a time when our land and history are becoming more fully acknowledged by the wider society. Our own unique system of reliability, validity, and dialogue brings a new wisdom and leadership into the system and service delivery of education and mental health care.

With an increased understanding of Indigenous methods and collaborative dialogue, professionals can be guided by the leadership of Indigenous people. Care and respect for our clients, community, land, and ethics can lead to shared learning and shared celebrations of wisdom. The bald eagle feather is a signature emblem of our North American Indigenous methodology. We see the *flight of eagles* as a symbol of our Native collective experience that, as such, gives credence to our work with our community. Within many Native or Indigenous North American traditions, the bald eagle feather is honored and represents cultural knowledge and a voice from the land. The work with our people operates at many levels and requires skill, ethical sensitivity, and cultural understandings. Sharing our cultural focus honors our own history, our racial pride, and our place in the North American narrative.

What is referred to as the "eagle dance," in this chapter and in our school project, is when several eagles literally fly above a community. We had nine different school sites using common methods of intervention, and the successes of our endeavors were honored through our celebration of the 22 eagles we counted over the time of our project that flew in the sky around our school and community. The eagle dance represents, symbolically and in reality, the integrity of work and the joy of community.

DOI: 10.4324/9781003124061-16

The Flight of Eagles Public School Project

Background and Scope of the Project

While I was employed by Edmonton Public Schools in Alberta, at the request of the school district I identified two primary needs: Helping Native students to remain in school and addressing issues around trauma experienced by the students. My work with the school system led to what is called an *Indigenous intervention*. Our Indigenous intervention was formulated to include the essential research indicator of bald eagles, which fly regularly in the skies over our schools, our communities, and our nations. Bald eagles are unique to North America, and they are a real presence in our lives and a symbol to Native people. While the field of psychology and research include statistical indicators (or explanatory context), the bald eagle fills this role in Indigenous North America. In statistics and research design, an indicator is a value and the presence or absence of a variable that can be observed. The concept of an Indigenous indicator represents, for us, the ethics and integrity of Native culture. Therefore, as an employee and researcher, I marshaled the eagle as a core element in the methodology to support Native students to gain a sense of belonging in their public schools. Integrating an Indigenous eagle dance into the curriculum acknowledges the Native students' cultural heritage and is a sign or emblem marking the success of our project's efforts. I describe later how we translated our school project into a new research paradigm.

Participants

The work began with the request of Native students enrolled in the Edmonton W. P. Wagner High School. The participants included from 102 Native students ages 14–18, and the project was designed to extend over 3 years. The method we chose aligned with our cultural practices: A collaboration with students through dance rhythm, sound, and the visual arts representing a return and connection to our land. This method is explained below.

Staff were trained in our plan, and some volunteered to attend and observe the student-led sessions. Our teaching and administrative staff was primarily non-Native. From just two Native high school graduates prior to the program, to many more today, the model became an example of collaborative leadership of students, staff, and administration. The initial school, a school of 1,600 students with a small Native population, achieved an extraordinary result: after the 3 years of our program, 100% of the Native students remained in school. The students began a leadership model for celebrating Natives who graduate from the 12th grade that continues to this date. This new graduation ceremony now includes all the high school Native students within Edmonton Public Schools. One unique aspect of this experience is that the initial groups of students from the high school were Native students from many Northern communities, Eastern communities, and the regional Nations: Cree, Nakota, Dené and Métis, and Inuit. This work was recognized with the 2002 Emory Crown award for the promotion of community wellness.

After the success of the first high school program, another school in the district requested that we work with Native students diagnosed with severe conduct disorder. The school with students diagnosed with severe conduct disorder had approximately 110 students ages 6–18, with 55 Native students. Generally, about half of the students who were attending the school for students with severe conduct disorder were Native. The relationship between behavior and trauma is often difficult to discern. We introduced an Indigenous peace process (described later in this chapter) to the school. One hundred percent of the Native students were successful with their grade 12 courses and were eligible to join the district-wide Native graduation ceremony. The program subsequently documented the success of Native students in this school over a 5-year period.

Expansion of the Project

Following the completion of the initial program, a group of schools in the West End of the city chose to adapt this collaborative model with students, incorporating an Indigenous approach in working with trauma. These West End schools with 200–300 students had a significant percentage of Native students, averaging 15–20% of the school population. The schools grouped within the West End of Edmonton also decided to work collaboratively with each other. We engaged an impressive multi-disciplinary team of professionals and community members to work with nine school sites over 3 years. Our teams included speech pathologists, teachers, psychologists, psychiatrists, school leaders, cultural leaders, guardians, singers, and educational assistants. One school within the group was an identified Native school within the district. The school leadership collaboration model developed previously at W. P. Wagner High School was fundamental to our project and to the success of this initiative. During this process, I was invited into this initiative to share our Native methods.

Soaring of Eagles: The Native Voice in Our History

The eagle feather represents the Indigenous voice of North American people to our community. A Native status card is a card registered with the federal government, and it applies to First Nations,

Métis, and Inuit people within Canada. A Native person with a status card has certain legal rights not granted to non-Natives. One legal right is the permission to carry an eagle feather, to use the feather in Native ritual, to share it with others, and to speak as a holder of that feather. These rights inherently include the protection of eagles. Our community recognizes it as an important time when *a Native person speaks with an eagle feather, the native person then explains the meaning and the context of the eagle feather and the teachings that are shared*. In our culture, the wisdom of an Indigenous leader resides with their voice, their place amongst many Indigenous nations, within their Native language, and alongside non-Indigenous peoples. Their wisdom reflects their experience of their land, language, Indigenous history, and learning. As an example, the Sioux word *Mahetuya* is defined as a deep and profound love that acknowledges Indigenous history and acceptance of human rights alongside non-Indigenous peoples. Today, there are many Indigenous North American peoples with their own ways of expressing love of land, language, and history and their own unique voice and identity. The Native American voice carries a *position of privilege* in our culture through the symbol of the eagle feather. During my work, the presence, flight, and respect for eagles were central in many different locations across Alberta. However, it is essential to acknowledge the existence of different wisdoms and symbols found in diverse communities (Blume, 2020; Garcia & Tehee, 2014).

Longitudinal Success: How Did We Accomplish This?

School Support for Change

The school district's administrators were openly supportive of a project addressing Native student retention and Native student trauma. At the high school, the statistics on the Native students at the school were shared, and the staff were encouraged to identify the Native students within their classes and to take time to connect with each student. As a Native teacher within the school, I was also present to assist the staff with any questions or concerns that they may have had. As I reflect on the limited training of the staff around Native culture, I am surprised that our success has come through efforts in building relationships with the students and the commitment made by the staff at W. P. Wagner High School. I had long believed in the high quality of the teaching staff, and the Native students frequently spoke about how nice it was of the staff to show their support. When I asked the students to describe their past schooling experience, in each case the positive memories of their schooling came when a teacher had built a relationship with them and showed support for their cultural ways.

The school professionals worked collaboratively with the community, governments, businesses, families, and nations. The student-led work was observed by our staff and administrators, and this was important to the work of collaborative wisdom sharing. The results of our project were observable through student-led implementation at the graduation cere- mony and the ongoing sharing dialogue.

The two goals of our project—Native student retention (also known as "school engagement") and addressing Native student trauma—are dis- cussed below. The immediate trauma that occurred for youth during this study was a massive forest fire in May 2016, that occurred to the north of the city. For the West End schools, eight schools of 200–300 students, trauma became a central focus. The school leadership was strong in their commitment to address this problem collaboratively. Case Study 1 describes how we engaged the students in their educational process. Case study 2 describes the Indigenous peace process used with students.

Case Study 1: School Engagement

The Edmonton Public School Board decided to confront the two problems of Native student retention and Native student trauma. W. P. Wagner High School was a school of 1,600 at the time, and only 3% of these students were Native. Native students represented a small, silent minority that for years had quietly left the world of high school. When this school district reviewed the dropout rates of their Native students, it was found that, generally one-third of beginning high school students had left by September and another third by January, and only the final third of Native students remained in school to graduate.

In 1998, when the study began, only two Native students graduated from W. P. Wagner High School. Then, the following year, 1999m 14 Native students graduated, and in the 2001 school term, 20 Native stu- dents were scheduled to graduate . The school then boasted a 0% dropout rate among the Native students. What caused this amazing turnaround? How could one school create such a rapid change in just three years? The school leadership team was strong in their commitment to the work. As the lead researcher in this study, I identified the following findings as important to understanding the pathway to success for Native students.

Native Approach to Research

To make the study acceptable to the Native students, I was able to use traditional Native research methods as a part of the study. These methods involved talking circles and vision quests that all focussed on the question, "Why do Native students leave school early?" (Leaving school early is the locally used expression for dropping out of school.)

These methods of research were used to make the research authentic and valuable to Native people. Frequently, the students mentioned how pleased they were to be a part of a study that honored traditional Native ways. *I am grateful for the district's support of these traditional Native ways of doing research.*

Regular Meetings with Native Students

From the beginning of the study, I chose to meet with the Native students on a regular basis. The students were pleased to meet and were surprised at the large number for they had felt very lonely within the large school. The students were asked for their views on why Native students dropped out of school and for suggestions on how the school could improve their practices to better assist the Native students. One suggestion that continued to be stressed by the students was the inclusion of Native programming, and the students led this change.

Factors Leading to Native Students Dropping Out

When I met with the Native students, I asked them why Native students dropped out, and they identified the following factors:

1 Relationships with their teachers
2 Racism
3 Peer pressure
4 Poor family support
5 Counseling needs
6 Personal wellness
7 Drugs and alcohol
8 Delinquency
9 Jobs
10 Few Native staff
11 Teen pregnancy

I then asked the students what changes needed to happen within the school to better meet the needs of the Native students, and they listed the following:

1   Native programming
2   Curriculum changes to include more Native culture
3   A teaching process that builds better relationships with the students
4   Native counseling
5   Bridging programs to improve racial understanding

Identification of Native Students

For this study, it was important to accurately identify the Native students within the school. The district information was not always accurate because the Native students were cautious about declaring themselves as Native. The Native students, staff, and parents assisted us in obtaining a more accurate count of Native students within the school. This process was repeated during each of the three terms. It was also clear that providing the staff with the current data on the retention of Native students made the staff proud of our collective success. The teaching and leading staff within most of the schools were mostly non-Native. There were Native support professionals and community leaders. The Native school was the exception; it had a higher number of Native school leaders and staff.

Assistance in High School Registration

Historically, one-third of the Native students dropped out within the first month of high school. So, I chose to assist many of the Native students with the registration process in September. In September 1999, two Native students dropped out, and in September 2000, not one Native student left school. It was clear that by providing support during this important time of transition, the school was able to reduce the number of Native students dropping out. Some Native students come from a reserve and are not accustomed to a large urban school. These times of transition can be extremely frightening for the Native students, and so special care was taken to help all the students to feel comfortable within the school.

Student Leadership

The Native students met with the school administration and asked for a Native Studies course. The Edmonton public school district had already developed an approved curriculum for such a course, and it was later approved by the provincial government. The students then met and offered suggestions for the course. The students had to give up their lunchtimes and weekends for such a course because the school year had already begun. I introduced the Edmonton curriculum and shared this with the students, and I offered core curriculum questions that the students could use in assisting with the course development. The focus questions came directly from the expected outcomes and requirements of the curriculum. The students also initiated the first Native graduation ceremony. The administration wholeheartedly supported this initiative. It was clear that allowing Native students to lead the changes was important to the successes within the school.

Support for At-Risk Students

Greater assistance for the at-risk Native students was needed. This assistance included tutoring, contacting parents, regular attendance monitoring, inviting community support, counseling, and advocacy for the students. In order to help Native students to remain in school, we targeted students who had tested with lower IQ scores, students with learning disabilities, and students with lower marks on exams. About 20% of the Native students were at risk, and I met with these students individually to encourage them and to assist them with any difficulties that they may have had. My roles with the students were tutor and attendance monitor.

Family Support

One great surprise was the tremendous support of parents, grandparents, and siblings. On a regular basis, families would come together to take part in the Native Studies course. Historically, Native families had not been involved in school activities, and this development was strongly encouraged by the students themselves. It was most surprising to see high school students wanting their parents, grandparents, and even siblings to be involved in the program. In each case, these families have continued to be involved 3 years later.

Involving Non-Native Students

One concern mentioned by the students was a need for programs that would help to bridge the differences between Native and non-Native students. The students decided to open the Native studies course to non-Native students, and a growing handful of non-Native students took part in the courses that have been offered over the past 2 years. This transition to include non-Native students also happened during a time when the Native student retention rate went up. It is difficult to fully understand the impact of the non-Native students, yet, significantly, I notice that students are more comfortable with each other and the Native students appear to be more confident now that this has occurred.

As a result of these interventions over all our programs, there have been significant reductions in the number of Native students who transferred from the school, were expelled, or dropped out. During the study, the number of expulsions was reduced from 10% to 0%, the transfer rate from 20% to 4%, and the dropout rate to 0%. Such a tremendous turnaround is a tribute to the commitment of the Native students to be successful in school and the many levels of support that have occurred within the school community.

Core Indigenous Methodology

Strategic interventions involved games played with the youth. These games used drawing paper, graphs, grids, and protractors for students draw out their problems to find solutions. For example, drawing could help youth draw their view of leadership and collaboration. Writing their ideas could further their vision.

Methodology: Song, Voice, Vowels, Breath, and Rhythm

The medium of song, voice, vowels, breath, and rhythm through an Indigenous soft shoe dance and visual arts brought vitality to helping students. These concepts and terms are defined as follows:

> The concepts of *land, the pause, quickness*, and *timing and rhythm* constituted optimal aspects of our strategic intervention.

Land was described as *love of the land*, as represented by the eagles. We began to count how many eagles flew around our schools. The eagles became our "language" for discussions and guided how to intervene and how to celebrate. We talked about how to "earn the privilege" of eagles. The eagles often flew overhead in groups as we were working outside in what seemed like significant moments.

The pause represented the need to honor the complexities of needs that require support and a pause. Taking a pause leads to solutions. Can we use a song when we need a pause? The Native songs are traditional songs sung in a traditional Native language and can be translated by the song keeper. The songs that I sang were about the forest, the animals, and the peace that exists alongside the wildlife. These are some of the lyrics:

> As the forest awakes as the sun breaks open a new day the animals join us around our schools.
>
> The eagles fly, the hawks fly, the rabbits hop and the geese fly by.
>
> Singing, drumming, dancing this story of the forest allows me to share this joy with others.
>
> Time to sing out the songs and share this joy.
>
> You too can join or add your own songs as we share this joy with the community.
>
> I invite you to sing, drum, and dance with me.
>
> We are telling the story of the life around our school.

These experiences became part of classroom discussions shared among Native and non-Native students.

The notion of *quickness* was created through time frames. These were the times it would take students to learn these methods: 5 minutes to learn the Indigenous soft shoe dance, 15 minutes to learn rhythm, and 50 minutes for a whole community to lead and participate in the Native school graduation celebration. The planning for school celebrations took place during our Native class time that the schools allowed to happen while classes were continuing. The gathering times of the Native students were done within the school schedule and routines.

Routine and rhythm are natural Indigenous ways, from round dance to goose dance to voice and turtle dances, to learn Indigenous soft shoe methods. Why soft shoe? The soft shoe or moccasin foot in a traditional Indigenous dance is unique amongst the many Indigenous nations. Communities often use this as a rhythm of welcoming. Rhythm was used to ease our students' fear. This nonverbal communication was used when initially meeting with students. The youth would practice with me in the hallways, moving slowly, quickly, slowly, and sometimes jump dancing. The trauma of coming to school was reduced through soft shoe methods of entrance and of dance. We then wanted to weave shawls of the land with the limited supplies that we could find to use in celebrations with the community and school.

Writing could also be included in the school day, allowing the youth to write their complex thoughts and questions. By adding an action word to the beginning of the sentence, the rhythm could be combined in their learning the skill of written expression. *Walking upon the earth, I could hear the geese as they flew by. Soaring into the air and above our community, the eagles danced in the skies. How do I lead?*

I chose the *vowel* for breathing, derived from a technique used by experts in trauma diagnosis. The youth would sing vowels to the trees as a gentle breeze would go by. We would practice singing vowels instead of what is a common response to traumatic experiences—the fight or flight of fear. The vowels in a Native dialect can be different. When the students would join me outside, we would practice singing with the land. As a Native person, when I say the vowel "a" my mouth opens wider, the vowel "e" resonates with the top of my mouth, the vowel "i" resonates fully with the top of my mouth, and the vowel "u" when soft comes from the diaphragm up through my voice and when long can form into the "oo" sound that grows into the song of the elk, wolf, or caribou. The land requires strategic intervention as well, so we would rub the ground with sage and let the youth decide if the earth was happy where we sat. When we agreed, we would continue to learn. The life around us was part of our world as the geese and eagles and hawks flew above. Can we sound aloud vowels when we need to open our voices? When walking indoors and outdoors, the land was there to greet our day. Sometimes ducks, geese, or eagles would fly nearby. The eagles spoke the language of leading.

Another method of sharing with others and with the professions through a nonverbal dialogue was through the *visual arts*. The love of land, language, land, learning, and leadership needed a method of translation, so we used art methods.

Many of the students, though obviously capable, could experience frustration in communication, so their art began to be a form of telling a story through *drawing* the story of the land through a process I call "drawing inside and outside of the shape, the story inside and outside." Students were given paper to express nonverbally the conversation about qualities, skills, and wholeness. Drawing the story could allow the youth to write their views of leadership. Their work also could be made into a shawl, added to a dance, and then shared with the community. The pattern of leadership within Indigenous youth had qualities of ethics, rhythm, caring, and responsibility to school, the community, and others. Nature provided the purpose, a living wholeness. Professional observations included those by teachers, speech pathologists, psychologists, liaison workers, assistants, and the systems around the youth adapted to the new wisdom of the day, a joy.

How does a student demonstrate that their development and progress with wholeness is an aspect of Indigenous health? When presented with grid paper, students would draw a design or illustrate their sense of self in a holistic context. Then the student would take time to explain to schoolmates and staff their artwork and its meaning. The meaning could be transposed to the required curriculum as the student's skills developed. Their work could also be connected to the context of the family or home and life within the community. The teaching staff and other professionals could learn about the student's progress and have a framework for dialogue.

The student drawings reflected traditional themes of wholeness and were unique to each student. Figures 11.1–11.3 represent one student's evolving view of himself and the world. His progression starts with a drawing of collective and cosmic wholeness and evolves into an internal, private experience. The feather represents a voice for the land, the moon's stages represent the universe and its phases, and the animals are the shared inhabitants in the land. Figure 11.1 shows the open, permeable relationship between the personal (inside) and the universe of land, animals, and cosmos (outside). The cosmos is drawn as the moon and the cycles of the moon, and, as the day begins, life continues. The soaring eagle and eagle feather represent the voice of the land (wolf), waters (turtles), and skies (soaring eagles). This figure shows the land and what is beyond oneself.

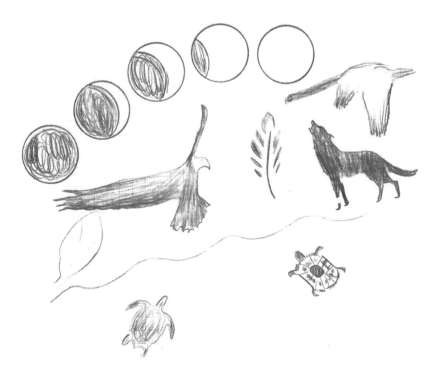

Figure 11.1 Student drawing: Open relationship of personal and universe.

The student's next drawing (Figure 11.2) shows wholeness as a shape (a circle or mandala), both *within* the individual and the natural life of the earth and *without/around* the person. This picture displays the wholeness and a sense of joy from life with the environment, symbolized by the soaring eagle.

The student's third drawing (Figure 11.3) shows the wholeness of life within the private self (the circle) and the awkwardness of oneself speaking to others, keeping to oneself, not being confident with the outside world yet still contextually aware. It shows the rhythm of life and the moon contained *within* the individual.

The student explained the artwork to the staff and other professionals, who listened and dialogued with him. This method allows the youth to discuss Indigenous wholeness through their artwork and explain their perceptions of Indigenous culture. The staff and other involved professionals gain knowledge about each individual youth and expand their understanding of the culture.

The drawing process allows the youth to connect to the rhythm, dialogue, and ethics of their life and growth in their own language; it helps

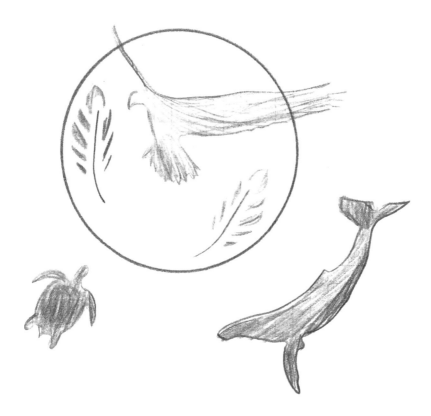

Figure 11.2 Student drawing: Personal within and universe without.

them to develop skills, ask profound questions, and take the lead in this process. Subsequent dialogue around their art allows them to expand their sentence structure and language development in English and to communicate with others. It allows younger students the opportunity to have a voice and demonstrate success. These activities allowed for further discussions among the students. Their self-expression and understanding led to positive behaviors and problem-solving (Michie, 2014).

Art and Design: Understanding Numbers and Dimensions

Indigenous languages are highly contextual, and so I introduced the concept of three-dimensional design. Geometric designs as shapes on grid paper were the conceptual building blocks for parks, buildings, rooms, and workplaces. The youth seemed to naturally understand these shapes as buildings or park designs. We used these drawings as a

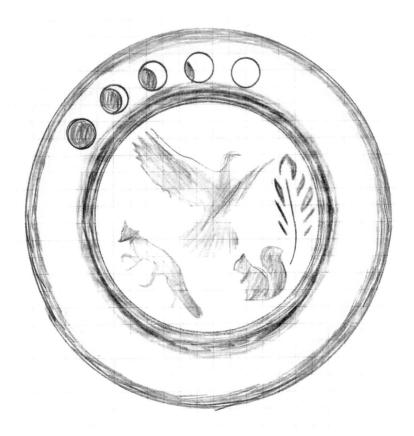

Figure 11.3 Student drawing: Privacy of the self.

launching point to talk about safe spaces within the school and community. Youth could share their perspectives about collaboration and leadership and care for each other.

What Do the Shapes Mean?

The geometric blocks seen in Figure 11.4 were of different types of thickness. As the youth drew their own blocks on paper, their designs were often a building in a structure for a workplace. They began to think about architecture, or how best to organize a space in a workplace. For older students, these seemingly simple geometric shapes could include thinking about business and collaborative leadership. The students appreciated that their work could be seen as contributing to collaborative

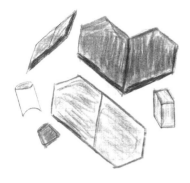 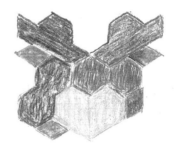

Figure 11.4 Design shapes.

leadership and social responsibility. The conversations around geometric shapes and mathematics guided them in expanding to community meaning and collaborative leadership in the workplace. Older students could develop their communication skills to share with others, including talking to visitors. As the success of the students was shared, more visitors arrived and wanted to meet the students.

Learning Research Methods from Eagles

As the dialogue extended past the student learning into traditional or professional dialogues, some of the non-Native staff would come to work and report the joy of seeing an eagle or two flying near their homes. When others were with me as we saw the eagles overhead, we could talk about eagles in the context of learning. The number of eagles we spotted grew over time, and we eventually were able to count up to 40 eagles around the schools. The work that began in the school district in 1999 has now, in 2021, grown to a point that whenever a bald eagle arches over the school district office or above the Treaty Six and Métis flags above the school district office, everyone present joins in this common understanding of community and our collaborative efforts. One day, as I stood below the flags with other district staff, the staff were proud of the new accomplishment as the bald eagle arrived that day literally *above the flags*. Our confidence in our methods of collaboration grew over the 5 years of developing the first student-based interventions and then expanding to more schools. These interventions are characterized by the students defining themselves for themselves, allowing for an expanded language and communication leading to demonstrated life skills. These holistic methods should provide new insights to professional educators. This hands-on project leads to a new contribution to humanistic psychology and grounded theory research methods.

The successful results of our Indigenous intervention methods highlight the need for collaborative research and ethics methods. Our older students began to build community, to design the first Indigenous graduation ceremony that continues today, and to attend post-secondary education. The students who were diagnosed with severe conduct disorder were able to attend that year's Indigenous graduation ceremony.

The focus of our work included land trauma, behavior, learning, wisdom sharing, and ethics with the land. Through multiple gatherings of professionals involved with Indigenous inclusive care, the students addressed the skills of dialogue and the language of diplomacy. Indigenous inclusive care involves building access to care and relationships with Indigenous people who have been underrepresented in history. In order to do this, I developed a working definition of our process for the students and practiced this working definition. Common to Indigenous diplomacy is what we call the peace process—a working definition derived from an Indigenous North American concept of finding solutions collaboratively through a traditional practice characterized by respectful sharing, protection of a holistic perspective, and a connection to the natural world. Celebrations and conversations can be led by young people, by students. While the working definition of the peace process originates within Indigenous Native teachings and the locale where it is practiced, the students can take the concepts and travel outside the school and out to the community. Taking time and offering these concepts can create a dialogue with professionals, schools, and communities. The rhythm and style of this dialogue can vary, as can the celebrations. Within urban and rural settings, the language may be different among Indigenous nations. The focus on our land, recognizing the rhythm of language, the fluency of life, and wisdom can include more "signs": actual visitations of geese, ducks, hawks, cranes, rabbits, robins, foxes, chickadees, and eagles. This work in each case led to student-led celebrations of diplomacy within the community. The students were encouraged to demonstrate their leadership skills and skills of diplomacy. These skills can be applied to multiple systems, including law, health, family, and community. These can be models for provincial, national, and international projects. Ethics of health and human rights in service delivery are now being defined at a global level (Blume, 2020), and work within research can include Indigenous North American indicators. Wholeness is integral to Indigenous culture and fundamental to Indigenous research (Garcia & Tehee, 2014; Hains, 2001).

Impact of the School Project

Learning this peace process and sharing it forward with Native students and students of other cultural backgrounds led to 100% of Aboriginal students remaining in school (Hains, 2013). Within the schools, there were successes in ethics, engagement, retention, and achievement, as measured by district data. Youth who had been identified as having extremely violent behaviors taught the working Indigenous peace process to others. Many problems were solved along the way using this method. The idea of "giving back," giving back or exchanging, did take place in many ways rather spontaneously, even when I didn't include it in the teachings. Quietly, I had shared the question, "Is it possible that our most troubled youth understand peace?" and I found that the answer was a deep and resounding yes. It worked!

I came to learn that the medium of rhythm and the ritual of soft shoe dance can help students with the fear of entering a school for the first time, away from home. At times, I would meet a Native student at the doors of the school, pause for 15–20 minutes with a dialogue of care and soft shoe dance, walking with the student to the classroom. Other times, the Native students would gather spontaneously during school times for 50 minutes and we would begin the teaching and learning times. These times would lead to opportunities for the students to practice their leadership skills. On specified occasions, the Native students would lead community celebrations of graduation, of learning, or of the seasons and the stories, songs, and dances of the land. The 15–20 minutes or the 50 minutes were also the timing used for the important collaboration with the Indigenous peace process. The students became so familiar with the steps that they could initiate the Indigenous peace process on their own. The 15–20 minutes built the confidence of the students in their capacity to find solutions collaboratively within that amount of time. A longer time period was used if the working peace process involved other professionals or family members. The time period built confidence in the student's capacity to design and implement collaborative solutions. The student-led and land-led implementation now included a rhythm—both spontaneous (when needed) and prescribed (for planned events). Perhaps our complex world could learn from this as well. The peace process became part of the Indigenous research process that assisted with conflicts using Indigenous ethics (Hains, 2013). It allowed us to use this as a way of understanding the original questions we asked about student behaviors, trauma, and pathways to success.

Directions for Indigenous Research Methods

Our work and Indigenous methods and the protection of cultural knowledge were presented to the Society for Indian Psychologists (Hains, 2001,

2013, 2021). The second set of presentations included work with the Social Sciences and Humanities Research Council of Canada and with the Canadian Institute for Health Research in 2006 and 2015. As a member of an Aboriginal Ethics Working Group for the Canadian Institute of Health Research, I was asked to present again in 2015 on the protection of cultural knowledge. Another working group was the Society of Indian Psychologists and their work with an Ethics Commentary on Ethical Principles for the American Psychology Association (Garcia & Tehee, 2014).

Our methods of Indigenous research (Blume, 202; Garcia & Tehee, 2014; Hains, 2001, 2013, 2021) are based on the grounded theory method. This method begins with a question and often with the collection of qualitative data. Ideas and concepts then emerge from the data in contrast to the deductive process of starting with a theory or idea to be proven. This method allows for a deeper understanding of Indigenous wisdom and the utilization of Indigenous indicators.

Directions for Indigenous Psychology

Grounded theory is implicit in the field of humanistic psychology, and strategic intervention is a term commonly used in humanistic fields. As Native professionals, we employed the term Indigenous intervention emerging from the theory of strategic intervention. The eagle feather as a representation of Native voices and indigenous intervention can be shared with other professionals and organizations. The eagle feather (and the right to carry it) currently is recognized as a right for Native North American Native peoples and has a central and privileged place within many workplaces, schools, communities, institutions, and nations.

Indigenous psychology is a strong and growing field of knowledge and research (Blume, 2020; Garcia & Tehee, 2014; Hains, 2001, 2013, 2021). The field works with both the ethics of psychology and Indigenous ethics. Indigenous psychology retains an international focus in indigenous methodologies aligned with and offering a transformative paradigm for social science and psychological research.

Case Study 2—An Underlying Philosophy: The Peace Process

Our Indigenous research emerged during a time when Indigenous ethics was being defined in the field of cultural psychology. How do we explain peace in research terms to other professionals? The wisdom on Indigenous research methods and Indigenous ethics methods has grown since I first began this work in 1999. Over 22 years of study using Indigenous research, the stages of student-led implementation have grown to include the peace process, and as the research knowledge supported by the work within the school district developed, a working definition of a peace process emerged. The working Indigenous peace process was a workable process that students understood and could be transposed both to Native and multicultural settings. Part of our definition is that it is a process that is operational cross-culturally. There are many ways to define peace within each of us and within our communities. When applying Indigenous research to a variety of Indigenous settings, the peace process emerged as a variable within Indigenous research in each setting. In my research into Aboriginal methods, I reaffirmed that there is a common history of Native people with regard to the land and colonization. Though there are many different nations in Canada, there are similar threads in our history. Each Native culture may dwell in their own collective dialogue with the land. As a professional, I was able to observe the land and work alongside Native and non-Native professionals and youth. When traveling with some of the professionals, we practiced the eagle dance in many places throughout our journey.

Traditional Native research methods emphasize the responsibility of knowledge. Within the traditional ways of knowing, there is a sacred place for the sharing of peace that can only be shared internally and privately. While understanding that the teachings of peace are considered sacred knowledge within many Native communities, the vital question was, "How could the sacred space of peace be protected while also allowing for the teaching about peace to go forward in research and ethical practice?" This is another way that Indigenous culture favors a definition of and balance between what is inner and private and what is outer and collectively shared.

The peace process incorporates the principles of *sovereignty*, *accountability*, and *wisdom gathering*. Sovereignty, as the ethics of peace, begins in a sacred place on the land. Sovereignty and accountability involve ownership and responsibility for one's life and community. This becomes a sacred time for traditional knowledge. The place of peace for me must begin with my own sovereignty, accountability, and wisdom gathering. The ethics of peace begins as a personal journey for me in a sacred place on the land. I discover new ways of working within this complex world. The ethics of peace goes with me as I go forward into this complex world. Years ago, I learned that people from other non-Native cultures or teachings could also locate themselves and be in dialogue with the land. Therefore, the peace process involves inclusivity whenever possible. As professionals became aware of the importance of sighting eagles near their homes, they could share their experience and enthusiasm with both Indigenous and non-Indigenous school district staff.

Wisdom gathering is a time when we sit in a circle and greet each other with peace. We can then share and gather wisdom from each other.

The qualities of this sharing are guided by the ethics of doing no harm and by remaining within an ethical place of dialogue. An ethical place is one where the Indigenous wisdom of Native people is both protected and allowed to be shared. We share, with respect, the sovereignty of each person in the circle and allow them to speak their truth. When there is a question or a problem that we choose to focus on, we all share equally in finding the solution during that time. We are respectful of the impact of that gathering on the community around us.

When working with groups, these are the steps we follow and have found to be helpful:

1   Sovereignty in preparation
2   Choosing to be responsible
3   Identifying the problem/topic
4   Allowing a sovereign voice
5   Wisdom gathering to the place of finding the solutions
6   Committing to go forward in peace
7   Accepting responsibility for peace outside the circle
8   Sovereignty when the process of peace takes time

Implications of the Peace Process

This second case study introduced diplomacy to government representatives, family, community, professionals, and our youth. The *wisdom* of leadership met the moments of *diplomacy*. The youth designed and implemented a wisdom Indigenous leadership with professionals, and they designed the 12th-grade graduation ceremony. After this wise design, the implementation with *diplomacy* was the only step missing. The students developed a drumming circle, a Native graduation ceremony with family, and shared the peace process within case conferences with other professionals and family. The results included the Native students leading the high school graduation ceremony as well as leading school and community occasions with songs, dances, and art displays. This implementation makes visible important qualities of wholeness—of health, land, and leadership. Implementation is not a demonstration, but a lived experience of diplomacy shared with many. The wholeness in their teaching is within school, family, community, and nations.

Professional observation included psychologists, counselors, teachers, assistants, community representatives, and government leaders. The surprise to me was the number of professionals who came to observe alongside other professionals while the youth continued to lead. The implementation of the inner wisdom of leadership then continued with the school district, a legacy forward of success.

Broader Implications for Psychology

Dialogue of Diplomacy

The dialogue of diplomacy can become a way of remembering and incorporating our history in the service of problem solving (Michie, 2014). The Indigenous wisdom of inclusion and acceptance (Garcia & Tehee, 2014) is intrinsic to diplomacy and guides problem solving in a context of cultural uniqueness. In my work, I chose a variety of methods—art, dance, design, pauses in dialogue—to demonstrate diplomacy. These methods reflect an acknowledgment of land-based ethics. Behavior can be culturally guided within land-based ethics and shared more widely (Hains, 2001, 2013, 2021). This system of ethics translates to the larger systems: Law, education, other professions, culture, community, and Indigenous projects.

The dialogue of Indigenous peace (Hains, 2013) is essential to health and well-being, behavior, trauma, research, and psychology, and indicators can now take their place within Indigenous student leadership and demonstrations of diplomacy. Psychologists, in turn, can bring this dialogue to relationships with their clients.

The Native Voice: Indigenous Terminology

Humanistic psychology now acknowledges the uniqueness of many peoples, communities, and nations. Each Indigenous nation is unique (rather than a sole global construct) in terms of its language, culture, and wisdom. Indigenous diplomacy (Hains, 2001, 2013, 2021) requires a deep understanding (Blume, 2020; Garcia & Tehee, 2014) of the need to work alongside other professions while maintaining levels of care in Native communities.

The Context for Health

Indigenous psychology as a robust field within psychology has begun to be defined and implemented. Through collaborative professional work, Indigenous wisdom can be shared responsibly. Common aspects include both non-Native and Native aspects: Indigenous voice, rhythm, observation, dialogue, leadership, and implementation.

Postscript: Origin of the Study

In 1999 the Edmonton Public School Board decided to focus on improving program delivery for Aboriginal students and on improving educational outcomes for disadvantaged students at risk of not completing their schooling. The assistant superintendent, Shirley Stiles, then encouraged a study to be done on why Native students dropped out of school. I was fortunate to be able to lead this study as a part of my doctoral research; however, without the district's commitment and support, this study would not have been possible. Any single school's success must be viewed within the collective direction of the school district.

As an Indigenous person in Canada, I chose to study psychology with a humanistic lens and used the study (Hains, 2001) to assist with the defining of Indigenous research methods. When I began the process of defining Aboriginal research methods for my dissertation, I met with another Elder, listened to other Aboriginal researchers, read research done by Aboriginal people, and then applied the process to my own research. In my research process, I prayed, met with people, listened in talking circles, fasted for four days twice, came back to my findings, and shared my findings with those who were involved in the research. After this was done, I came to the following conclusions:

1   Indigenous history of Native North American peoples has its origin in land and wisdom and moves from colonization to attempts at assimilation to a deep truth, the truth of acceptance of others. This truth, *Mahetuya*, a Sioux word, represents a deep and profound truth of the acceptance amongst other races and cultures during the farm trade and fur trade years. In many different Indigenous nations, collaboration is the common wisdom that came from years of Indigenous North American diplomacy. Any study done using traditional Native research methods is a part of the greater history of acceptance.
2   The traditional ways are holistic and incorporate all ways of knowing. These ways are not the same as the ways that separate science from other ways of knowing.
3   Traditional Native research methods emphasize the responsibility of knowledge. This responsibility extends beyond any specific point of knowledge to the impact of the knowledge on the community. Interdependence emerges when responsibility is accepted for the knowledge gained and for the impact of the knowledge on the community. Such knowledge is earned through the disciplined work of the researcher. The wisdom within the speaker is represented with an eagle feather.
4   Traditional Native research implies action as well as reflection.
5   Traditional Native research is about service. The skills of academic research are viewed as earned and are to be used to assist the community.
6   Traditional Native research involves many ways of listening, which include prayer. In my research, I used prayer (typically not part of

mainstream research practice), and this practice was accepted by "traditional" academic researchers.

7 Traditional Native research involves personal honesty. This honesty includes not only reflection but also the upfront facing of biases and the influence of personal experiences.

8 Traditional Native research comes from the knowledge of traditional Native epistemology. This includes the great history of Native people within Canada, valuing a sacred dialogue with the land. Native culture influences all aspects of a Native person's life and life view.

9 The role of the Elder is essential.

10 Traditional Native research involves focusing on a problem with the intention of finding a deeper understanding that will provide insight into a solution (Hains, 2001).

11 These principles allow for the dialogue of differences. For example, a Native person from North America with an eagle feather and specific wisdom can examine the principles of ethics, psychology, and education alongside a non-Native person and explain the differences in understanding. For example, the Native person might explain the following terms in these ways:

a Voice—I can use an eagle feather and speak to the findings with a unique wisdom, love, land, language, and history.

b Implementation—From this position of privilege, I can suggest concerns during moments of professional collaboration.

c Observation—I have a unique perspective on issues and can share this through dialogue.

d Need—The time of speaking as a Native person is based on the need during times of professional collaboration while knowing that there has been work done to allow for this within my country or region.

e Skills—The skills that I need are added to in learning and speaking as a Native professional.

f Wisdom—The wisdom when shared is protected by the respected place that the eagle feather, wisdom, and voice have within the country or region.

g Research—Indigenous research can be validated by a Native person, and one commonly known indicator is the flight of eagles over a community, nation, or region while using the Native position of privilege to present findings and wisdom.

h Ethics—The ethics of land, language, and learning become whole with the flight of eagles and that ethic takes its place within research.

i Unique conclusions—The conclusions that I find are uniquely interpreted from the Native wisdom within me.

Then, the Native person might ask the non-Native person, "Now, as a non-Native person, are the meanings of these words the same for you?"

a   Voice
b   Implementation
c   Observation
d   Need
e   Skills
f   Wisdom
g   Research
h   Ethics
i   Unique conclusions

Then, the professional dialogue can allow for a time of explaining how these simple terms can have unique meanings.

Conclusion

Allowing student-led dialogue and learning how to engage in responsible cross-cultural dialogue required me as a psychologist to develop the skills of professional collaboration and a growing cultural awareness with the specificity of context and explanations. Issues of behavioral causes, trauma, learning, and language development are complex and require a context of wholeness and an understanding of the uniqueness of each student. Systems of support require many professionals who can meet together to discuss these complex needs. Understanding the context of culture and race is necessary and instrumental to professional dialogue. This work is meant to encourage further collaborative professional work in the context of Indigenous psychology.

References

Blume, A. (2020). *A new psychology based on community, equality, and care of the Earth*. Praeger.

Garcia, M., & Tehee, M. (2014). *Society of Indian psychologists commentary on the American Psychological Association's (APA) ethical principles of psychologists and code of conduct*. Society of Indian Psychologists.

Hains, S. (2001). *An emerging voice: A study using traditional Aboriginal research methods*. Saybrook University.

Hains, S. (2013). Defining of a peace process within Indigenous research, Indigenous ethics and the implications in psychology. *Journal of Indigenous Research, 1*, Article 8. https://digitalcommons.usu.edu/kicjir/vol1/iss2/8

Hains, S. (2021). Indigenous utmost care. *Journal of Indigenous Research, 9*, Article 3. https://digitalcommons.usu.edu/kicjir/vol9/iss2021/3

Michie, S. A. (2014). *The behavior change wheel*. Silverback.

Chapter 12

The Interface: Western Tools and the Mental Health and Wellbeing of Aboriginal and Torres Strait Islander Peoples

*Helen Milroy, Monique Platell,
and Shraddha Kashyap*

In this chapter, we begin by outlining the historical, political, social, and environmental contexts which impact the health and wellbeing of the Indigenous peoples of Australia; Aboriginal and Torres Strait Islander peoples. We then discuss the current state of assessing psychological outcomes among Aboriginal and Torres Strait Islander peoples. Our aim is to help the reader understand the limitations of using the Western lens of mental health and psychological measures among Aboriginal and Torres Strait Islander peoples. We will provide examples of culturally appropriate and responsive ways of working with Aboriginal and Torres Strait Island peoples. Aboriginal and Torres Strait Islander peoples view health as a holistic concept, encompassing the social, emotional, and cultural wellbeing of the individual and the community. Therefore, capturing an accurate picture of wellbeing involves much more than what is assessed within a Western paradigm of mental and physical health. To understand the need for culturally appropriate psychological assessment and support, we must first appreciate the historical and cultural contexts which have shaped and continue to shape the health and wellbeing of Aboriginal and Torres Strait Islander communities.

The Indigenous peoples of Australia comprise two groups: Aboriginal peoples from mainland Australia and Torres Strait Islander peoples originating from the islands in the Torres Strait. Although the two groups share similar experiences in history, there are distinct ethnic and cultural differences between Aboriginal and Torres Strait Islander societies (Dudgeon, Wright, et al., 2014).

Australia's Aboriginal cultural traditions have a history and continuity unrivalled in the world. Aboriginal peoples have been in Australia for between 50,000 and 120,000 years and were hunter-gatherer peoples who had adapted well to the environment. Before British arrival in 1788, there were between 300,000 and 950,000 Aboriginal peoples living in Australia, with approximately 260 distinct language groups. Aboriginal peoples lived a semi-nomadic lifestyle with family groups living in defined

DOI: 10.4324/9781003124061-17

territories. Family groups were governed by complex kinships systems which placed each person securely in relationship to every other person in the group and determined the behaviour of an individual to each person. Aboriginal peoples experience the land as a richly symbolic and spiritual landscape rather than only a physical environment. According to Aboriginal beliefs, the physical environment of each local area was created and shaped by the actions of spiritual ancestors. Religion was based on a philosophy of oneness with the natural environment, with land not being owned but with one belonging to the land (Dudgeon, Wright, et al., 2014).

Torres Strait Islander peoples were sea-faring peoples with cultures based around subsistence farming and fishing. At the time of first colonial contact, the Torres Strait Islander population was estimated around 3,800. There are 270 islands in the Torres Strait; however, today Torres Strait Islander peoples live permanently in 20 communities on 17 of the Torres Strait Islands, and there are two main language groups. In 1863, the first European settlement was established in the Torres Strait, and between 1872 and 1879 the Torres Strait Islands were annexed to become British Crown lands (Shnukal, 2001).

This chapter is largely based on content related to the cultures of Aboriginal peoples and so may not capture the nuances associated with Torres Strait Islander peoples. Indeed, Aboriginal and Torres Strait Islander peoples have rich and diverse cultures and a history of resilience and resistance against the impacts of colonisation. It is therefore important to understand contemporary issues faced by Aboriginal and Torres Strait Islander peoples through the lens of historical, socio-cultural, and political contexts as well as through an Aboriginal and Torres Strait Islander lens of health and wellbeing. In this way, we propose that this chapter is broadly applicable to Aboriginal and Torres Strait Islander peoples of Australia.

In summary, we first outline determinants of health and wellbeing among Aboriginal and Torres Strait Islander peoples. We then discuss the current state of psychological measurement and propose a way forward for mental health professionals.

Determinants of Health and Wellbeing

Social and Emotional Wellbeing (SEWB)

Aboriginal and Torres Strait Islander peoples view health as the social, emotional, and cultural wellbeing of the whole community. These beliefs and values have been conceptualised under the Social and Emotional Wellbeing (SEWB) model (Gee et al., 2014). This model results from a network of relationships between individuals, family, kin and community, and recognises the importance of connection to land, culture, spirituality, and ancestry and their impacts on wellbeing (Gee et al., 2014) (Figure 12.1).

The seven social and emotional wellbeing domains (body, mind, and emotions, family and kin, community, culture, country, and spirituality and ancestors) are optimal sources of wellbeing and connection that support a strong identity grounded in a collective perspective (Gee et al., 2014). These connections are influenced by social (e.g., education, employment, housing, life stress), historical (past government policies, oppression, and cultural displacement), and political determinants of SEWB (land rights, control of resources, cultural security, and the right to self-determination) (Gee et al., 2014; Zubrick et al., 2014).

Social and Emotional Wellbeing is a multidimensional concept of health, of which mental health is one part; SEWB and mental health interact to influence each other (Gee et al., 2014). For example, systemic problems such as social and economic disadvantage are also risk factors for numerous mental health problems (Gee et al., 2014). Therefore, from an Aboriginal and Torres Strait Islander perspective, the development of mental health problems would be a symptom of a larger SEWB disturbance (Parker & Milroy, 2014).

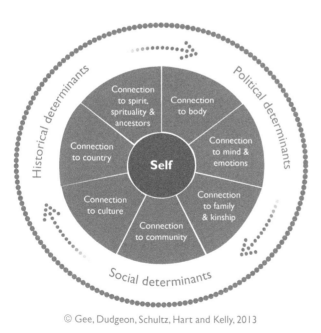

© Gee, Dudgeon, Schultz, Hart and Kelly, 2013

Figure 12.1 Social and emotional wellbeing model.

Historical and Political Determinants of Social and Emotional Wellbeing

The health and wellbeing of Aboriginal and Torres Strait Islander peoples have been shaped by the historical and continued impact of colonisation. Colonisation, and the subsequent genocide of Aboriginal and Torres Strait Islander peoples led to sustained and profound trauma over generations (Milroy et al., 2014). A stark example of the brutality of colonisation includes the forcible removal of Aboriginal and Torres Strait Islander children from their families and communities (Swan & Raphael, 1997). The 1997 *Bringing Them Home* report revealed that "the predominant aims of Indigenous child removals was the absorption or assimilation of the children into the wider, non-Indigenous, community so their unique values and ethnic identity would disappear" (Swan & Raphael, 1997). The nature of this trauma experienced by Aboriginal and Torres Strait Islander peoples can be discussed under three themes: (1) powerlessness and loss of control, (2) loss and disconnection, and (3) trauma and helplessness (Milroy et al., 2014). These concepts are key to understanding the challenges faced by colonised Aboriginal and Torres Strait Islander communities today.

Powerlessness and Loss of Control

Aboriginal and Torres Strait Islander peoples have experienced cumulative forms of control imposed over their lives that have undermined their connection to land, elders as custodians of culture, community, kinship, and children (Milroy et al., 2014). By the middle of the 19th century, Aboriginal and Torres Strait Islander communities had been dispossessed of their land. They were living in reserves or non-Indigenous settlements, often dependent on government rations, and suffering from malnutrition and disease (Dudgeon, Wright, et al., 2014). Colonial control, including massacres, slave labour, incarceration, race-based legislation, and an "apartheid" system diminished the rights of Aboriginal and Torres Strait Islander peoples in all aspects of society (Reynolds, 1990). The sense of degradation and humiliation at being treated as less than human remains a source of distress for many families (Swan & Raphael, 1997). Indeed, feelings of powerlessness and a lack of control have been linked to poor health and life outcomes (Brunner & Marmot, 2003; Marmot, 2004).

Loss and Disconnection

Post-colonisation, Aboriginal and Torres Strait Islander peoples have experienced profound loss, including loss of life, land, culture, heritage, ancestry, identity, language, and children (Milroy et al., 2014). The forcible removal of children from their families under government legislation (1900s–1970s) was the colonialist rule's largest attempt to assimilate Aboriginal and Torres Strait Islander peoples into the White community and effectively wipe out Aboriginal and Torres Strait Islander peoples and cultures (Swan & Raphael, 1997). Implicit in this policy was the idea that there was nothing of value in Aboriginal and Torres Strait Islander cultures (Human Rights and Equal Opportunity Commission, 1997). The loss of kinship networks made it difficult for many people to return home and to re-establish links to culture, and the resulting disconnection and isolation affected not only the removed children but also their families, and communities (Milroy et al., 2014). These policies had significant negative impacts on health and social and emotional wellbeing and continue to be experienced by successive generations (Menzies, 2019).

Trauma and Helplessness

Aboriginal and Torres Strait Islander peoples have experienced multiple atrocities and disproportionately high levels of trauma in numerous forms throughout colonial history (Menzies, 2019; Milroy et al., 2014; Swan & Raphael, 1997). They have also endured cultural and spiritual trauma experienced through denial and denigration of beliefs and practices, the mislabelling of behaviours and experiences, and the destruction and desecration of sacred sites, objects, and deceased persons (Menzies, 2019; Milroy et al., 2014). The consequences of such trauma are complex and intergenerational. Central to the experiences of overwhelming and sustained trauma is the sense of complete helplessness combined with ongoing fear and distress (Milroy et al., 2014). Trauma can also negatively impact a person's ability to cope with future adverse events and circumstances, such as through disruptions to emotional self-regulation (Milroy et al., 2014).

Social Determinants of Social and Emotional Wellbeing

Social determinants of health are the economic and social conditions that influence individual and group differences in health status such as education, employment, and housing (World Health Organization, 2020). In Australia, the health of Aboriginal and Torres Strait Islander peoples is affected by a complex interplay of environmental factors, behaviours, and biological factors together with social and cultural contexts (Australian Indigenous HealthInfoNet, 2020). For example, social determinants were found to explain more than one-third (34%) of the health gap between Aboriginal and Torres Strait Islander peoples and non-Indigenous Australians (Australian Institute of Health and Welfare, 2018b). For example, Aboriginal and Torres Strait Islander peoples who were most likely to report very good or excellent health in 2014–2015 lived in the highest socioeconomic areas, were employed, had higher educational attainment, and felt safe at home (Australian Institute of Health and Welfare, 2018b). Further, Aboriginal and Torres Strait Islander peoples who were employed were less likely to smoke, less likely to use illicit substances, and more likely to have an adequate daily fruit intake than those who were unemployed (Australian Institute of Health and Welfare, 2018b). Social determinants of SEWB are influenced by demographics and exposure to life stressors.

Demographics

Social, political, and historical determinants of health and wellbeing account for disproportionate suffering in terms of mental health problems and mortality. Our understanding is currently characterised by the Australian Bureau of Statistics, and some demographic factors are summarised below. Importantly, we note that issues of data governance and sovereignty mean that available data likely reflects White dominance and does not measure outcomes of value to Aboriginal and Torres Strait Islander peoples, such as the domain of SEWB.

In 2016, the estimated Aboriginal and Torres Strait Islander population was at 798,400 people and accounted for 3.3% of Australia's total population (Australian Bureau of Statistics, 2019b). More than one-third of Aboriginal and Torres Strait Islander peoples lived in major cities while 7% and 12% lived in remote and very remote locations, respectively (Australian Bureau of Statistics, 2018b, 2019b). The pattern of population distribution across the ages for Aboriginal and Torres Strait Islander peoples is predominantly young, with a median age of 20 in 2016 compared to 38 for non-Indigenous Australians (Australian Bureau of Statistics, 2018a; Australian Institute of Health and Welfare, 2019) (Figure 12.2).

In 2018, the age-standardised mortality rate for Aboriginal and Torres Strait Islander peoples was 927 per 100,000, which is around 1.7 times higher than the non-Indigenous rate (Commonwealth of Australia, 2020). Between 2015 and 2017, life expectancy at birth was 71.6 years for Aboriginal and Torres Strait Islander males (8.6 fewer years than non-Indigenous males) and 75.6 for Aboriginal and Torres Strait Islander females (7.8 fewer years than non-Indigenous females (Commonwealth of Australia, 2020).

This population pyramid reflects the ongoing impacts of colonisation. Colonisation has resulted in a severe lack of human capital to support families in Aboriginal and Torres Strait Islander communities. With there being more children than adults, the usual buffering for families through extended family members to assist parents and children is lacking

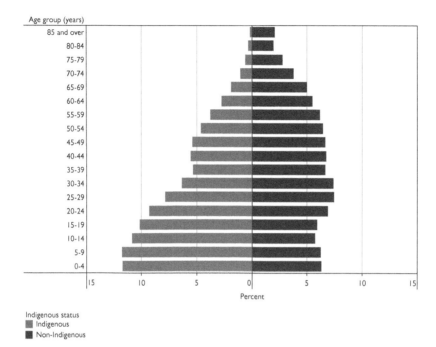

Figure 12.2 Population pyramid of Indigenous and non-indigenous populations.

(Milroy, 2008). This results in children and young people having reduced access to older, experienced people available for care, protection, cultural guidance, general life skills, and education (Hammill, 2001; Telethon Kids Institute, 2005).

Life Stressors

Aboriginal and Torres Strait Islander peoples are exposed to greater levels of life stress than non-Indigenous Australians (Australian Bureau of Statistics, 2016). The 2014–2015 National Aboriginal and Torres Strait Islander Social Survey found that 68% of Aboriginal and Torres Strait Islander peoples aged 15 years and over experienced one or more personal stressors in the 12 months prior to the survey (Australian Bureau of Statistics, 2016). The most commonly experienced stressors were the death of a family member or close friend (28%), not being able to get a job (19%), and serious illness (12%) (Australian Bureau of Statistics, 2016). The rates of experiencing life stressors are also high for Aboriginal and Torres Strait Islander children aged 4–14 years (67%) (Australian Bureau of Statistics, 2016). The most common stressors reported by children were death of a family member and close friend (25%), problems keeping up at school (23%), and being scared or upset by an argument or someone's behaviour (23%) (Australian Bureau of Statistics, 2016). Exposure to such life stress is a significant risk factor for developing mental health problems (Zubrick et al., 2014).

Psychological Measures and Interventions Among Aboriginal and Torres Strait Islander Peoples

Prevalence of Mental Health Problems

We initially discuss mental health problems in this section from the paradigm of Western psychology, acknowledging that this does not fully represent Aboriginal and Torres Strait Islander views on health and wellbeing. Taking this into account, the data suggests that Aboriginal and Torres Strait Islander peoples reported significantly higher levels of psychological distress than non-Indigenous Australians.

The 2018–2019 National Aboriginal and Torres Strait Islander Health Survey found that 31% of Aboriginal and Torres Strait Islander peoples aged 18 years and over reported high or very high levels of psychological distress in the 4 weeks prior to the survey. High levels of psychological distress were especially reported by Aboriginal and Torres Strait Islander adults who had been removed from their family and had relatives removed (Australian Institute of Health and Welfare, 2015). Indeed, descendants of the stolen generations were found to be 1.3 times more likely to report poor mental health than other Aboriginal and Torres Strait Islander peoples (Australian Institute of Health and Welfare, 2018a). Finally, rates of suicide among Aboriginal and Torres Strait Islander peoples were found to be at least two times higher than among non-Indigenous Australians (Australian Institute of Health and Welfare, 2020). In 2017, suicide was the leading cause of death for Aboriginal and Torres Strait Islander peoples aged 15–34 years and for children aged 5–17 years (Australian Bureau of Statistics, 2017, 2019a).

Measures

Psychology as a paradigm of science and as a clinical profession has had a significant impact on knowledge and perceptions about Aboriginal and Torres Strait Islander mental health (Dudgeon, Rickwood, et al., 2014). Psychology in Australia has a history of domination over Aboriginal and Torres Strait Islander peoples, which is still evident today (Dudgeon & Walker, 2015). This has occurred through the imposition of Western psychology and understandings of mental illness which have informed assessment, diagnosis, and treatment of mental health problems. The Western lens has largely ignored the knowledge and practices of Aboriginal and Torres Strait Islander peoples (Dudgeon & Walker, 2015). That is, the ethnocentric expertise of mainstream mental health practitioners and services has negated awareness of the unique needs of Aboriginal and Torres Strait Islander communities and the profound impact of colonisation. Indeed, Aboriginal and Torres Strait Islander peoples have experienced a long history of mistreatment by mainstream health and welfare services, and diagnoses of mental illness have been used to disempower and disadvantage those from marginalised groups (Dudgeon, Rickwood, et al., 2014). The historical experiences and ongoing trauma and distress, together with the fundamental differences in mental health constructs between Western and Aboriginal and Torres Strait Islander peoples, highlight the urgent need for culturally sensitive and appropriate assessment and testing tools (Adams et al., 2014).

The emergence of Aboriginal and Torres Strait Islander mental health professionals has led to increased recognition and prioritisation of holistic health and has promoted culturally informed approaches in psychological research and practice. These changes in perceptions have been underpinned by an approach to empowerment and self-determination in the provision of mental health services for Aboriginal and Torres Strait Islander peoples (Dudgeon & Pickett, 2000). Such perception shifts can be seen in the Australian Psychological Society's formal commitment to enabling the profession and discipline of psychology to acknowledge and support the SEWB of Aboriginal and Torres Strait Islander peoples, including the de-colonisation of psychology curriculums (Dudgeon, Rickwood, et al., 2014). The National Practice Standards for the Mental Health Workforce in Australia now require mental health practitioners working with Aboriginal and Torres Strait Islander clients to use culturally appropriate assessment instruments and techniques and to consider cultural issues that may impact upon the appropriateness of assessment, care, and treatment (Australian Government Department of Health, 2013). However, despite these acknowledgements of the unique needs and values of Aboriginal and Torres Strait Islander peoples, there is a paucity of widely accepted, culturally appropriate, and scientifically validated mental health measurement tools.

Psychological Diagnostic Tools

Establishing culturally safe and acceptable diagnostic tools is vital to identifying psychiatric morbidity in Aboriginal and Torres Strait Islander peoples and providing appropriate mental health care (Toombs et al., 2019). To date, various methods are employed to diagnose mental health problems in Aboriginal and Torres Strait Islander populations, including clinical assessment, self-report instruments, and diagnostic interviews

(Black et al., 2015). The variability in methods used is likely to contribute to inconsistencies in diagnoses and morbidity data (Black et al., 2015). Western assessment tools currently being used have several limitations when applied to Aboriginal and Torres Strait Islander peoples for mental health diagnosis.

Firstly, it must be considered how mental health problems may be expressed through different symptomology in Aboriginal and Torres Strait Islander populations compared with non-Indigenous populations, for whom these assessments were developed. For example, anger has been shown as a unique indicator of depression for Aboriginal and Torres Strait Islander peoples (Thomas et al., 2010). In addition, in remote and tradition-oriented populations, paranormal experiences (visions and voices) are expected in grieving and traditional activities (Hunter, 2014). Sorcery is also commonly used to explain illness or death, especially if it is unanticipated (Hunter, 2014). Such occurrences can be difficult to differentiate from psychosis for practitioners who do not have an understanding of Aboriginal and Torres Strait Islander culture (Hunter, 2014). Therefore, the reliability of psychological diagnoses among Aboriginal and Torres Strait Islander peoples relies heavily on the cultural capacity and opinions of clinicians (Adams et al., 2014; Dingwall & Cairney, 2010). However, clinicians have reported low levels of confidence in using many of the existing tools with their Aboriginal and Torres Strait Islander clients (Adams et al., 2014). As a consequence, the nature and extent of mental health problems among Aboriginal and Torres Strait Islander peoples can remain unrecognized, undiagnosed, and untreated (Dingwall & Cairney, 2010).

Finally, most research into appropriate diagnostic tools for Aboriginal and Torres Strait Islander peoples is based around determining the applicability of Western tools to this population. Predominantly, these tools are based on a Western medical model and on criteria from either the *Diagnostic and Statistical Manual of Mental Disorders* (5th ed.; DSM-5; American Psychiatric Association, 2013) or the *International Classification of Diseases* (ICD; Adams et al., 2014; Black et al., 2018). Such criteria focus on the individual's level of functioning and on the labelling of mental health problems and ultimately ignore Aboriginal and Torres Strait Islander peoples' holistic view of mental health as one part of SEWB (i.e., including the physical, social, emotional, and spiritual wellbeing of an individual and their community; Adams et al., 2014; Black et al., 2018; Social Health Reference Group, 2004).

Psychological Screening Tools

In contrast to diagnostic tools, numerous examples of screening tools have been designed to be used with Aboriginal and Torres Strait Islander peoples (see Appendix A) (Black et al., 2018). However, there does not appear to be an agreed-upon standardised definition or procedure for cultural validation. This has led to varying degrees of participation of Aboriginal and Torres Strait Islander researchers, clinical experts, and community members in the development and testing of tools in the current literature. The Centre of Best Practice in Aboriginal and Torres Strait Islander Suicide Prevention define a tool as culturally validated when "development was led by or involved Aboriginal or Torres Strait Islander clinical or cultural experts in the study and the tool were validated for use with Aboriginal and Torres Strait Islander people" (Centre of Best Practice in Aboriginal and Torres Strait Islander Suicide Prevention, 2020).

Outcome Measures

Research on mental health outcome measures for Aboriginal and Torres Strait Islander peoples remains limited. One example is Trauer and Nagel (2012), who attempted to explore the feasibility and practicality of using a national outcome measure in a sample of Aboriginal and Torres Strait Islander adults in far Northern Queensland. This research applied the Health of the Nation Outcome Scales (HONOS; Trauer & Nagel, 2012), which collects information about a person's mental health and social functioning. Guidelines were developed to encourage practitioners to assess clients within their cultural contexts, involve informants to gain a more accurate view of the true extent of the consumer's difficulties, and understand the complex issues of Aboriginal and Torres Strait Islander identity, wellbeing, and mental health (Haswell-Elkins et al., 2007; Trauer & Nagel, 2012). However, based on practitioner responses to the use of the scales, more than half of the 496 assessments completed (58%) did not include any of the recommended additional informants (Trauer & Nagel, 2012).

Case Study 1: Aboriginal Community Controlled Health Services

Aboriginal Community Controlled Health Services (ACCHS) have been established in Australia as primary health facilities that are both built and run by local Aboriginal and Torres Strait Islander communities. ACCHS strives to provide medical and mental health services that are responsive to, and respectful of, the needs of their Aboriginal and Torres Strait Islander clients. The psychological screening and assessment tools used by these services represent varying degrees of cultural validation, and this highlights the complexities involved in discerning between the need for measurement and service evaluation and the availability of culturally valid measures.

One challenge facing these services is the paucity of psychological tools which accurately capture the context and realities of Aboriginal and Torres Strait Islander peoples' lives, their languages, and their experiences and expressions of psychological wellbeing. In light of the overwhelming burden of suicide among Aboriginal and Torres Strait Islander communities, it is vital that mental health workers and researchers understand and document the needs and challenges of Aboriginal and Torres Strait Islander peoples seeking support.

Indeed, the use of psychological tools by ACCHS that have been specifically developed for use with Aboriginal and Torres Strait Islander peoples (e.g., the iBobbly self-help app[1] and the Youth Social Emotional Wellbeing assessment[2]) represents a movement away from Western-developed psychological measures, which do not measure SEWB or account for the historical, social, and political contexts of colonisation and structural racism which continue to impact the lives of Aboriginal and Torres Strait Islander peoples today. Such culturally valid measures reject the universality of definitions of mental health and wellbeing offered by Western psychology and focus on social and emotional wellbeing and strength-based models. However, few of these tools have been widely validated.

Therefore, working with Aboriginal and Torres Strait Islander communities to co-design culturally valid measures of mental health and wellbeing (i.e., SEWB) should be a major priority for mental health researchers and clinicians.

A Way Forward for Psychological Assessments

In summary, the quality of psychological tools currently being used with Aboriginal and Torres Strait Islander peoples depends heavily on the abilities and skills of the clinician and their ability to use these tools in a culturally responsive way (Dingwall & Cairney, 2010). Cultural responsiveness refers to health care services and professionals who are respectful of the health beliefs, health practices, cultures, and linguistic needs of Aboriginal and Torres Strait Islander consumers and communities (Australian Health Ministers' Advisory Council, 2016; Department of Health and Human Services, 2011). For mental health practitioners, this is the capacity to respond to the health care issues of Aboriginal and Torres Strait Islander communities (Department of Health and Human Services, 2011). It is a cyclical and ongoing process requiring the ability to identify and challenge one's own cultural assumptions, values, and beliefs while also recognising the importance of acknowledging the influence of culture, ethnicity, racism, and other contextual factors in the experiences of individuals and communities (Department of Health and Human Services, 2011; Walker et al., 2014).

To begin to develop cultural responsiveness, a necessary first step is a foundation of cultural awareness, which is defined as a basic understanding of Aboriginal and Torres Strait Islander histories, peoples, and cultures (Australian Health Ministers' Advisory Council, 2016). Through cultural awareness and responsiveness, mental health services may become culturally safe (Australian Health Ministers' Advisory Council, 2016). Cultural safety means that health consumers are safest when health professionals have considered power relations, cultural differences, and patients' rights. The presence or absence of cultural safety is determined by the experiences of the health consumer and not by the caregiver (Australian Health Ministers' Advisory Council, 2016). Without improvements in the cultural awareness and responsiveness of the mental health workforce and wider mental health system, the effectiveness of culturally validated tools will be undermined.

Australian Indigenous Psychology Education Project

The Australian Indigenous Psychology Education Project (AIPEP) was formed to develop frameworks, guidelines, and strategies to increase the capabilities of the psychology workforce and graduates to work appropriately and effectively with Aboriginal and Torres Strait Islander peoples (Dudgeon et al., 2016). The Workforce Capabilities Framework developed under this initiative establishes principles for the knowledge, skills, and values required of psychologists working with Aboriginal and Torres Strait Islander peoples, in line with the Psychology Board of Australia core capabilities. This framework was developed out of the concerns of practitioners who felt ill equipped to work with Aboriginal and Torres Strait Islander peoples, including how to engage, build, and maintain positive working relationships (Carey et al., 2017). The formation of AIPEP and the workforce framework is an example of decolonising the discipline of psychology to recognise Aboriginal and Torres Strait Islander cultural views, conceptual frameworks, and practices based on holistic concepts of health and wellbeing (Carey et al., 2017).

Dance of Life (Helen Milroy)

To assist practitioners in exploring Aboriginal and Torres Strait Islander values, experiences, and understandings in a systematic and culturally appropriate way, a framework entitled the Dance of Life was developed by Helen Milroy (2006). This framework was based on a series of six paintings by Milroy, each depicting a dimension of health and wellbeing (physical, psychological, social, spiritual, and cultural). The last picture in the series depicts the bringing together of these dimensions to reflect the delicate balance of life within the universe (Milroy, 2006). The subsequent framework outlines the physical, psychological, social, spiritual, and cultural dimensions that must be considered when understanding Aboriginal mental health in assessments and treatment decisions (Adams et al., 2014; Milroy, 2006). Within this framework, each dimension is explained in terms of the historical context, the traditional and contemporary views as well as gaps in knowledge (Adams et al., 2014; Milroy, 2006). It is imperative to recognise that the incorporation of historical and cultural perspectives is essential to enhancing mental health practitioners' skills to provide a meaningful and respectful cross-cultural exchange with their Aboriginal clients (Figure 12.3).

Cultural Safety

Providing a culturally safe environment is fundamental to the practice of cultural responsiveness. According to the *Cultural Respect Framework 2016–2026*, cultural safety identifies that health consumers are safest when health professionals have considered power relations, cultural differences, and patients' rights. Cultural safety is not defined by the health professional but by the consumer's experience of the care they are given and their ability to access services and to raise concerns (Australian Health Ministers' Advisory Council, 2016).

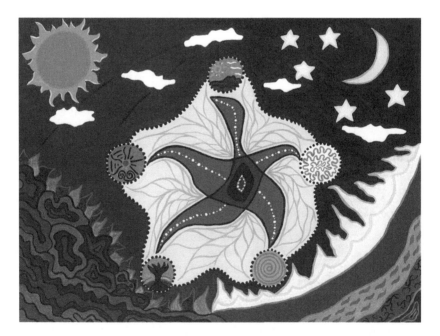

Figure 12.3 Dance of life.

Involving Aboriginal and Torres Strait Islander mental health workers and Traditional Healers when providing mental health services is one example of cultural safety (Sheldon, 2010). Aboriginal and Torres Strait Islander peoples' health and social and emotional wellbeing are bound to their collective rights, which include cultural practices, and the maintenance and application of traditional knowledge (Hunter et al., 2012). The *National Practice Standards for the Mental Health Workforce 2013* specifies that mental health practitioners should work collaboratively with Aboriginal and Torres Strait Islander mental health workers and Traditional Healers (Australian Government Department of Health, 2013). Currently, no national data is available on the use of cultural advisors or Traditional Healers in the psychological assessment process, and there is a lack of programs that combine traditional treatments with Western medical approaches to treat the wellbeing of the whole person (Dudgeon, Walker, et al., 2014). The practice standards state that such collaboration with Aboriginal and Torres Strait Islander mental health workers and traditional healers should be included "where appropriate" (Australian Government Department of Health, 2013). Such language indicates that collaboration is at the discretion of the practitioner and may result in inconsistent application of these practice standards. For example, evidence from the *Mental Health Advocacy Service Inquiry into Services for Aboriginal and Torres Strait Islander People and Compliance with the Mental Health Act 2014* showed that only two of the 11 metropolitan hospitals with authorised mental health wards in Perth, Western Australia, had Aboriginal mental health workers. It was also highlighted that in Western Australian hospitals Aboriginal mental health workers were generally not routinely available outside of business hours, and therefore many Aboriginal consumers receiving mental health assessments, examinations, and admissions may not able to access their full rights under the Mental Health Act (Mental Health Advocacy Service, 2020). If practitioners are not educated on how such collaboration looks in practicality or on the benefits of such a practice, this may create resistance to incorporating Aboriginal and Torres Strait Islander mental health workers into mainstream mental health services. Further research is needed to form an evidence base to help advocate for including Aboriginal and Torres Strait Islander mental health workers and traditional healers.

Indeed, mental health practitioners need to employ new models and approaches to screen, diagnose, and provide care for Aboriginal and Torres Strait Islander clients outside of Western health models (Gee et al., 2014). The development of such new models needs to be embedded within Aboriginal participatory action research, which prioritises genuine community collaboration and consultation designed to provide the community with control over the research processes and outcomes

(Dudgeon et al., 2017). Such methodology has the potential to balance power differentials, which have long been present between researchers, mental health practitioners, and Aboriginal and Torres Strait Islander peoples, by ensuring the views and experiences of all participants are recognised and valued (Dudgeon et al., 2017).

From the literature, it is evident that strength-based models based on Aboriginal and Torres Strait Islander SEWB in psychological tools are lacking.

Case Study 2: AIMhi

One attempt to fill this gap in practice is the Aboriginal and Islander Mental Health Initiative (AIMhi), which includes culturally adapted resources and training to support a client-centred and strengths-based approach to assessment and early intervention for Aboriginal and Torres Strait Islander peoples. One resource created by the initiative is the AIMhi Stay Strong care plan, which is a culturally appropriate approach to brief therapy that has been translated into an e-mental health resource. The AIMhi Stay Strong care plan is based on the stress vulnerability model, which posits that a person's wellbeing is a result of resilience factors and risk factors which constantly interact (Mueser et al., 2002; Nagel et al., 2012). Therefore, the key message to clients is that there is a need to balance strengths and stressors to increase resilience and reduce the risk to developing mental health problems (Mueser et al., 2002; Nagel et al., 2012). The AIMhi Stay Strong care plan has some key differences to other brief therapies; it is culturally adapted for Aboriginal and Torres Strait Islander peoples and presents a holistic model of mental health and wellbeing (Nagel & Dingwall, 2014). The care plan also uses colourful pictures to support conversations about areas of stress and uses metaphors from daily life to promote engagement and understanding (Nagel & Dingwall, 2014).

Central to the AIMhi Stay Strong care plan approach is the Grow Strong Tree, which represents to clients the balance of strengths and stressors. The Grow Strong Tree depicts four root systems and four leaves representing the SEWB domains of spiritual, physical, family and social and work, and mental and emotional (Nagel & Dingwall, 2014). Through collaboration between practitioners and clients, the Grow Strong Tree is used to guide discussions about social connections to family and friends that keep the client strong as well as identifying the client's individual strengths, stressors, and goals under each of the four SEWB domains. The AIMhi approach to therapy emphasises that any mental health assessments must only be included after discussions of self-identified strengths, stressors, and goals for change have been completed. The initiative focuses on working from the client's understandings

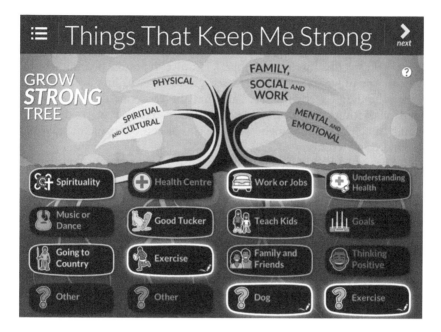

Figure 12.4 Grow strong tree.

of their concerns and what the client might want to do differently. By planning, supporting, and reinforcing healthy and rewarding behaviours, it is hoped to promote resilience, improve wellbeing, and increase self-efficacy for Aboriginal and Torres Strait Islander clients (Nagel & Dingwall, 2014) (Figure 12.4).

Case Study 3: "Tom"

This is a hypothetical case study and thus is not based on an actual person. "Tom" is a 16-year-old Aboriginal adolescent from a small remote community who lives with his grandmother and siblings. Tom speaks three traditional languages, and English is his fourth language.

Tom was exposed to domestic violence as a child and was sexually abused by an uncle when he was 8 years old. He was not sleeping well and had recently become aggressive towards his family. Tom had also been using marijuana quite heavily over recent months. His family noticed that he would sometimes talk to himself and that he spent a lot of time alone in his room. Once, he threatened to kill them if they didn't leave him alone. His grandmother took him to the health centre, and he was involuntarily admitted to an adolescent mental health inpatient unit in the nearest city for assessment for psychosis under the Mental Health Act.

In the ward, he was quiet and guarded, mostly staring at the floor. He did not speak much with the mental health staff and said that he wanted to go home. At times, Tom would punch the walls and burn his arms with a lighter, to the point where he needed medical care for his injuries. Tom said he did this to feel relief. He also reported hearing several voices, one of which was his deceased grandfather calling his name; the others he didn't recognise. He said that the voices he didn't recognise said nasty things about him and his family. He was worried he was going to be punished at night when he was asleep but couldn't say what he had done wrong.

Tom said he had not been feeling good for a few months and that he used the marijuana to try to feel better, but things appeared to get worse. He said he often thought about how he could end his life, and said that he didn't really have much hope for the future.

Aboriginal Community Controlled Health Services

In this case study, it is important to recognise the cultural factors which can influence symptom formation and meaning. In cases like Tom's, it is important for Aboriginal Community Controlled Health Services and mainstream mental health services to work in partnership to promote culturally safe mental health care. For example, Tom being able to speak to a mental health worker in any of the three languages he is more comfortable with than English would allow him to express his distress and needs and feel more confident that the service provider would understand him. Indeed, if mainstream mental health services employed more Aboriginal and Torres Strait Islander mental health workers, then the opportunity for Tom to speak in one of the three traditional languages would be more likely. Second, it is common for Aboriginal people to hear voices of their relatives when they are experiencing distress, so Tom hearing his grandfather's voice may not be a symptom of psychosis. However, the unknown voices that Tom is experiencing may be psychotic in nature and/or influenced by his heavy marijuana use. Tom's fear of punishment from the unknown voices may also be real if he has broken traditional law. This can cause considerable distress, and he may not be able to speak about this issue outside of his cultural group. Aboriginal and Torres Strait Islander Mental health and SEWB workers would understand these cultural issues and would be essential in determining what is culturally appropriate for Tom's care. Even if the phenomena Tom is experiencing are psychotic in nature, they may still have a cultural dimension that requires understanding from Tom's personal cultural orientation (Parker & Milroy, 2003). A balance between psychopathology and cultural aspects is needed to ensure neither is overlooked in Tom's treatment and long-term management (Parker & Milroy, 2003). An Aboriginal mental health professional and/or Aboriginal Community Controlled Health Services will be able to consult with Tom's treatment team at the inpatient unit on these cultural aspects and engage with Elders in Tom's local community. In this way, connecting Tom with Aboriginal mental health workers, Elders, traditional healers, and family members can help differentiate the cultural norm regarding symptoms and behaviour changes. Finally, an intervention based on an SEWB framework would not only focus on Tom's symptoms but would also consider his strengths and help build his resilience.

AIMhi

The use of the culturally appropriate AIMhi Stay Strong care plan can help clinicians understand Tom's current state of mind. Since English is Tom's fourth language, the strong visual elements of the Stay Strong plan provide an alternative to paper-based Western diagnostic tools and can help to overcome issues of English literacy. In addition, with Tom's traumatic developmental history, he may have difficulty expressing his strong emotions and may be "acting out" with the substance abuse in response to his trauma. The strength-based focus of the Stay Strong plan can help build Tom's sense of mastery and his life skills and restore a sense of purpose and hope. Engaging Tom in conversation using the Grow Strong Tree about family and strengths can help identify networks for healing and what Tom perceives as strong in his life. The SEWB focus of the Grow Strong Tree relating to spiritual and cultural, physical, family, social, work, and mental and emotional aspects can also help Tom recognise what aspects of his life are taking away his strengths. Recognising factors contributing to and taking away from Tom's SEWB can provide valuable information for additional SEWB-focused programs that can be incorporated into his care and facilitate ongoing engagement.

Summary

There is a complex interplay between cultural and psychological phenomena that Western psychological tools do not adequately account for. Viewing Tom's presentation through a Western clinical lens alone would not account for his hearing his grandfather's voice or his worry around a broken rule. Further, as mentioned previously in this chapter, there are few diagnostic tools that are derived from the SEWB framework, and so interventions which do not take SEWB into account are less likely to build on Tom's strengths and build his resilience in a culturally appropriate and safe way. Western-trained clinicians working with Aboriginal and Torres Strait Islander peoples presenting with mental health issues need to understand the cultural behaviours and, individual responses to trauma as well as the prevailing burden of disadvantage and loss to avoid misdiagnosing and mislabelling. If an Aboriginal or Torres Strait Islander person seeks support from a mainstream service, then there should be a pathway for them to access Aboriginal and Torres Strait Islander mental health workers within the service as well as Aboriginal and Torres Strait Islander-run health and mental health services. This would enable Aboriginal and Torres Strait Islander consumers to be provided with culturally safe support and interventions.

Reflection Questions

- Thinking about your own education in mental health and psychology, in which paradigm was this training based and would this approach be suitable for all your clients?
- What tools do you use for assessment, and are these measurements valid for all clients you work with?
- How can you work or practice in a more culturally safe way?

Conclusion

In this chapter, we have outlined the historical, social, and political contexts as well as the determinants of health and of social and emotional wellbeing among Aboriginal and Torres Strait Islander peoples. We discussed the current state of psychological screening, assessment, and outcome measures being used with Aboriginal and Torres Strait Islander peoples and highlighted the limitations that need to be considered when applying a Western lens of psychology and mental health to Aboriginal and Torres Strait Islander peoples. The historical and continued impacts of colonisation and the fundamental differences in mental health constructs reinforce the need for rigorously developed psychological measures and interventions that are culturally sensitive and appropriate. While positive advancements in the field of culturally validated psychological measures have been made, research on culturally valid psychological assessment, screening, and outcome measures remains limited. Furthermore, the development of culturally validated measures should be only one component of a wider culturally responsive assessment, treatment, and outcomes process. This highlights the need to improve cultural awareness and responsiveness among practitioners to support the effectiveness of culturally validated tools and culturally safe mental health care for Aboriginal and Torres Strait Islander peoples. This needs to occur within a paradigm of Aboriginal and Torres Strait Islander holistic views of social and emotional wellbeing.

Notes

1 Black Dog Institute, iBobbly [app], https://www.blackdoginstitute.org.au/research/digital-dog/programs/ibobbly-app
2 Royal Australian College of General Practitioners, *National Guide to a Preventive Health Assessment for Aboriginal and Torres Strait Islander People* (3rd ed.), appendix, 2018, https://www.racgp.org.au/clinical-resources/clinical-guidelines/key-racgp-guidelines/view-all-racgp-guidelines/national-guide/chapter-4-the-health-of-young-people/appendix#app2

References

Adams, Y., Drew, N., & Walker, R. (2014). Principles of practice in mental health assessment with Aborginal Australians. In P. Dudgeon, H. Milroy, & R. Walker (Eds.), *Working together: Aboriginal and Torres Strait Islander mental health and wellbeing principles and practice* (pp. 271–288). Commonwealth of Australia.

American Psychiatric Association. (2013). *Diagnostic and statistical manual of mental disorders* (5th ed.). https://doi.org/10.1176/appi.books.9780890425596

Australian Bureau of Statistics. (2016). *National Aboriginal and Torres Strait Islander Social Survey, 2014–15*. American Bureau of Statistics. https://www.abs.gov.au/AUSSTATS/abs@.nsf/DetailsPage/4714.02014–15?OpenDocument

Australian Bureau of Statistics. (2017). *Causes of death, Australia, 2017*. ABS. https://www.abs.gov.au/ausstats/abs@.nsf/Lookup/by%20Subject/3303.0~2017~Main%20Features~Intentional%20self-harm%20in%20Aboriginal%20and%20Torres%20Strait%20Islander%20people~10

Australian Bureau of Statistics. (2018a). *Estimates of Aboriginal and Torres Srait Islander Australians, June 2016*. Retrieved October 21, 2020, from https://www.abs.gov.au/statistics/people/aboriginal-and-torres-strait-islander-peoples/estimates-aboriginal-and-torres-strait-islander-australians/latest-release

Australian Bureau of Statistics. (2018b). *Estimates of Aboriginal and Torres Strait Islander Australians, June 2016*. Retrieved October 21, 2020, from https://www.abs.gov.au/statistics/people/aboriginal-and-torres-strait-islander-peoples/estimates-aboriginal-and-torres-strait-islander-australians/latest-release#data-download

Australian Bureau of Statistics. (2019a). *Causes of death, Australia, 2018*. https://www.abs.gov.au/statistics/health/causes-death/causes-death-australia/latest-release

Australian Bureau of Statistics. (2019b). *Estimates and projections, Aboriginal and Torres Strait Islander Australians*. Retrieved October 21, 2020, from https://www.abs.gov.au/statistics/people/aboriginal-and-torres-strait-islander-peoples/estimates-and-projections-aboriginal-and-torres-strait-islander-australians/latest-release

Australian Government Department of Health. (2013). *National practice standards for the mental health workforce 2013*. Victorian Government Department of Health. https://www.health.gov.au/resources/publications/national-practice-standards-for-the-mental-health-workforce-2013

Australian Health Ministers' Advisory Council. (2016). *Cultural Respect Framework 2016–2026 for Aboriginal and Torres Strait Islander health*. http://www.

coaghealthcouncil.gov.au/Portals/0/National%20Cultural%20Respect%20Frame
work%20for%20Aboriginal%20and%20Torres%20Strait%20Islander%20Health
%202016_2026_2.pdf

Australian Indigenous HealthInfoNet. (2020). *Overview of Aboriginal and
Torres Strait Islander health status, 2019*. https://healthinfonet.ecu.edu.au/
learn/health-facts/overview-aboriginal-torres-strait-islander-health-status/

Australian Institute of Health and Welfare. (2015). *The health and welfare of
Australia's Aboriginal and Torres Strait Islander peoples*. AIHW. https://www.
aihw.gov.au/getmedia/584073f7–041e-4818–9419–39f5a060b1aa/18175.pdf.
aspx?inline=true

Australian Institute of Health and Welfare. (2018a). *Aboriginal and Torres Strait
Islander stolen generations and descendants: Numbers, demographic characteristics and selected outcomes*. AIHW. https://www.aihw.gov.au/getmedia/
a6c077c3-e1af-40de-847f-e8a3e3456c44/aihw-ihw-195.pdf.aspx?inline=true

Australian Institute of Health and Welfare. (2018b). *Australia's health 2018*. AIHW.
https://www.aihw.gov.au/getmedia/7c42913d-295f-4bc9–9c24–4e44eff4a04a/
aihw-aus-221.pdf

Australian Institute of Health and Welfare. (2019). *Profile of Indigenous
Australians*. AIHW. https://www.aihw.gov.au/reports/australias-welfare/profile-
of-indigenous-australians

Australian Institute of Health and Welfare. (2020). *Suicide and intentional self-
harm*. AIHW. https://www.aihw.gov.au/reports/australias-health/suicide-and-
intentional-self-harm

Black, E., Ranmuthugala, G., & Kondalsamy-Chennakesavan, S. (2015). A sys-
tematic review: Identifying the prevalence rates of psychiatric disorder in
Australia's Indigenous population. *Australian & New Zealand Journal of
Psychiatry*, *49*(5), 412–429. https://doi.org/10.1177/0004867415569802h

Black, E., Toombs, M., & Kisely, S. (2018). The cultural validity of diagnostic
psychiatric measures for Indigenous Australians. *Australian Psychologist*, *53*,
383–393. https://aps.onlinelibrary.wiley.com/doi/pdf/10.1111/ap.12335

Brunner, E., & Marmot, M. (2003). Social organisation, stress and health. In
M. Marmot & R. G. Wilkinson (Eds.), *Social determinants of health*. Oxford:
Oxford University Press.

Carey, T., Dudgeon, P., Hammond, S., Hirvonen, T., Kyrios, M., Roufeil, L., &
Smith, P. (2017). The Australian Psychological Society's apology to Aboriginal
and Torres Strait Islander people. *Australian Psychologist*, *52*, 261–267.

Centre of Best Practice in Aboriginal and Torres Strait Islander Suicide Prevention.
(2020). *Screening and assessment tools*. Retrieved October 27, 2020, from
https://www.cbpatsisp.com.au/our-research/screening-assessment-tools/

Commonwealth of Australia, Department of Prime Minister and Cabinet (2020).
Closing the Gap Report 2020. Department of Prime Minister and Cabinet. https://
ctgreport.niaa.gov.au/sites/default/files/pdf/closing-the-gap-report-2020.pdf

Department of Health and Human Services. (2011). *Cultural responsiveness framework – Guidelines for Victorian health services*. Rural and Regional Health
and Aged Care Services. https://www2.health.vic.gov.au/about/publications/
policiesandguidelines/Cultural-responsiveness-framework---Guidelines-for-
Victorian-health-services

Dingwall, K., & Cairney, S. (2010). Psychological and cognitive assessment of Indigenous Australians. *Australian & New Zealand Journal of Psychiatry, 44*(1), 20–30. https://journals-sagepubcom.ezproxy.library.uwa.edu.au/doi/full/10.3109/00048670903393670#articleCitationDownloadContainer

Dudgeon, P., Harris, J., Newnham, K., Brideson, T., Cranney, J., Darlaston-Jones, D., Hammond, S., Herbert, J., Homewood, J., Page, S., & Phillips, G. (2016). *Australian Indigenous Psychology Education Project Workforce Capabilities Framework.* University of Western Australia.

Dudgeon, P., & Pickett, H. (2000). Psychology and reconciliation: Australian perspectives. *Australian Psychologist, 35*(2), 82–87.

Dudgeon, P., Rickwood, D., Garvey, D., & Gridley, H. (2014). A history of Indigenous psychology. In P. Dudgeon, H. Milroy, & R. Walker (Eds.), *Working Together: Aboriginal and Torres Strait Islander mental health and wellbeing principles and practice* (pp. 39–54). Commonwealth of Australia.

Dudgeon, P., Scrine, C., Cox, A., & Walker, R. (2017). Facilitating empowerment and self-determination through participatory action research: Findings from the national empowerment project. *International Journal of Qualitative Methods, 16*(1). https://doi.org/10.1177/1609406917699515

Dudgeon, P., & Walker, R. (2015). Decolonising Australian psychology: Discourses, strategies, and practice. *Journal of Social and Political Psychology, 3*(1), 276–297. https://jspp.psychopen.eu/article/view/126/html

Dudgeon, P., Walker, R., Scrine, C., Shepherd, C., Calma, T., & Ring, I. (2014). *Effective strategies to strengthen the mental health and wellbeing of Aboriginal and Torres Strait Islander people.* Issues paper no. 12. https://www.aihw.gov.au/getmedia/6d50a4d2-d4da-4c53-8aeb-9ec22b856dc5/ctgc-ip12-4nov2014.pdf.aspx?inline=true

Dudgeon, P., Wright, M., Paradies, Y., Garvey, D., & Walker, I. (2014). Aboriginal social, cultural and historical contexts. In P. Dudgeon, H. Milroy, & R. Walker (Eds.), *Working together: Aboriginal and Torres Strait Islander mental health and wellbeing principles and practice* (pp. 3–24). Commonwealth of Australia.

Gee, G., Dudgeon, P., Schultz, C., Hart, A., & Kelly, K. (2014). Aboriginal and Torres Strait Islander social and emotional wellbeing. In P. Dudgeon, H. Milroy, & R. Walker (Eds.), *Working together: Aboriginal and Torres Strait Islander mental health and wellbeing principles and practice* (pp. 55–68). Commonwealth of Australia.

Hammill, J. (2001). Granny rights: Combatting the granny burnout syndrome among Australian Indigenous communities. *Development, 44*(2), 69–74.

Haswell-Elkins, M., Sebasio, T., Hunter, E., & Mar, M. (2007). Challenges of measuring the mental health of Indigenous Australians: Honoring ethical expectations and driving greater accuracy. *Royal Australian and New Zealand College of Psychiatrists, 15*, S29–S33. https://doi.org/10.1080/10398560701701155

Human Rights and Equal Opportunity Commission. (1997). *Bringing them home: Report of the national inquiry into the separation of Aboriginal and Torres Strait Islander children.* Human Rights and Equal Opportunity Commission. https://humanrights.gov.au/our-work/bringing-them-home-report-1997

Hunter, E. (2014). Mental health in Indigenous settings: Challenges for clinicians. *Australian Family Physician, 43*(1), 26–28. https://www.racgp.org.au/afp/2014/januaryfebruary/mental-health-in-indigenous-settings/

Hunter, E., Milroy, H., Brown, N., & Calma, T. (2012). Human rights, health and Indigenous Australians. In M. Dudley, D. Silove, & F. Gale (Eds.), *Mental health and human rights: Vision, praxis and courage* (pp. 448–464). Oxford University Press.

Marmot, M. (2004). *The status syndrome*. Henry Holt.

Mental Health Advocacy Service (2020). Mental health advocacy service inquiry into services for Aboriginal and Torres Strait Islander people and compliance with the Mental Health Act 2014: Final Report July 2020.

Menzies, K. (2019). Understanding the Australian Aboriginal experience of collective, historical and intergenerational trauma. *International Social Work, 62*(6), 1522–1534.

Milroy, H. (2006). *The dance of life*. Retrieved November 16, 2020, from https://www.ranzcp.org/practice-education/indigenous-mental-health/aboriginal-torres-strait-islander-mental-health/the-dance-of-life

Milroy, H. (2008). Children are our future: Understanding the needs of Aboriginal children and their families. In A. S. Williams and V. Cowling (Eds.), *Infants of parents with mental illness: Developmental, cultural and personal perspectives* (pp. 121–140). Australian Academic Press.

Milroy, H., Dudgeon, P., & Walker, R. (2014). Community life and development programs: Pathways to healing. In P. Dudgeon, H. Milroy, & R. Walker (Eds.), *Working together: Aboriginal and Torres Strait Islander mental health and wellbeing principles and practice* (pp. 419–436). Commonwealth of Australia.

Mueser, K., Corrigan, P., Hilton, D., Tanzman, B., Schaub, A., Gingerich, S., Essock, S., Tarrier, N., Morey, B., Vogel-Scibilia, S., & Herz, M. (2002). Illness management and recovery: A review of the research. *Psychiatric Services, 53*(10), 1272–1284.

Nagel, T., & Dingwall, K. (2014). *AIMhi Stay Strong planning: Brief treatment manual*. Menzies School of Health Research. https://www.menzies.edu.au/icms_docs/250130_Brief_Treatment_Manual.pdf

Nagel, T., Hinton, R., & Griffin, C. (2012). Yarning about Indigenous mental health: Translation of a recovery paradigm to practice. *Advances in Mental Health, 10*(3), 216–233. https://doi.org/10.5172/jamh.2012.10.3.216

Parker, R., & Milroy, H. (2003). Schizophrenia and related psychosis in Aboriginal and Torres Strait Islander people. *Aboriginal and Islander Health Worker Journal, 27*(5), 17–19.

Parker, R., & Milroy, H. (2014). Aboriginal and Torres Strait Islander mental health: An overview. In P. Dudgeon, H. Milroy, & R. Walker (Eds.), *Working together: Aboriginal and Torres Strait Islander mental health and wellbeing principles and practice* (pp. 25–38). Commonwealth of Australia.

Reynolds, H. (1990). *The other side of the frontier: Aboriginal resistance to the European invasion of Australia*. Penguin.

Sheldon, M. (2010). Reviewing psychiatric assessment in remote Aboriginal communities. In N. Purdie, P. Dudgeon, & R. Walker (Eds.), *Working together: Aboriginal and Torres Strait Islander mental health and wellbeing principles and practice* (pp. 211–222). Commonwealth of Australia.

Shnukal, A. (2001). Torres Strait Islanders. In M. Brandle (Ed.), *Multicultural Queensland 2001: 100 years, 100 communities, a century of contributions.* Department of Premier and Cabinet. http://www.multiculturalaustralia.edu.au/doc/shnukal_torres_strait.pdf

Social Health Reference Group. (2004). *National Strategic Framework for Aboriginal and Torres Strait Islander Peoples' mental health and social and emotional wellbeing 2004–2009.* Australian Department of Health and Ageing.

Swan, P., & Raphael, B. (1997). *Bringing them home: Report of the national inquiry into the separation of Aboriginal and Torres Strait Islander children from their families.* https://humanrights.gov.au/our-work/bringing-them-home-report-1997

Telethon Kids Institute. (2005). *The Western Australian Child Health Survey: The health of Aboriginal children and young people.* https://www.telethonkids.org.au/our-research/aboriginal-health/waachs/

Thomas, A., Cairney, S., Gunthorpe, W., Paradies, Y., & Sayers, S. (2010). Strong Souls: Development and validation of a culturally appropriate tool for assessment of social and emotional well-being in Indigenous youth. *Australian & New Zealand Journal of Psychiatry, 44*(1), 40–48. https://doi.org/10.3109/00048670903393589

Toombs, M., Nasir, B., Kisely, S., Ranmuthugala, G., Gill, N., Beccaria, G., Hayman, N., Kondalsamy-Chennakesavan, S., & Nicholson, G. (2019). Cultural validation of the structured clinical interview for diagnostic and statistical manual of mental disorders in Indigenous Australians. *Australasian Psychiatry, 27*(4), 362–365.

Trauer, T., & Nagel, T. (2012). Outcome measurement in adult Indigenous mental health consumers. *Advances in Mental Health, 11*(1), 106–116.

Walker, R., Schultz, C., & Sonn, C. (2014). Cultural competence: Transforming policy, services, programs and practice. In P. Dudgeon, H. Milroy, & R. Walker (Eds.), *Working together: Aboriginal and Torres Strait Islander mental health and wellbeing principles and practice* (pp. 195–220). Commonwealth of Australia.

World Health Organization. (2020). *Social determinants of health.* Retrieved October 20, 2020, from https://www.who.int/social_determinants/en/

Zubrick, S., Shepherd, C., Dudgeon, P., Gee, G., Paradies, Y., Scrine, C., & Walker, R. (2014). Social determinants of social and emotional wellbeing. In P. Dudgeon, H. Milroy, & R. Walker (Eds.), *Working together: Aboriginal and Torres Strait Islander mental health and wellbeing principles and practice* (pp. 93–107). Commonwealth of Australia.

Appendix A: Screening Tools Designed to Be Used with Aboriginal and Torres Strait Islander Peoples

Indigenous Risk Impact Screen (IRIS)

Schlesinger, C. M., Ober, C., McCarthy, M. M., Watson, J. D., Seinen, A. (2007). The development and validation of the Indigenous Risk Impact Screen (IRIS): A 13-item screening instrument for alcohol and drug and mental health risk. *Drug and Alcohol Review*, *26*(2), 109–117. https://doi.org/10.1080/09595230601146611

Kimberley Assessment of Depression of Older Indigenous Australians (KICA-dep)

Almeida, O. P., Flicker, L., Fenner, S., Smith, K., Hyde, Z., Atkinson, D., Skeaf, L., Malay, R., & LoGiudice, D. (2014). The Kimberley Assessment of Depression of Older Indigenous Australians: Prevalence of depressive disorders, risk factors and validation of the KICA-dep scale. *PLOS One*, *9*(4), Article 94983.

Adapted 9-item Patient Health Questionnaire (aPHQ)

The Getting It Right Collaborative Group (2019). Getting it right: Validating a culturally specific tool for depression (aPHD-9) in Aboriginal and Torres Strait Islander Australians. *Medical Journal of Australia*, *211*(1), 24–30.

Here and Now Aboriginal Assessment tool (HANAA)

Janca, A., Lyons, Z., Balaratnasingam, S., Parfitt, D., Davison, S., & Laugharne, J. (2015). Here and Now Aboriginal Assessment: Background, development and preliminary evaluation of a culturally appropriate screening tool. *Australasian Psychiatry*, *23*(3), 287–292.

Kimberley Mum's Mood Scale (KMMS)

Marley, J., Kotz, J., Engelke, C., Williams, M., Stephen, D., Coutinho, S. & Trust, S. (2017) Validity and acceptability of the Kimberley Mum's Mood Scale to screen for perinatal anxiety and depression in remote Aboriginal Australian health care settings. *Plos One*, *12*, Article 0168969.

Youth Social Emotional Wellbeing Assessment (SEW)

Nori A., Piovesan, R., O'Connor, J., Rigney, D., McMillan, M. M., & Brown, N. (2014*). 'Y Health – Staying Deadly': An Aboriginal youth focussed translational action research project.* Canberra: ANU. https://openresearch-repository.anu.edu.au/handle/1885/140086

Strong Souls Assessment Tool

Thomas, A., Cairney, S., Gunthorpe, W., Paradies, Y., & Sayers, S. (2010). Strong Souls: Development and validation of a culturally appropriate tool for assessment of social and emotional well-being in Indigenous youth. *Australian and New Zealand Journal of Psychiatry, 44*(1), 40–48.

Aboriginal and Islander Mental Health Initiative (AIMhi) Brief Wellbeing Screener

Menzies School of Health Research. Brief Wellbeing Screener. http://www.menzies.edu.au/icms_docs/161345_Brief_Wellbeing_Screener.pdf

Index

For Product Safety Concerns and Information please contact our
EU representative GPSR@taylorandfrancis.com Taylor & Francis
Verlag GmbH, Kaufingerstraße 24, 80331 München, Germany